OSSEOINTEGRATED IMPLANT
— A MANUAL —

Department of Oral Implantology
The Nippon Dental University

Ishiyaku EuroAmerica, Inc.
St. Louis • Tokyo

Copy Editor : Brian W. Cochran M.F.A. } English Edition

Ishiyaku EuroAmerica, Inc.
716 Hanley Industrial Court, Brentwood, Missouri 63144, U.S.A. and
1-43-9 Komagome, Toshima-ku, Tokyo 170, JAPAN

Library of Congress Catalogue Card Number 92-54542

OSSEOINTEGRATED IMPLANT—A MANUAL

ISBN 1-56386-014-7

Printed in Japan

Contributors

Yasushi Hiraga
Instructor
Dept. of Partial and Complete Denture
Dept. of Oral Implantology
School of Dentistry
The Nippon Dental University

Hiroshi Kamezawa
Assistant Professor
Dept. of Crown and Bridge
Dept. of Oral Implantology
School of Dentistry
The Nippon Dental University

Kyuichi Kamoi
Professor and Chairman
Dept. of Periodontology
School of Dentistry
The Nippon Dental University

Hiroshi Kobayashi
Periodontist
Tokyo, Japan

Yoshinori Kobayashi
Professor and Chairman
Dept. of Partial and Complete Denture
School of Dentistry
The Nippon Dental University

Hiroyuki Miyata
Assistant Professor
Dept. of Periodontology
School of Dentistry
The Nippon Dental University

Atsushi Nomura
Assistant Professor
Dept. of Oral and Maxillofacial Surgery
Dept. of Oral Implantology
School of Dentistry
The Nippon Dental University

Masato Sumitomo
Associate Professor
Dept. of Anesthesiology
School of Dentistry
The Nippon Dental University

Hitoshi Takamori
Associate Professor
Dept. of Oral and Maxillofacial Surgery
Dept. of Oral Implantology
School of Dentistry
The Nippon Dental University

Yoshitaka Takeda
Assistant Professor
Dept. of Partial and Complete Denture
School of Dentistry
The Nippon Dental University

Minoru Uchida
Professor and Chairman
Dept. of Oral and Maxillofacial Surgery
School of Dentistry
The Nippon Dental University

Kaichi Watanabe
Associate Professor
Dept. of Crown and Bridge
Dept. of Oral Implantology
School of Dentistry
The Nippon Dental University

Takashi Yosue
Associate Professor
Dept. of Radiology
Dept. of Oral Implantology
School of Dentistry
The Nippon Dental University

FOREWORD for the First Japanese Edition

Rehabilitation of partial and complete edentulism according to the osseointegration principle involves creation of permanent functional coexistence between bone and mucoperiosteum at the biologic side of the interface and titanium and titanium oxide on the synthetic side.

Extreme precision in manufacturing and handling the hardware and gentle preparation technique in the treatment of the biologic tissue is a prerequisite for prognostic predictability. It is therefore of utmost importance that the clinical and technical procedures which create and maintain osseointegration are described and demonstrated in detail to those who intend to use osseointegration as a clinical rehabilitation procedure.

The present publication is a good example of the mode of information that over the years has proven successful in providing a reliable longterm prognosis as documented by training courses and clinical activities at Nippon Dental University.

Göthenburg, March 22, 1989

Per-Ingvar Brånemark
Professor, M.D., Ph.D., O.Dhc.

PREFACE

Patients who have lost their teeth naturally seek treatment which will enable them to eat normally again.

Under some conditions and with certain patients, however, satisfaction is low even when excellent prosthetic techniques are employed. Dental implants are especially useful in such cases. Treatment using implants has a long history, but many obstacles have had to be overcome in finding suitable implant materials and proper techniques for attaining natural function.

From the results of a number of basic studies, Professor Brånemark of Göteborg University devised the concept of an implant in direct contact with the bone, i.e., an osseointegrated implant. He also established safer and more secure operative procedures, and has reported high rates of success based on long-follow-up observations. His method has been introduced to great acclaim in various countries, and his concepts and methods have garnered an ever-growing body of scientific evidence in their favor.

At our Nippon Dental University Hospital, the Brånemark implant was introduced in 1985, and an implant team comprised of various specialists was initially established. Then in January 1991, the Department of Oral Implantology was formed. Basic training courses have been given at the hospital since 1988. One reason for the favorable results we have consistently achieved in terms of safety and security, has been that all steps including examination, diagnosis, surgical procedure, prosthetic procedure and maintenance are supported by training courses, the contents of which are uniform and systematized. We have produced a manual the illustrates the techniques used in each step, so that practitioners in the training courses can be sure to gain mastery of the techniques involved. Since our first edition was published, we have been asked to translate the manual into English and make it available abroad. We have taken this opportunity to publish a revised edition and translate it into English. While this manual is a guide to osseointegrated technique in toto, different specialists have been responsible for individual sections of the manual. We also feel confident that this book will prove to be applicable to the actual clinical cases. In the section on hands-on training, details involved in various methods and precise instructions on how to use various devices are given clearly, so that even assistants will be able to understand them. We hope that this book will come into wide use.

In publishing this manual, we express our gratitude to chairman of the board of directors Soh Nakahara and Director Kazu Itoh for their kind understanding and help. We also thank Professor Lekholm, chairman of the Brånemark Clinic for his kind efforts in reviewing the manuscript and giving constructive suggestion.

May 1993

Department of Oral Implantology
The Nippon Dental University

Recommendations

Oral implant treatment has worldwide become an accepted therapy in dentistry of today, much due to the introduction of the Brånemark implant procedure. However, in order to be successful, the technique must be performed the correct way, and consequently, before starting to use the procedure clinically, there is a need for good instructions. As in all training, the education must be based on both theoretical as well as practical elements, in order to be able to transmit the knowledge from one generation of clinicians to the next one. Besides the use of good textbooks, there is also a need for manuals, summarizing the information on how to perform the procedure.

The present manual, being based on several years of clinical and teaching experience of the osseointegration technique by the team of the Nippon Dental University, is a good contribution to the educational literature. The reader will here find a step by step description of the method, including preoperative examinations and treatment planning, surgical and anaesthesia techniques, prosthetic procedures, and technical laboratory handling. The manual deals mainly with the edentulous jaw but presents also information on theatment of the partially edentulous situation. Furthermore, it contains descriptions on recommended maintenance care, as well as it gives information on how to deal with some clinical problems that might occur, when using the technique. All parts of the manual are based on excellent pictures, being combined with short-term text information. The quality of the illustrations is very high, and the pictures give a good overview of how to perform the procedure. The manual ought to be helpful for all trainees going through basic education courses and when starting to use the technique clinically.

At a time when there is an explosion of publications within the field of implant treatment, it is a pleasure to recommend the manual to all members of the treatment team as a suitable introduction to how to use the osseointegration procedure ad modum Brånemark.

Göteborg, December 20, 1992

Ulf Lekholm, DDS, PhD
Professor and Chairman
of the Brånemark Clinic
Göteborg, Sweden

From the Chairman

The Nippon Dental University School of Dentistry has been expanding and reorganizing in accordance with its long-term plans. New buildings have already been constructed for the Dental Technicians and Hygienists School. Further, construction of a new university hospital convenient to a railway station has finally been realized, more than 50 years after first planned.

But new or remodeled buildings are meaningless if the functioning of the hospital itself remains unchanged. Our team working on osseointegrated implants (as part of the university hospital) is also being reorganized to take on new responsibilities. Oral implants are expected to play an important role in clinical practice during the 21 st century, when the percentage of elderly among the total population will be high. Standardized materials, academically established surgical procedures, feasible methods that can be used by all dentists, and an accumulation of clinical trials will be required before implants are applied clinically.

To cope with the coming "old-age society," large numbers of dentists will need to have the knowledge and experience necessary to perform implant procedures. Hospitals attached to dental school will be expected to provide information and services pertaining to implants for the benefit of dentists and patients alike.

On November 1, 1990, our university hospital was authorized by the Ministry of Health and Welfare as a medical institution for advanced implant dentures. On January 21, a Department of Oral Implantology was established in the hospital. At present, only a few universities in Sweden, and New York University in the U.S. have a similar capacity. In Japan, we have taken a futuristic perspective on implantology by establishing our implant clinic. We believe that this decision will open a new era in dentistry. Our university hospital expects to serve as an implant center with connections to dentists throughout the nation.

As we enter Japan's new *Heisei* era, I have great hopes for the progress of our university hospital and its implant clinic.

May 1993

Soh Nakahara

Soh Nakahara, D.D.S., M.D., D.D.Sc., D.M.Sc.
Chairman of the Board of Directors
The Nippon Dental University

TABLE OF CONTENTS

I. THE CLINICAL APPLICATION OF OSSEOINTEGRATED IMPLANTS

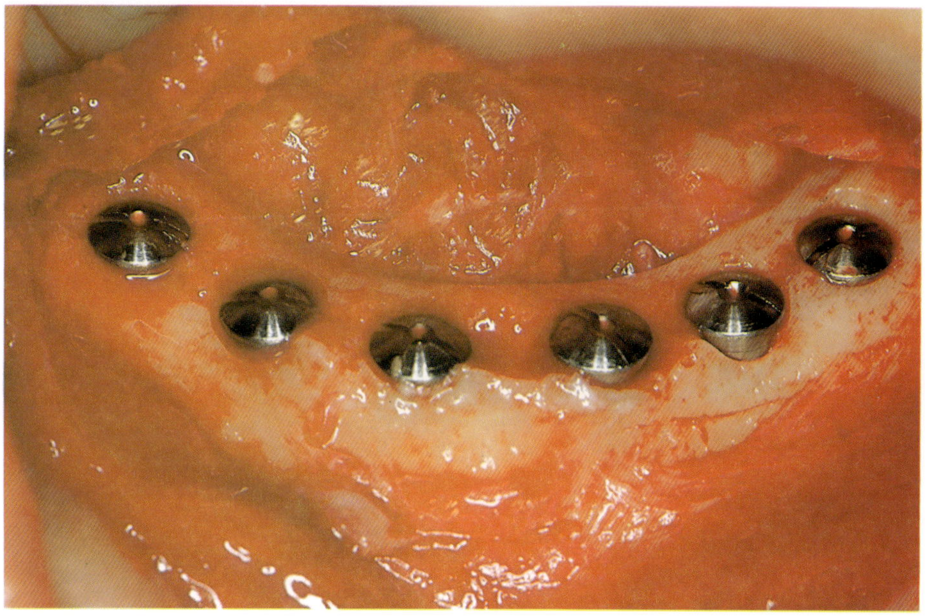

CHAPTER I

EXAMINATIONS, DIAGNOSIS AND TREATMENT PLANNING

The department of Oral Implantology of the Nippon Dental University has been using Brånemark implants under a teamcentered approach. In this chapter, the basic concepts involved with implants and the basic procedures for examination, diagnosis, assessment of indications, and treatment planning-as used at our implant clinic-will be presented briefly. Because this chapter illustrates a team approach at a university hospital, some portions will not be directly applicable to private dental practices. Dentists engaged in private dental practice are urged to make the appropriate adjustments.

Fig. 1 outlines the basic steps used for the Brånemark implant procedure. One main characteristic of this implant system is its two-stage approach; i.e., Stage I Operation (fixture installation) and Stage II Operation (abutment connection). A healing period is required between the two operations, which has been shown to be of importance for the longterm prognosis, so this implant system requires more time than others. This has to be adequately explained to the patient to obtain his or her cooperation.

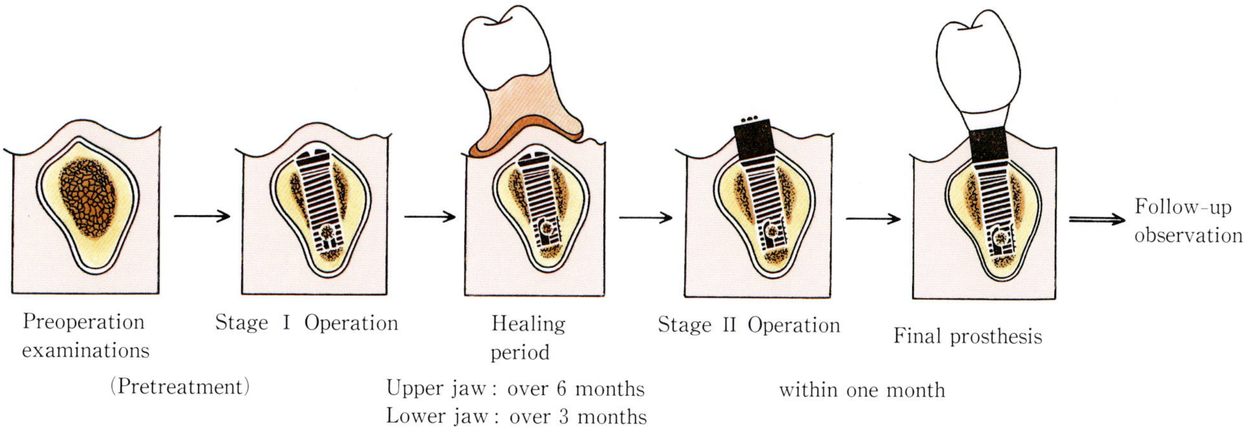

Fig. 1. Steps used for Brånemark implants

Initial Examinations

The initial examination should cover the following items:

(1) Chief complaint

The patient's reason for wanting an implant and his or her suitability for the procedure need to be determined. The dentist should assess whether an implant would address the patient's chief complaint. Implant should be avoided in cases where postoperative problems are anticipated.

(2) Patient history

Because patients who receive implants are usually elderly, their disease history has to be taken carefully.

(3) Present prosthetic condition

Information on the cause of tooth loss, past dental treatment, and current use of dentures is important in determining whether an implant will be successful.

(4) Present medical and oral health conditions

Because patients, receiving implants, usually have a high prevalence of disease, their systemic condition has to be evaluated. Physical constitution, nutritional state, and disease control status need to be assessed. In the oral cavity, the alveolar ridge, frenulum, remaining teeth and overall oral hygiene have to be evaluated as well.

(5) Stone cast model analysis

Using a study model, the relationship between the upper and lower jaws has to be assessed to judge the esthetic suitability of an implant for a given patient.

(6) Radiographic examinations

A rotating panoramic radiograph and lateral cephalograph have to be taken at the preliminary stage. See the supplement ("Radiographic Examination") at the end of this chapter for details.

(7) Final assessments and treatment planning

Patients who are indicated for implants on the basis of the above-mentioned preliminary examination are subjected to a more detailed examination after appropriate pretreatment.

Main Examination

The main examination should include the following:

(1) Facial appearance

Assessment of the facial profile, nasolabial groove and upper and lower lips is particularly important.

(2) Oral examination

① State of oral hygiene

② Degree of compression in the oral mucosa

③ Attachment point of frenulum

④ Properties of saliva

⑤ State of alveolar crest

⑥ Site and state of remaining teeth

(3) Existing denture

① Shape and size of the denture base

② Arrangement of artificial teeth

③ Occlusal relationship

④ Esthetic appearance

⑤ Phonation

(4) Stomatognathic function

① Check for abnormalities of the temporomandibular joint

② Palpate the masticatory muscles

③ Check for bruxism

④ Determine maximum mandibular movement

⑤ Trace the gothic arch

(5) Radiography

Sectional radiographs, CT, TMJ, etc., are used. See the supplement on "Radiographic Examination" which concludes this chapter.

(6) Mental examination

In some cases, mental status has to be examined by CMI (Cornell Medical Index), Y-G (Yatabe-Guilford test) or MAS (Taylor manifest anxiaty scale) test.

(7) Hematology, urinalysis, etc.

Hematological tests, urinalysis, and so on have to be performed for patients in whom the preliminary test suggests the presence of some disease. If the patient is under the care of another physician, he is asked to carry out these tests.

(8) Treatment planning

After the above-mentioned tests, a conference with members of the departments of oral surgery, prosthodontics, periodontics and radiology is held to devise a treatment plan for the patient.

Brånemark implants are applicable to all patients regardless of age or sex as long as the patient's bone mass is sufficient to allow implant insertion. Contraindications for implants are similar to those for general surgery. In addition, the following patients are contraindicated.

① Patients with mental disease

② Patients with drug or alcohol addiction

③ Patients whose major concern is esthetic improvement

④ Patients who expect too much of implants

⑤ Patients in whom an ordinary denture functions well

At this stage of preoperative examination, the patient's bone architecture and morphology have to be assessed with a rotating panoramic radiograph, lateral cephalograph, CT or sectional radiograph. Usually, the density of the bone trabecula on radiographs serves as an index of bone architecture. The study model and lateral cephalogram are important in assessing bone mass and the relationship between the upper and lower jaw. Figs. 2 and 3 outline bone quality and mass (including the relationship between the upper and lower jaw). Because these factors affect the operation, it is important that they be evaluated.

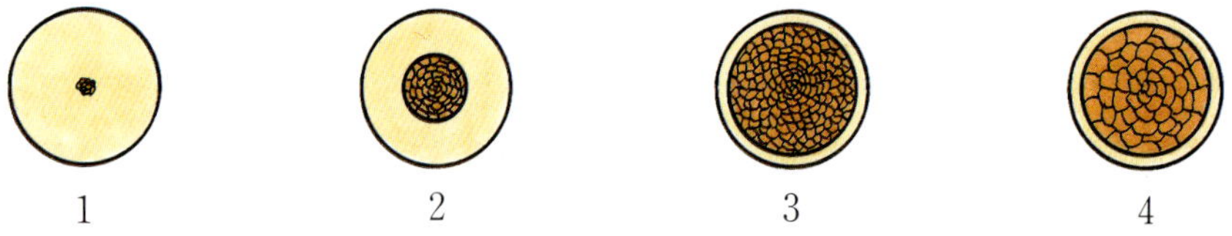

Fig. 2. Bone quality (Leckholm U. and Zarb G. A. Tissue-Integrated Prostheses)

1. Almost the entire jaw is comprised of homogenous compact bone
2. A thick layer of compact bone surrounds a core of dense trabecular bone
3. A thin layer of cortical bone surrounds a core of dense trabecular bone of favorable strength
4. A thin layer of cortical bone surrounds a core of low density trabecular bone

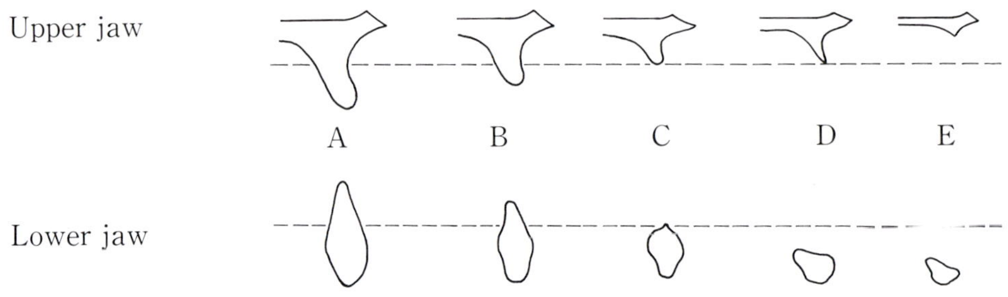

Fig. 3. Bone resorption (Leckholm U. and Zarb G. A. Tissue-Integrated Prostheses)

SUPPLEMENT

Radiographic Examination

Radiography is performed on the following four occasions:

(1) initial examination, (2) main examination, (3) abutment connection, and (4) upon completion of the prosthesis and at follow-up observation. The suitability of an osseointegrated implant for a given patient is determined at the first examination or the main examination. Because the prognosis for osseointegrated implants is affected by patient selection, examination and assessment on these two occasions are very important.

Table 1 shows the time, method and essential test points for radiography. Radiography may not be performed during the interval between the primary and secondary operation, because a high dose of secondary (scattered) x-ray irradiation to the peri-implant area might injure osteoblasts, which are important for healing.

Table 1. Radiography for Osseointegrated Implants

Time	Technique	Essential point of interpretation
Initial examination	Panoramic Occlusal Dental Cephalography Panagraphy	Bone quality; Bone architecture (resorption) Jaw height and shape Detailed check of remaining teeth Position of mental foramen Position of maxillary sinus, nasal cavity and incisive canal
Additional (main) examination	Tomography CT TMJ	Height and width of possible fixtures Designing of treatment denture Direction of fixture insertion Check of bone quality TMJ diagnosis
After secondary operation	Panoramic Dental	Check of abutment connection Check of marginal bone level
Upon completion of prosthesis and during observation	Dental	Check of abutment connection Check for marginal conditions State of osseointegration

Radiography at the Initial Examination

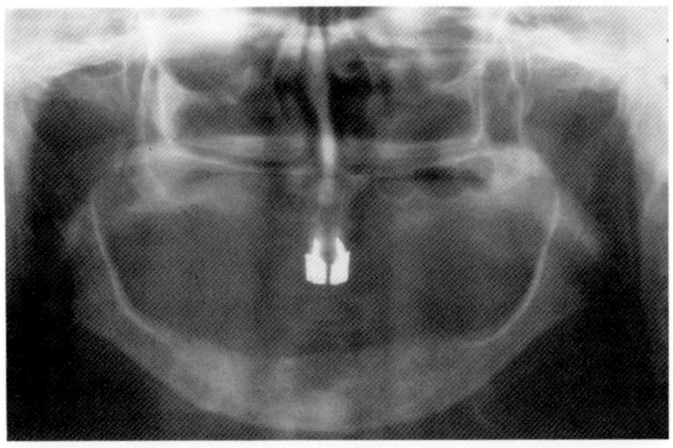

Fig. 4. Radiography plays an important role in preoperative examination. Its purpose is not only to check bone mass and quality but also to evaluate the arrangement of the mandibular canal, position of the mental foramen, maxillary sinus and nasal cavity base, and condition of the remaining teeth.

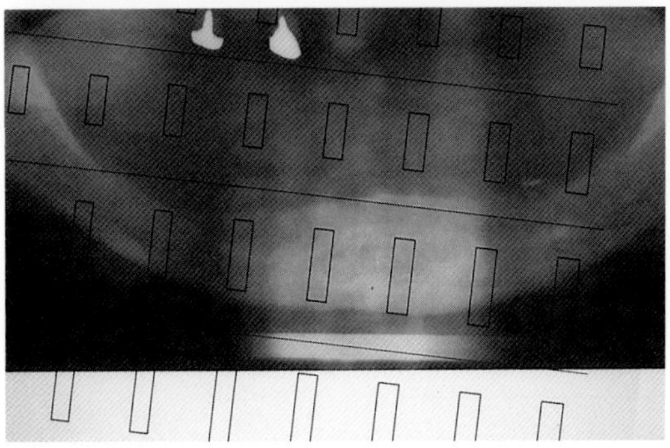

Fig. 5. Using a transparent scale, the acceptable number and length of fixtures are estimated on a rotating panoramic radiograph. Care should be taken to avoid overestimation of the height of the jawbone, bearing in mind that the magnification rate on the panoramic x-ray film is about 1.2~1.3.

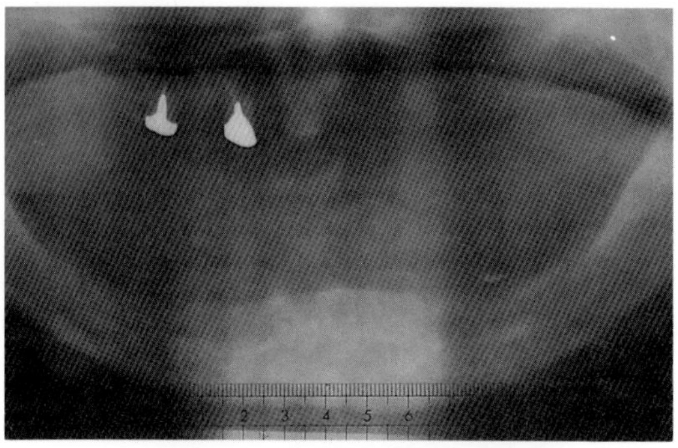

Fig. 6. The occlusion have to be evaluated with the use of a panoramic radiograph as well as a study model. For example, the distance between the alveolar crest and the occlusal plane of the opposite jaw have to be longer than the total length of the abutment and the gold cylinder. It is advisable to use a scale to estimate the distance.

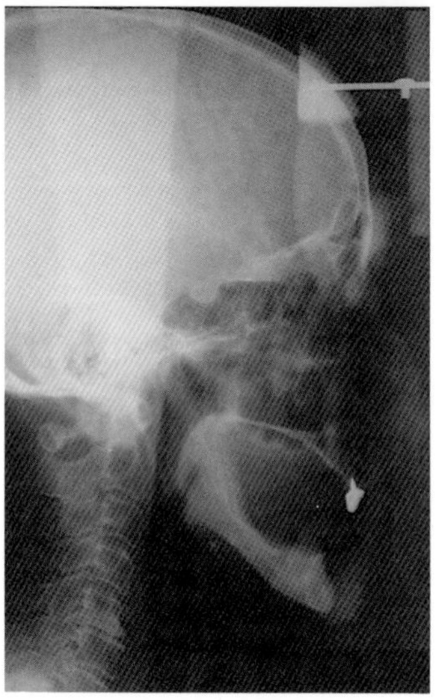

Fig. 7. Lateral cephalography is performed to assess the vertical and labiolingual morphology of the anterior teeth region of the mandible and to determine a maxillomandibular relationship. In estimating the length of the fixture to be used the magnification rate (×1.1) on the cephalogram has to be considered. This type of radiography also allows for the assessment of bone quality in the region to be operated.

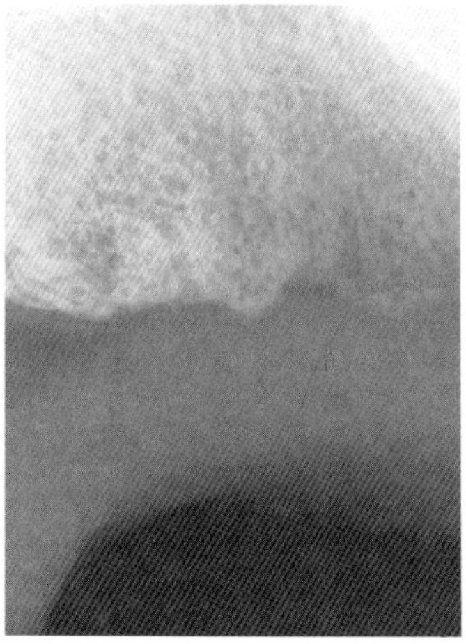

Fig. 8. If the implant is planned for the upper anterior teeth, the position of the nasal cavity base, alveolar crest and anterior wall of the maxillary sinus have to be assessed, irrespective of the presence/absence of teeth. Furthermore, the acceptable length and number of fixtures have to be estimated. For these purposes, paralleling dental radiography is needed. We make it a rule to take three radiographs (right and left canine regions and median region).

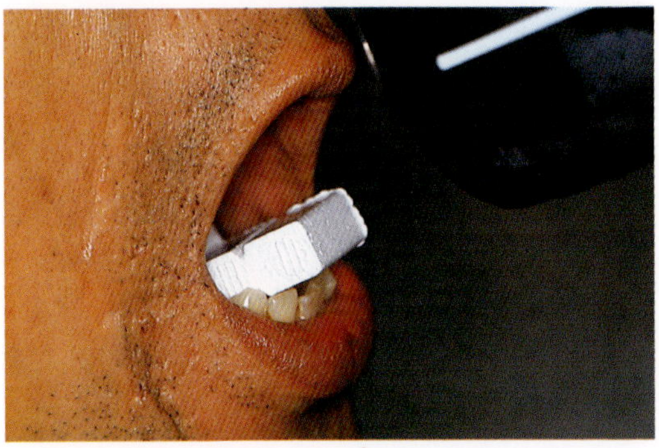

Fig. 9. The use of an Eggen holder has been recommended in the paralleling method. However, we use a Stabe disposable device, which is easier to retain in the oral cavity and is more hygienic. If the panoramic radiograph suggest marginal periodontitis or periapical lesions, detailed examination with routine dental radiography is necessary.

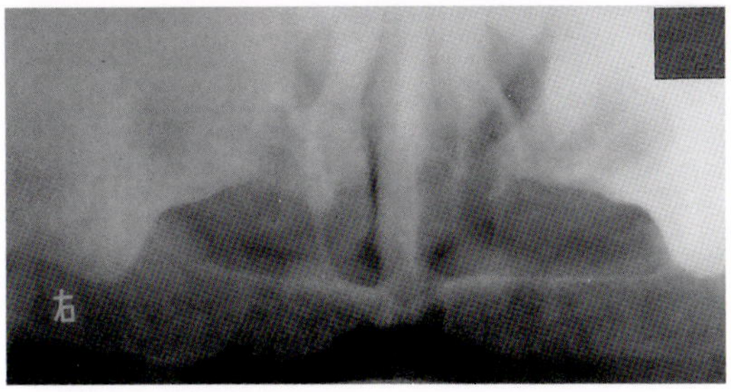

Fig. 10. Intracavitary panoramic radiography (panagraphy) is sometimes performed as a substitute for dental radiography or to obtain additional information on the anterior teeth region after rotating panoramic radiography. This technique provides higher resolution but causes more distortion than the rotating method.

Radiography During Additional Examinations

An additional examination is performed with patients judged suitable for implants on the basis of the first examination (x-ray and various examinations the oral cavity and other regions) and with those who wish to continue with the procedure. Although the anterior teeth region of the mandible does not require additional radiography after the initial examination, the other regions require precise examination to determine the length and width of the areas to be utilized for implant. For this purpose, tomography is needed.

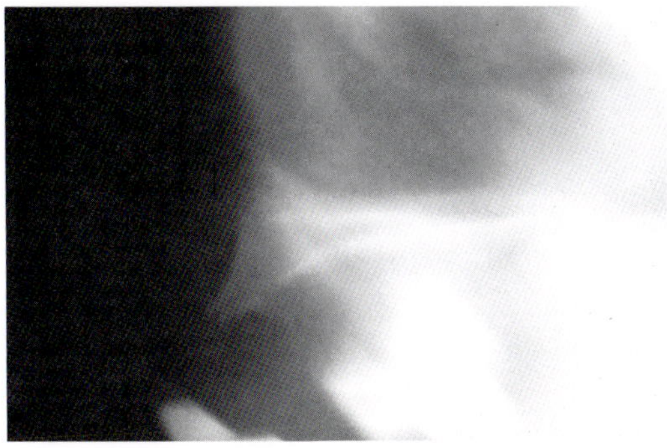

Fig. 11. If an implant is planned for the maxilla, it must be determined whether the bone in the canine fossa is wide enough for fixture insertion. A sectional radiograph taken after marking this region is shown here. The magnification rate has to be considered in interpreting the film. This technique can also be used to assess the mandibular canal arrangement.

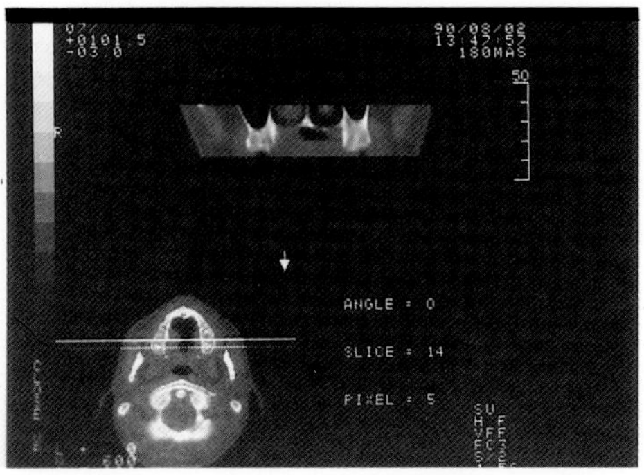

Fig. 12. The vertical thickness of the bone can be assessed by transverse CT-scan instead of tomography. Shown is a CT image with a 2 mm slice-thickness taken of a patient selected for an implant in the anterior teeth region of the maxilla. CT provides information similar to that provided by tomography.

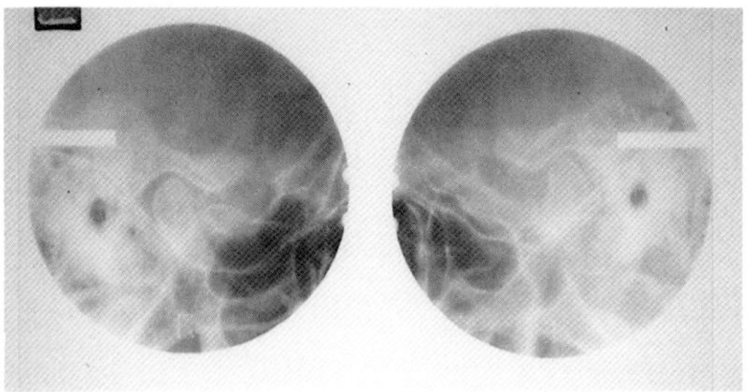

Fig. 13. In order for the implant to be stable and function well in the oral cavity, factors causing temporomandibular joint disease must be ruled out. Cephalometric radiography of the temporomandibular joint by lateral oblique projection is suitable for this, although it does not provide perfect evaluation.

CHAPTER II

SURGICAL PROCEDURES

Stage I Operation (Fixture Installation)

Here, the Stage I Operation is presented, taking as an example an edentulous mandible (a typical case of implant application).

The operation is performed under local anesthesia and intravenous sedation (see Chapter 3, "Systemic Management and Anesthesia" for details.)

Remark: At our university, general anesthesia is frequently used instead of local anesthesia in order to minimize the surgical stress for the patient.

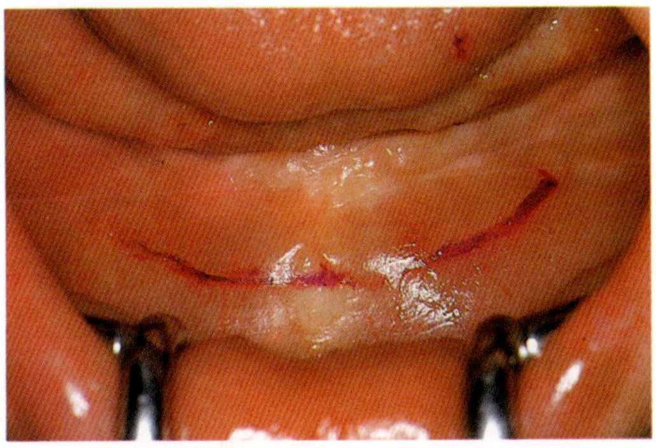

Fig. 14. Using a dissector, the incision line is marked in the buccal sulcus between the bilateral canines, parallel to the alveolar crest. The dissected line is deviated slightly towards the alveolar crest in the canine region to prevent injury to the mental nerve.

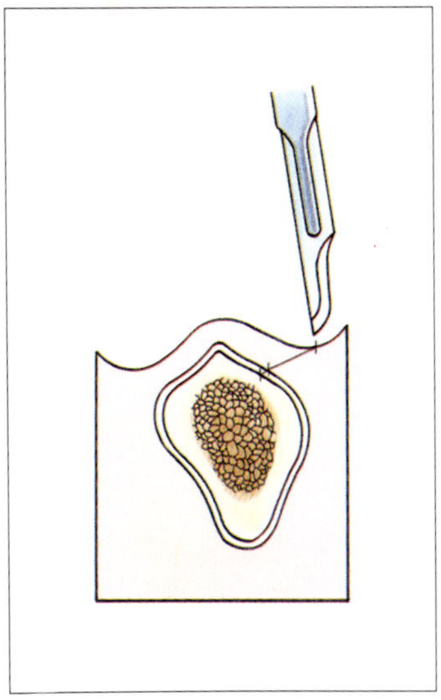

Fig. 15. The mucous membrane is incised with a No. 15 blade.

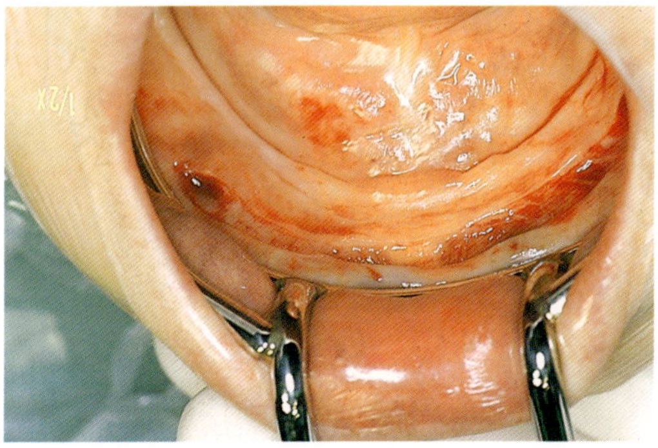

Fig. 16. Sharp incision of the mucosa alone is possible if the vestibule is sufficiently stretched by a lip retractor.

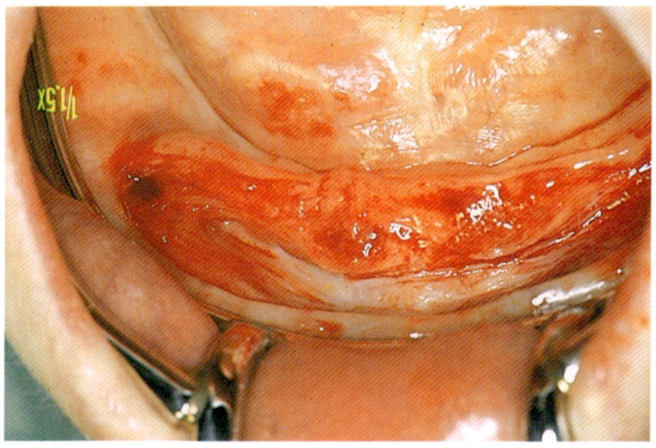

Fig. 17. A supraperiosteal flap is elevated in the direction of the alveolar crest. The periosteum is, then, incised 5–6 mm below the alveolar crest between the bilateral canines.

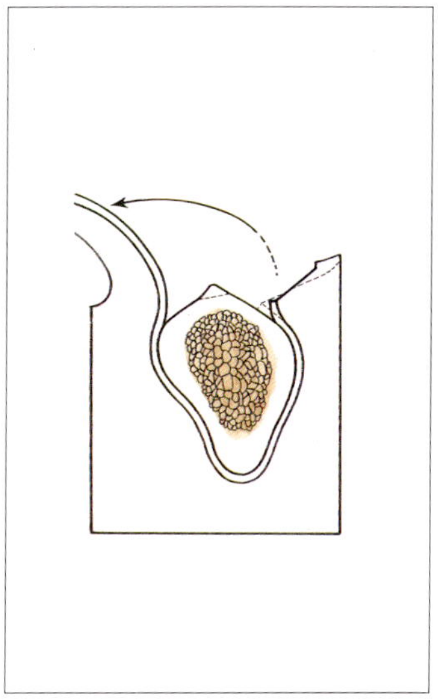

Fig. 18. Using a dissector or elevator, the alveolar crest is exposed. Fibrous connective tissue, which frequently covers the alveolar crest, is removed completely. If the alveolar crest forms a knife-edge, the crest is slightly reduced in height with a bone forceps.

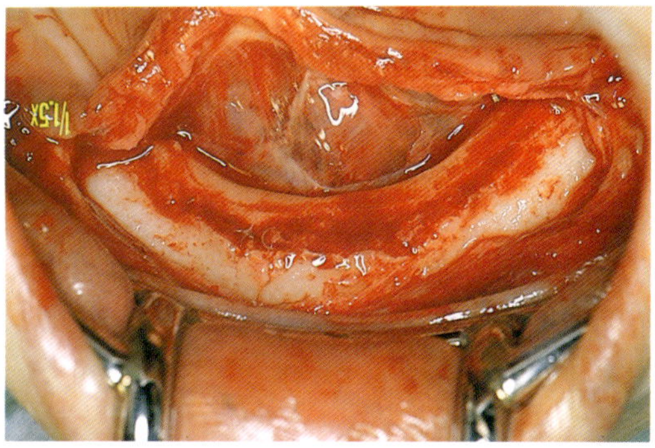

Fig. 19. With the elevated flap on the lingual side, care is taken to avoid perforation of the thin periosteum and mucosa. The morphology of the lingual side is examined with a dissector during this procedure.

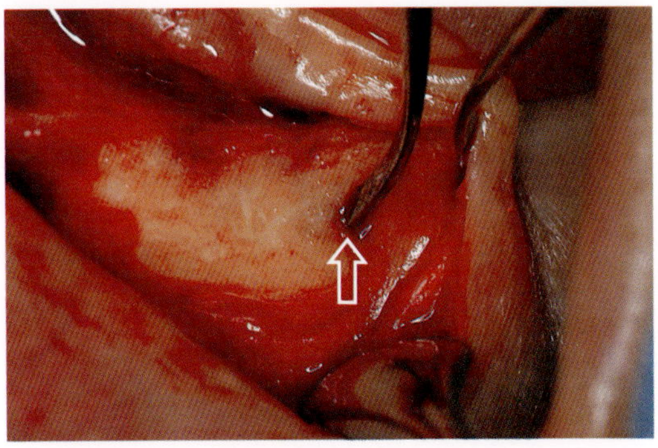

Fig. 20. The area from the canine to the premolar is freed, making a bag-like dissection. The mental foramen is confirmed. Taking care to avoid compressing the mental nerve, the mucosa and periosteum are gradually incised to expose the mental foramen. The dissector is, then, inserted into the mental foramen (*arrow*), in order to check the direction of the so-called mental loop.

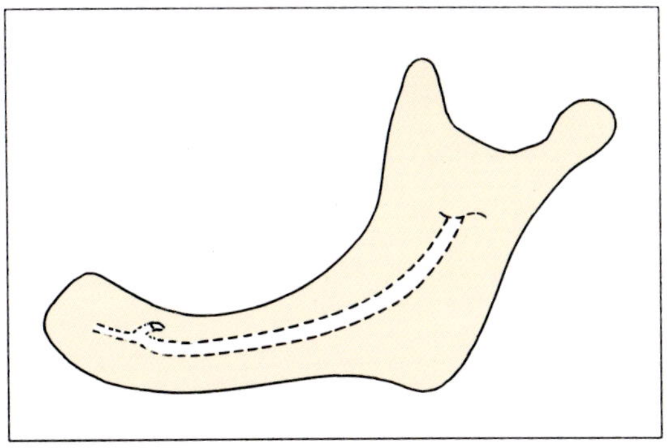

Fig. 21.

Remark: The direction of the mandibular canal near the mental foramen (mental loop) is shown in this picture. The mandibular canal sends out a branch, which curves in the posterior direction, and opens as the mental foramen.

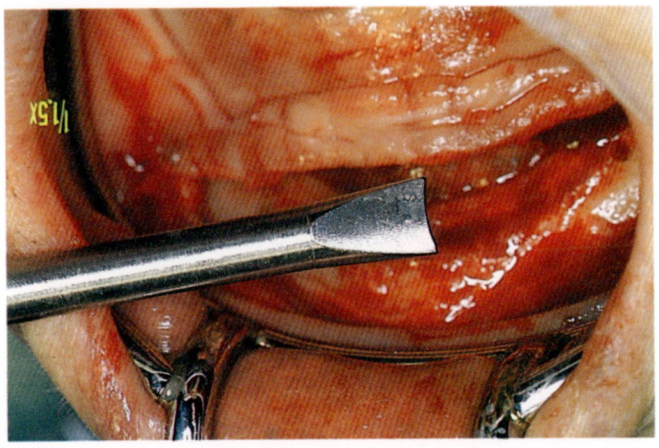

Fig. 22. Using the opposite end of the depth gauge, applied to a point about 5 mm ahead of the mental foramen, the position of an acceptable number of fixtures is determined. If a bridge prosthesis is planned, four to six fixtures need to be inserted.

Remark: Using a surgical stent (Fig.136), the direction of the sites is also predicted.

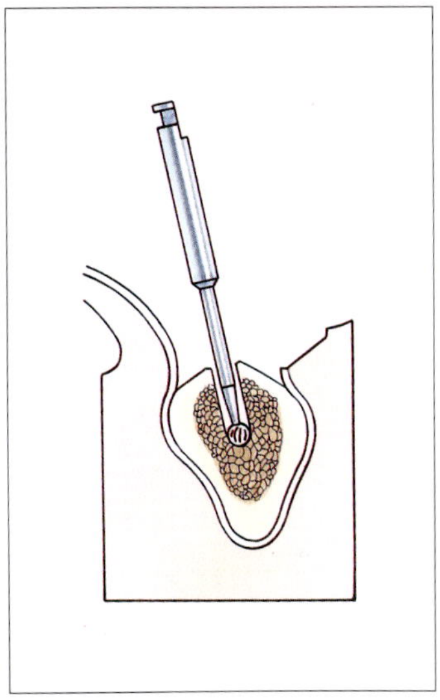

Fig. 23. The most distal fixture site, which is affected by the position of the mental foramen, is marked by drilling (through the cortical layer and a few millimeters into the cancellous bone) with a round bur at a site about 5 mm mesial to the mental foramen. Thereafter, the remaining implant locations are marked. At the same time, the thickness of the compact bone is examined. In subsequent steps, high speed rotation (2000 rpm at maximum) is used. (When utilizing a DEC 500 engine, the black point on the motor is matched to the blue point.)

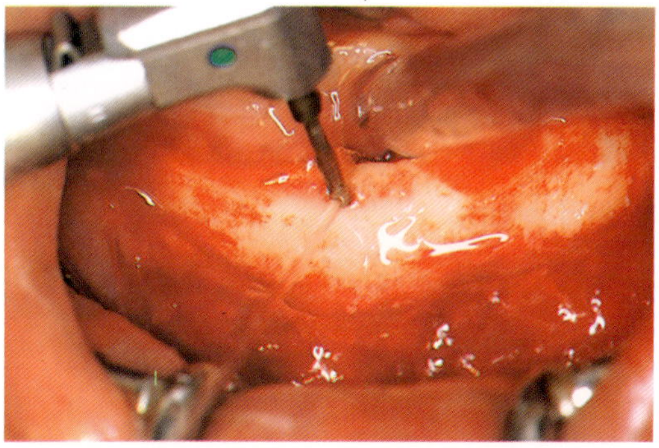

Fig. 24.

Remark: To prevent excess heat and thus minimize injury to bone tissue, saline should be profusely irrigated every time rotating instruments are used. During drilling, the bur should be moved up and down so the irrigation can remove bone chips from the drill groove.

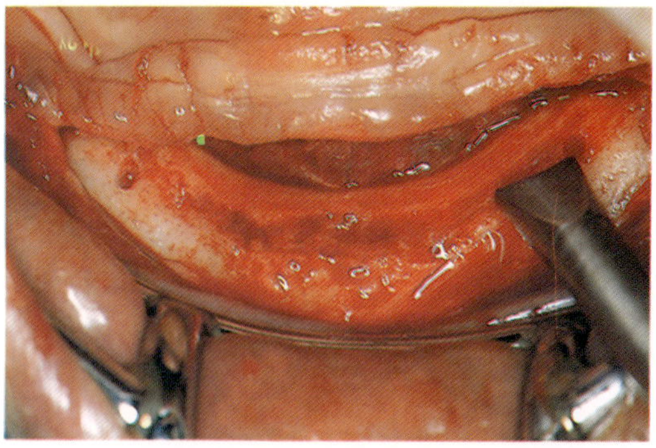

Fig. 25. The ideal distance between fixtures is equal to the diameter of the fixture (3.75 mm). Therefore, there is a distance of about 7.5 mm between the center of a fixture and the center of the neighboring fixture. The opposite end of the depth gauge is convenient for measuring the distance.

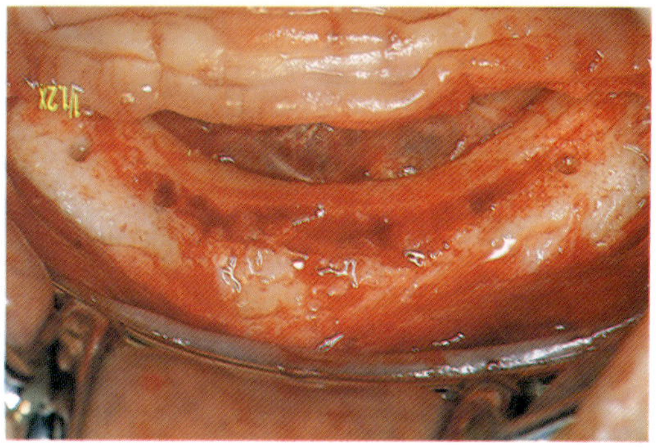

Fig. 26. This case allows for the installation of six implants. Therefore, six points are marked on the alveolar crest.

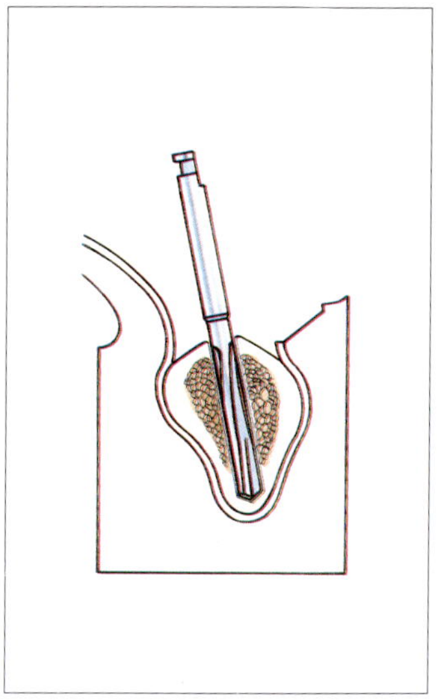

Fig. 27. First, the installation site close to the midline is prepared with a 2.0 mm diameter twist drill.

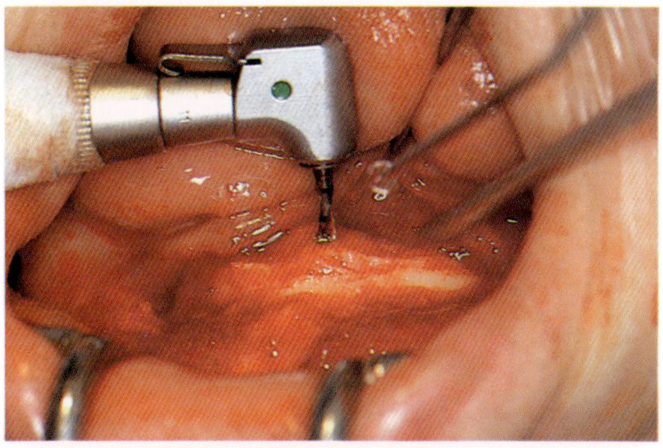

Fig. 28. This drilling direction serves as the standard for subsequent preparations. The direction of natural or artificial teeth on the opposite jaw should be taken into consideration. To ensure that the direction of the site is parallel to the midline, the direction is checked by the assistant or nurse from a different angle. A surgical stent can also be used in this step.

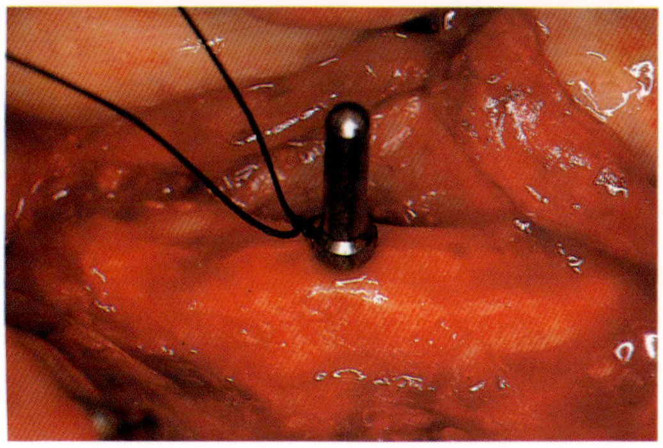

Fig. 29. When the preparation has been completed, the narrow end of a direction indicator is inserted into the site to carefully check the relationship between the upper and lower jaw and the parallelism to the midline.

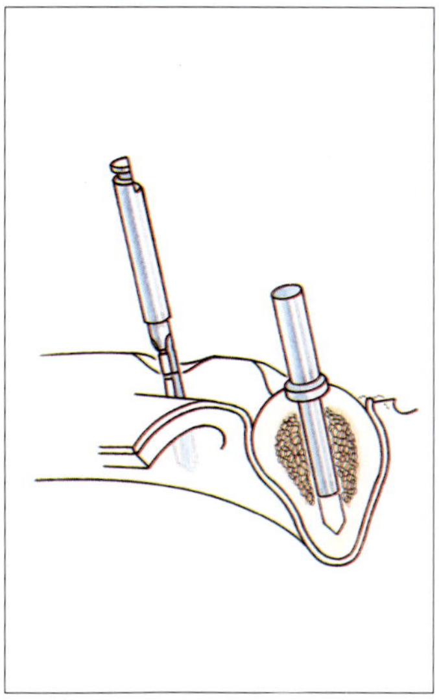

Fig. 30. The most distal site on the left (if the surgeon is right handed) is then prepared with a 2.0 mm diameter twist drill.

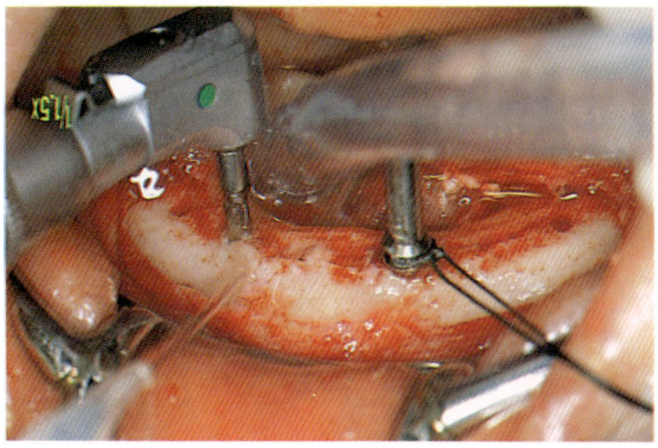

Fig. 31. Inserting the direction indicator into the prepared sites, step by step and from left to right, the drilling of the sites is continued.

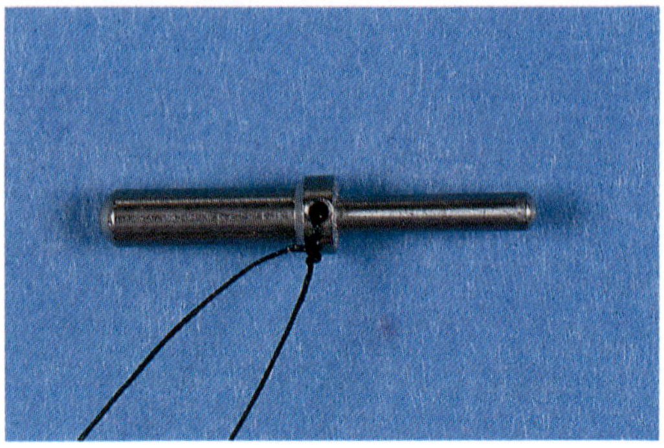

Fig. 32.

Remark: To avoid accidental swallowing of the direction indicator, a 4-0 silk suture is tied to the center hole.

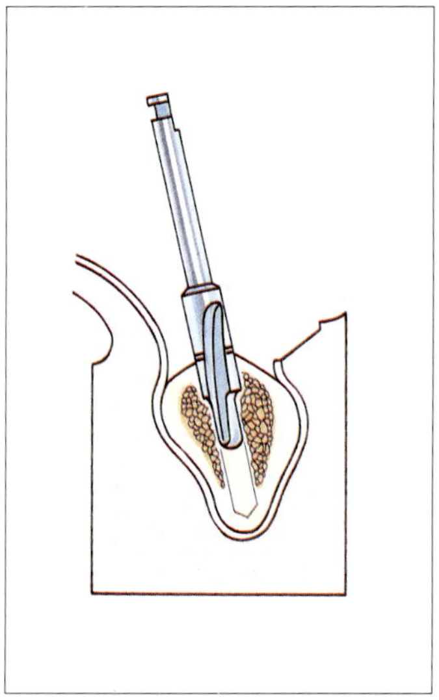

Fig. 33. From the right side towards the left, pilot holes for the 3.0 mm twist drill are created with a pilot drill, taking care to preserve parallelism. The pilot drill is inserted to the marking.

Remark: In this step, the direction can be modified to some extent. In later steps, modification of direction is impossible.

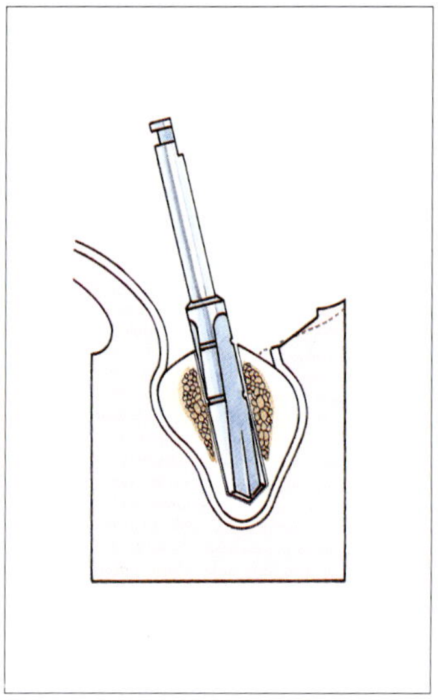

Fig. 34. Using a 3.0 mm twist drill, the canal created by the 2.0 mm twist drill and the pilot drill near the midline is widened, taking care to preserve the relationship between the upper and lower jaw and the parallel relationship to the midline.

Remark: Preparation is performed to the depth predicted by preoperative radiography.

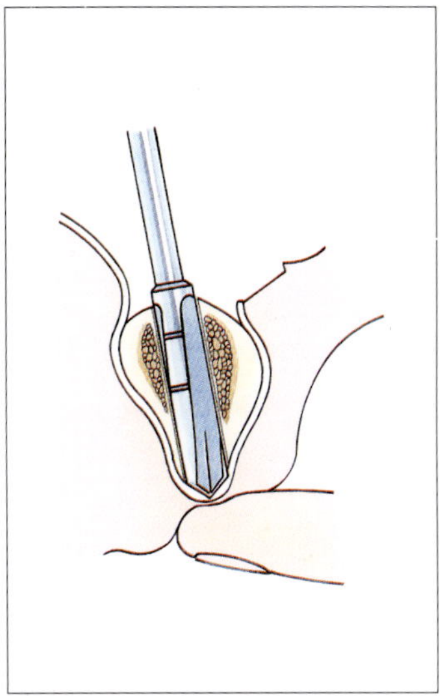

Fig. 35.

Remark: The base compact bone of the mandible may be penetrated intentionally, if the mandibular height is extremely low or if very poor bone quality is at hand. In such cases, the surgeon should press an index finger to the skin of the base of the mandible to palpate drill movements and thereby try to prevent injury to the periosteum.

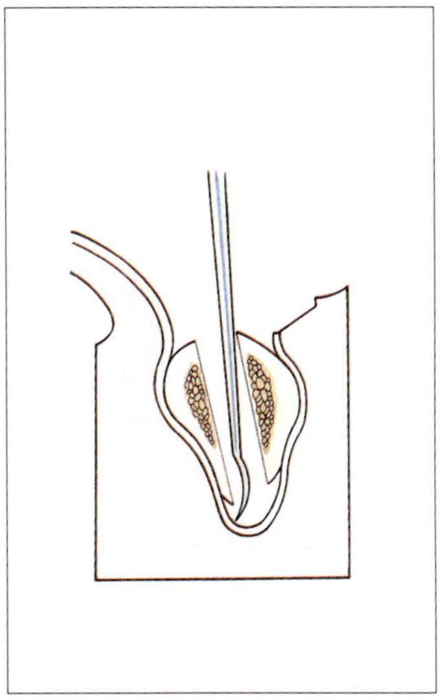

Fig. 36.

Remark: Using a dissector, the periosteum of the lower border is thereafter freed so that this area can be filled with blood, which might facilitate additional bone formation.

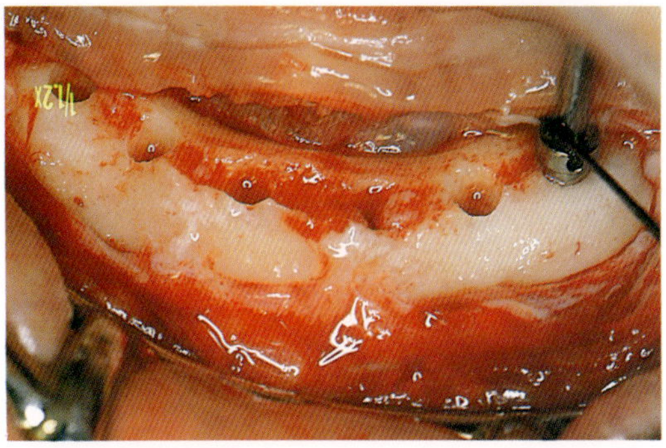

Fig. 37. Preparation with a 3.0mm twistdrill is performed from left to right, while inserting the thicker side of the direction indicator into the widened canal.

Remark: If bleeding from the perforated site occurs, i. e., bleeding of marrow origin, the direction indicator is left inserted to facilitate hemostasis.

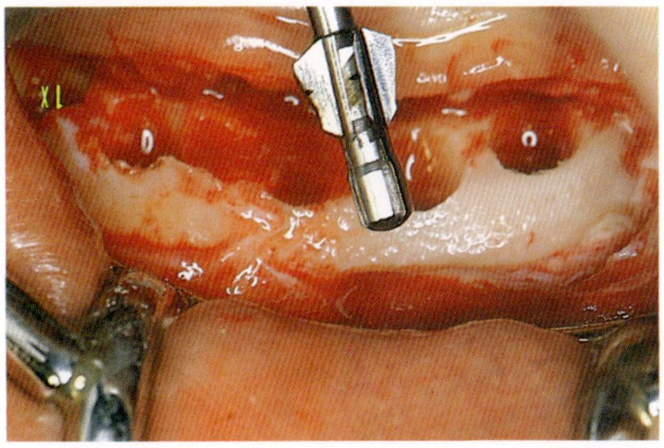

Fig. 38. The last stainless steel drill to be used is the countersink, which is inserted into the entrance of the canal. In this way, a countersink area (a shoulder) is created to receive the upper part of the fixture.

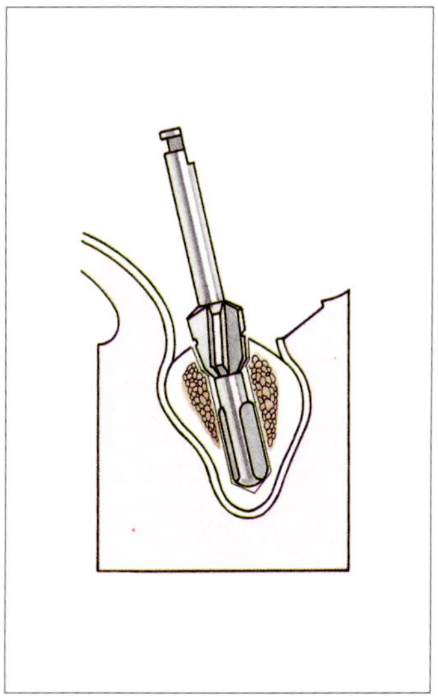

Fig. 39. In creating the shoulder, care needs to be taken that depth does not exceed half the thickness of the marginal compact bone.

Remark: In the molar region, perforation in the base compact bone is impossible, due to the inferior alveolar nerve canal. In this region, therefore, the installed fixture is only retained by the screw threads on the marginal compact bone, during osseointegration.

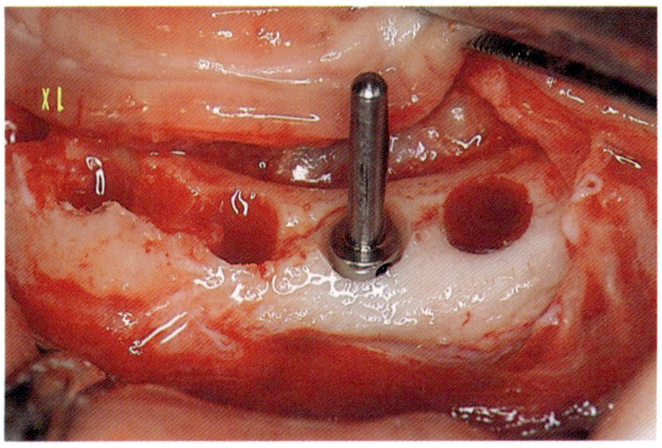

Fig. 40. The created shoulder is tested with a direction indicator. The upper plane of the mid ring of the direction indicator should correspond with the top of the alveolar crest.

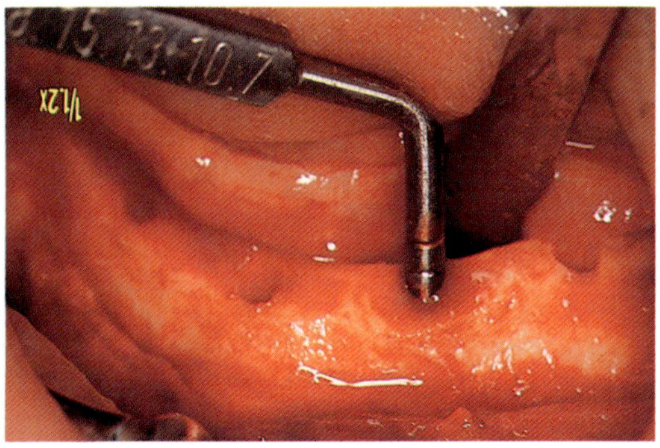

Fig. 41. The depth of the canal is measured with a gauge. The preferred depth is 1-2 mm deeper than the length of the planned fixture.

Remark: See Fig. 351 for the relationship between canal depth, depth gauge, countersink, tap, fixture mount and cover screw.

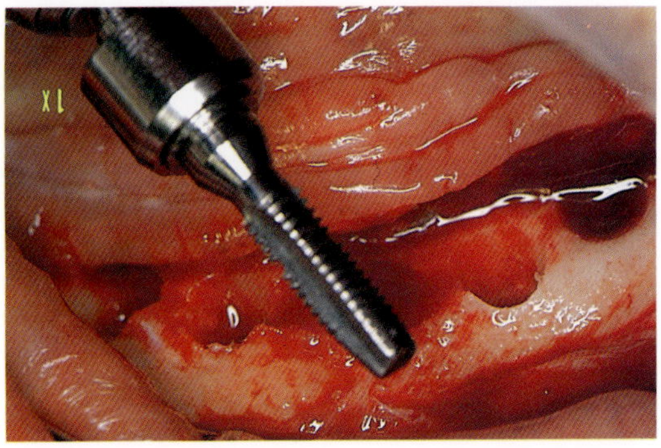

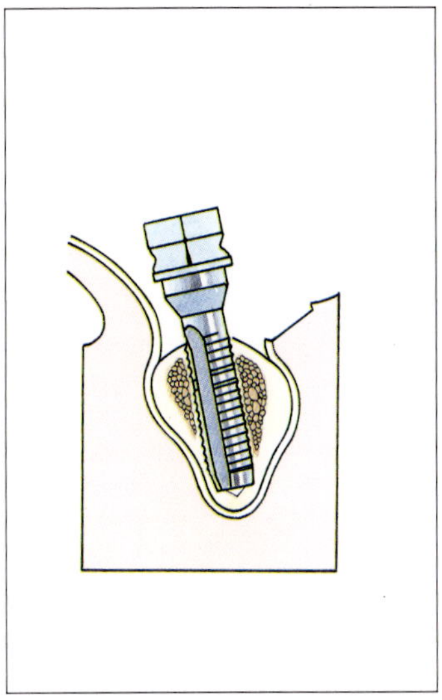

Figs. 42&43. A connection is attached to the contra-angle handpiece, and a screw tap ("tap") is attached, with which screw threads are created on the inside of the canal.

Remark: Subsequent steps are made using slow rotation (maximum 28 rpm). If a DEC 500 engine is utilized, the black point on the motor is matched to the green point. Instruments made of titanium should be manipulated with a titanium forceps. If the compact bone is too dense, and it is hard to create screw threads with the tap, a 3.15 mm twist drill should be used prior to tapping. If cancellous bone predominates over compact bone, the surgeon must be steady on hand while using the tap, because screw threads may otherwise be broken by improper movements of the instrument.

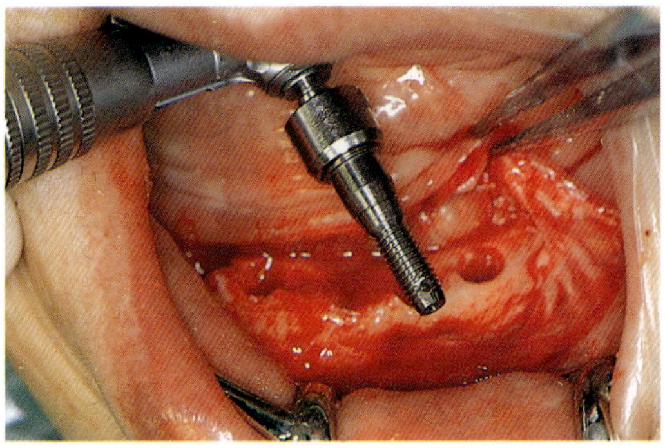

Fig. 44. After tapping the most distal site on the left site, the first fixture is inserted.

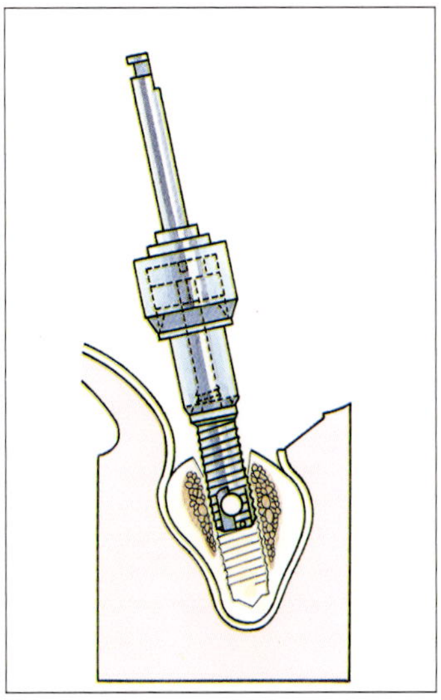

Fig. 45. To prevent saline from being pressed into the bone marrow by the fixture, irrigation should be avoided until the horizontal hole at the fixture tip has entered the bone site completely.

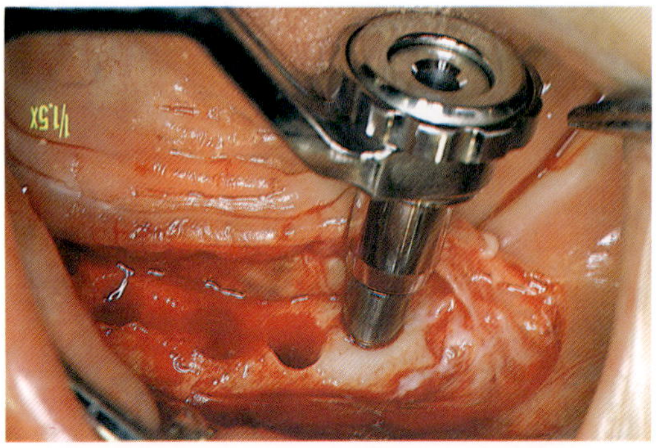

Fig. 46. After the rotation of the fixture mount has stopped, the connection is removed and final tightening is done with a cylinder wrench using profuse irrigation.

Remark: Tightening should be discontinued if high resistance is felt, or if the marginal compact bone begins to crack.

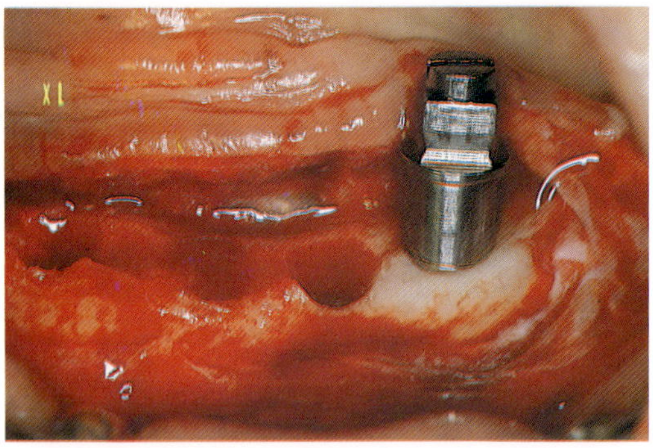

Fig. 47. The percussion sound is checked with a tap against the fixture mount, using a dissector. A high metallic sound indicates that the fixture is surrounded by a lot of bone.

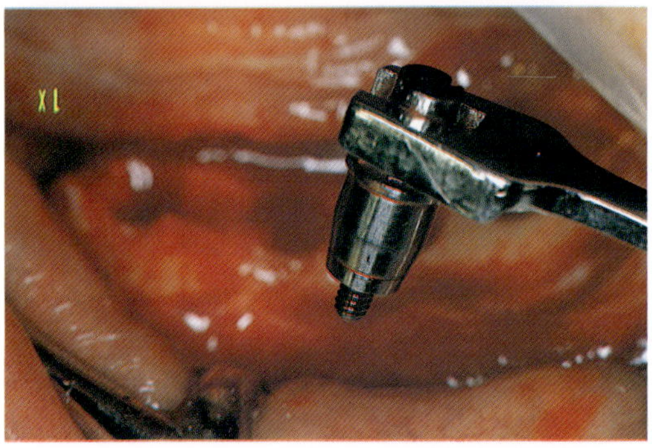

Fig. 48. An open-end wrench is attached to the square portion of the fixture mount, which is removed by rotating the machine screwdriver in reverse.

Remark: The wrench is used to avoid that the rotating force of the driver is transferred to the fixture. Even if a manual driver is employed, the wrench must be utilized.

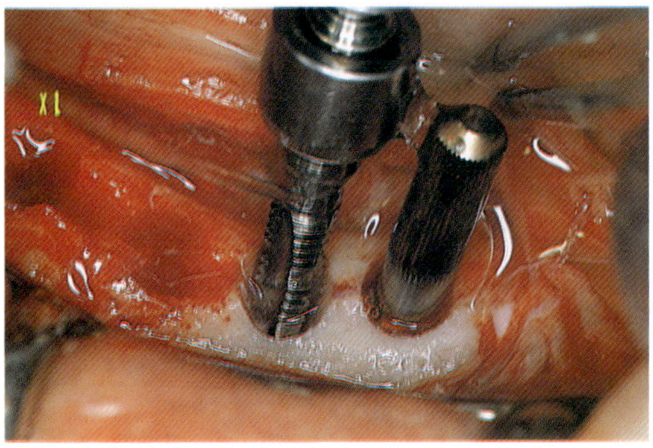

Fig. 49. The threading of the sites and the fixture insertions are repeated from left to right.

Remark: After fixture installation, the direction indicator for the fixture is inserted into the central canal to check the parallelism (errors of up to about 30 degrees do not cause serious problems).

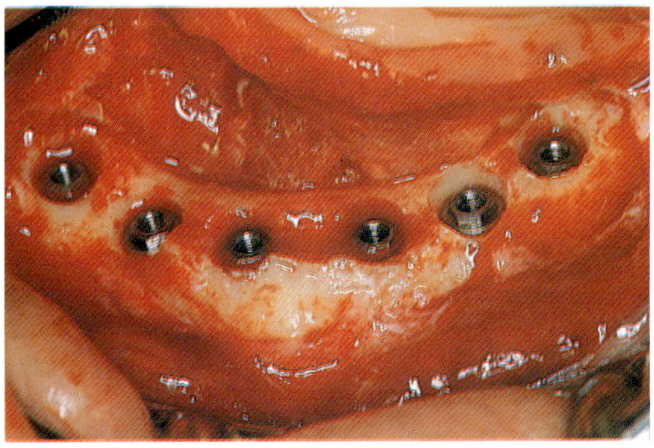

Fig. 50. Installation of six fixtures has been completed.

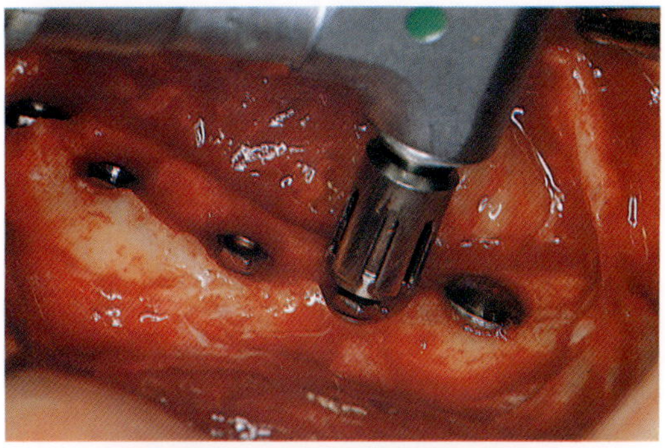

Fig. 51. Using a screw inserter, the cover screws are applied to the fixtures to prevent bone and soft tissue from growing into the internally threaded canal of the implants.

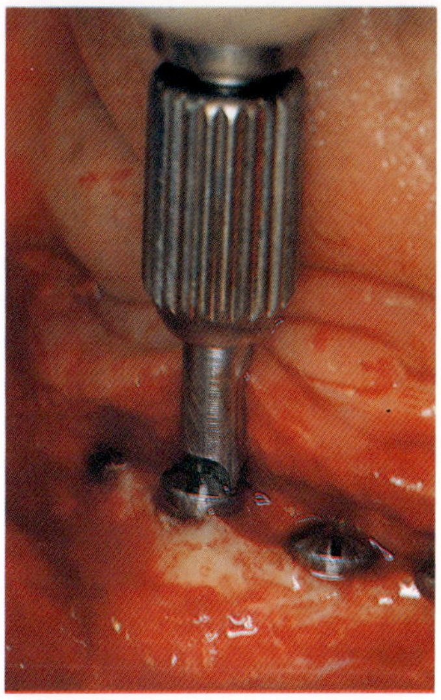

Fig. 52. After the cover screw has been applied to the fixture, it is smoothly tightened with a short manual screw-driver.

Remark: Even a small space between the cover screw and the fixture head can later cause infiltration of bone or soft tissues, making the secondary operation difficult.

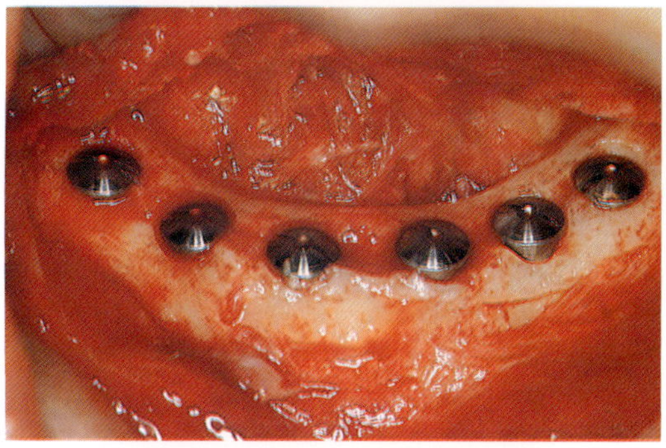

Fig. 53. After insertion of all the cover screws, the operative field is thoroughly flushed clean with saline solution.

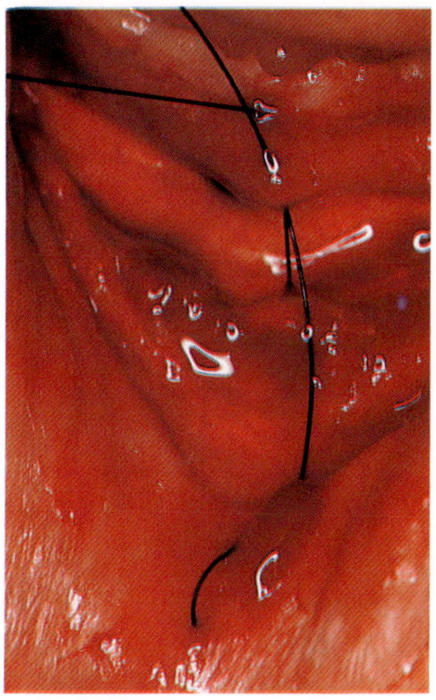

Fig. 54. Vertical mattress sutures using 3-0 nylon sutures are made starting in the midline. The knot should be placed on the lingual gingival side.

Remark: Vertical mattress sutures around the mental foramen may involve the nerve. Therefore, an simple interrupted suture is recommended to be used in this region.

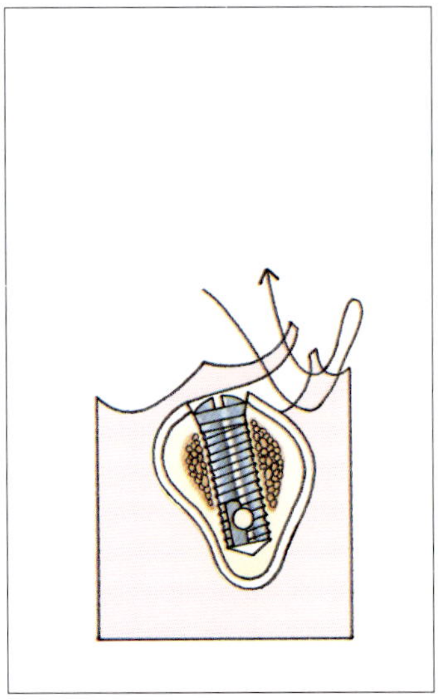

Fig. 55.

Remark: Vertical mattress sutures are used when a wound has to be closed securely. First, the needle passes a little deeper than usual through the mucosa flap on the lingual side and is then catching up the periosteum on the buccal aspect before being pulled out at a point slightly distant from the wound margin of the buccal flap. Second, the needle is passed through a shallower region nearer the wound margins of the two flaps.

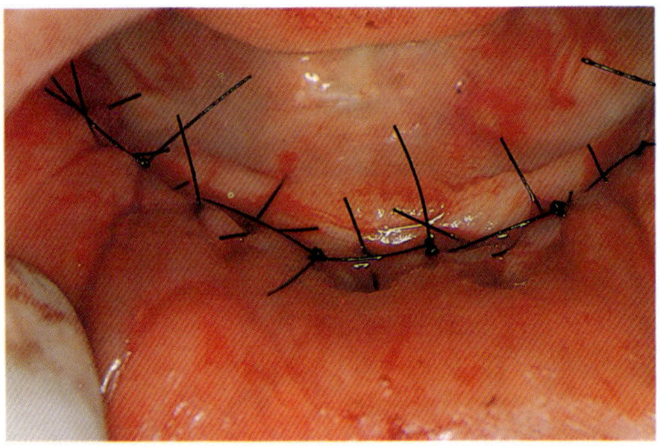

Fig. 56. Suturing is performed in such a manner as to allow complete closure of the wound, avoiding to put sutures directly over the cover screws.

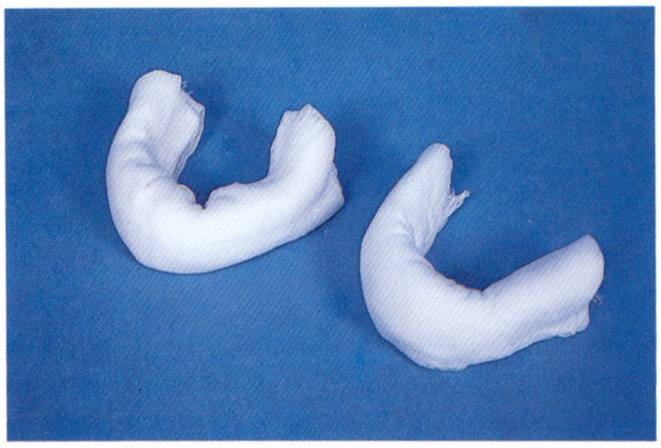

Fig. 57. Two saline-moistened gauze rolls are prepared.

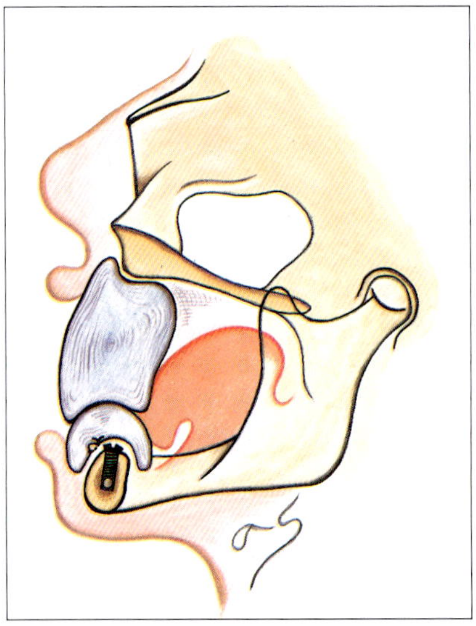

Fig. 58. One gauze roll is placed on the operated area; the another one, thick enough to fill the wide-opened mouth of the patient, is applied over the first one to achieve compression and hemostasis of the operation area.

Precautions after Stage I Operation

1. An analgesic 〔e.g., *Diclofenac* sodium (Voltaren®), 2 tablets×3〕, a synthetic penicillin which poses no risk of disturbing ossification (e.g., Lenampicillin, 1000mg/day for 3 days and 750mg/day for 7 days), and gargle 〔saline, or e.g., *Azulene* sulfonate sodium (*Azulene* Granules®), 3 packs/day for 14 days〕 are prescribed.
2. A cold pack is used for 2 days. Many patients develop swelling, accompanied by bleeding spots in the mucosa of the oral floor. Intense swelling may also be seen in the inferior region of the jaw or the chin.
3. Radiography is not performed during the healing period, because secondary (scattered) x-ray irradiation can impair the osteoblasts around the fixture.
4. The sutures are removed one week after surgery. With vertical mattress sutures, this procedure frequently requires local anesthesia. The sutures have to be completely taken away, if non resorbable material is used.
5. After surgery, detailed records have to be made regarding the diameter, length, position and direction of inserted fixtures, as well as of the type of cover screws used and of the bone quality. An example of this record form (taken from the manual of the Nobelpharma Co.) is shown on the next page.
6. The following instructions have to be given to the patient:

— Only liquid food can be taken during the first week. Depending on symptoms, an ordinary diet can thereafter gradually be resumed.

— Mouth rinsing should be performed after every meal.

— The denture must not be used before adjusted and relined. (The denture is better left at the hospital.)

7. See the chapter (see Figs. 138-140) on "prosthesis" for denture placement.
8. The stage II operation is normally performed 3 (for the lower jaw) to 6 months (for the upper jaw) after the stage I operation.

OPERATION REPORT

Date :

Patient : Date of birth :

Op : Jaw :

Surgeon / Assistant :

Preoperative medicine :

Anesthetics :

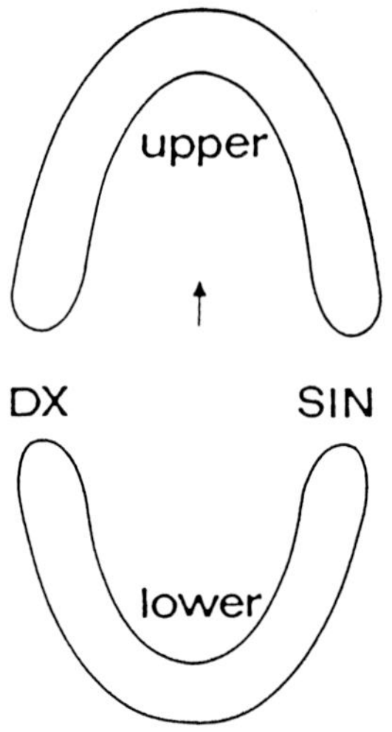

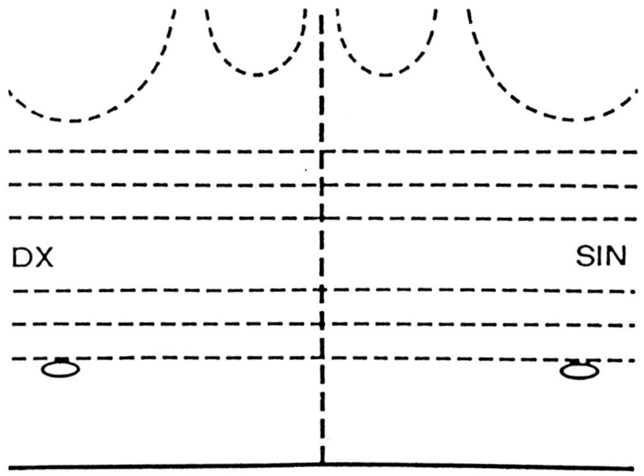

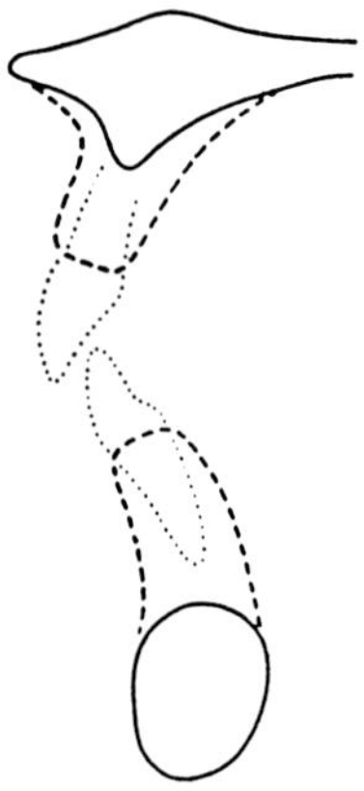

Resorption :	moderate, advanced, extreme		
Bone strength :	good,	moderate,	poor
Vascularization :	good,	moderate,	sparse

.... type of fixtures .... No : ....

Preparation : guide drill, twist drill ϕ 2 mm, pilot drill, twist drill ϕ 3 mm, countersink, screw tap, mechanical, manual.

Primary stability : excellent, good, uncertain

Flap :

Antibiotics :

Mineral and vitamins :

Remarks :

Stage II Operation (Abutment Connection)

The stage II operation is performed under local anesthesia combined with intravenous sedation. For details, see Chapter 3 ("Systemic Management and Anesthesia").

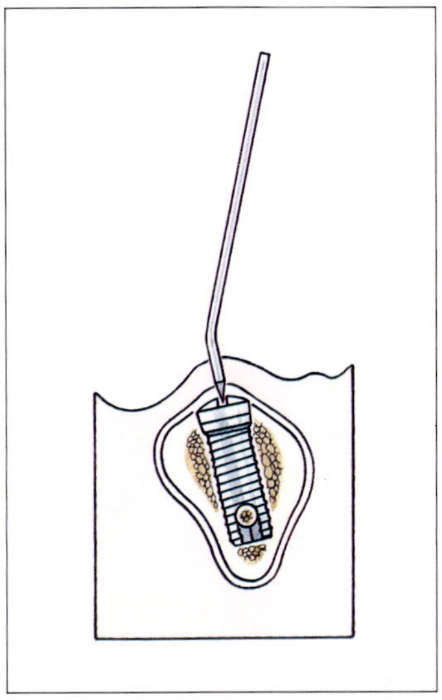

Fig. 59. Based on the records of the stage I operation and on palpation, the positions of the cover screws are identified. A probe is inserted into the central hole of the cover screw to check the position of the implant, by which the gingiva is marked by producing a bleeding spot.

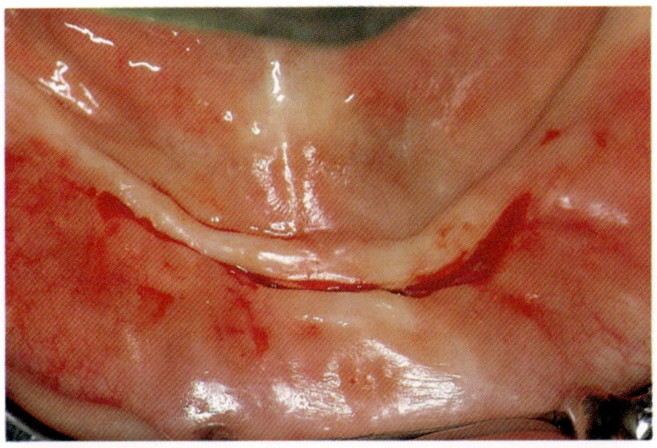

Fig. 60. A continuous crestal incision, connecting the bleeding spots in the gingiva, is made, passing over the cover screws.

Remark: It is also possible to place a mesiodistal incision of about 5 mm over each cover screw. However, a continuous crestal incision makes the subsequent steps easier.

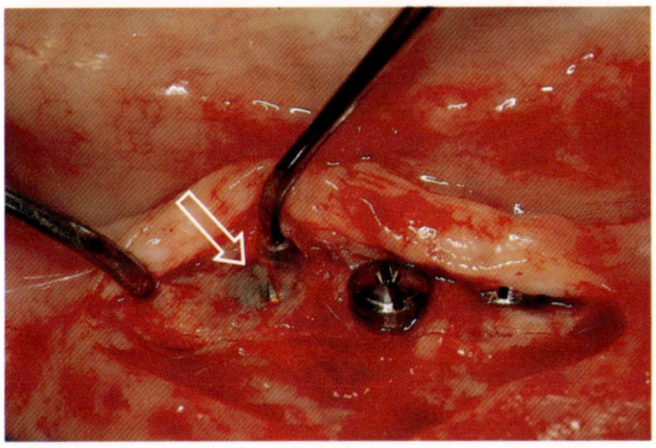

Fig. 61. The gingiva over the cover screws is freed with a dissector. The cover screws are frequently covered with fibrous connective tissue and bone (*arrow*). In such cases, the tissues are removed by inserting the guide peg of the punch through the central hole of the cover screw and pushing and rotating the punch blade.

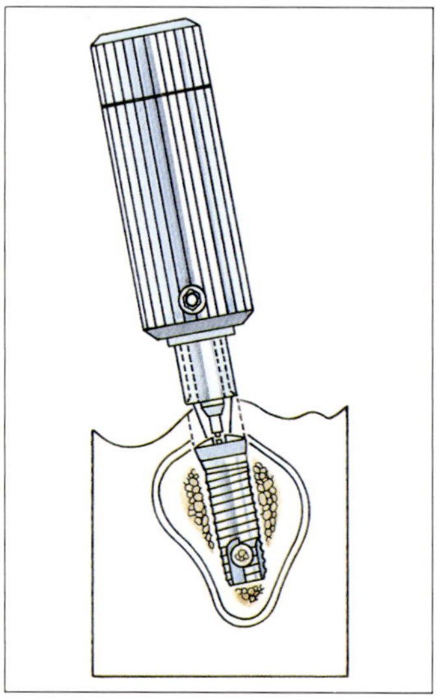

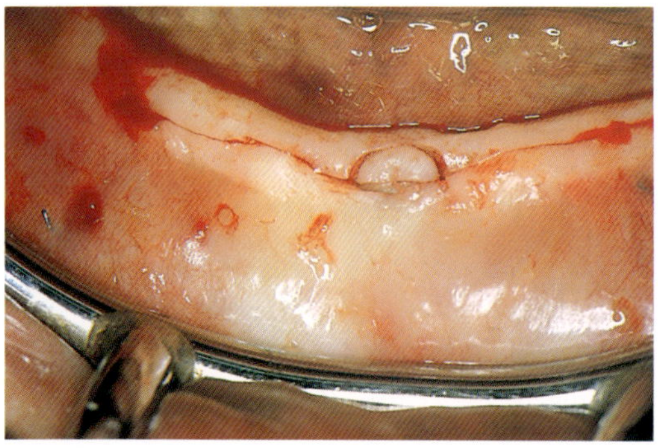

Figs. 62&63.

Remark: The gingiva and connective tissue over the cover screw can also be removed, using a cylindrical punch blade. However, punching should not be done, if the punch reaches the movable mucosal region.

If cutting out into the non-attached mucosa, the wound will be enlarged, later resulting in a less favourable attachment of the mucosa around the abutment.

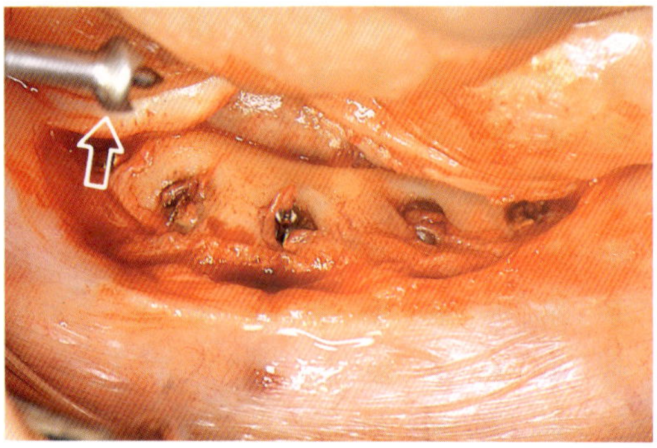

Fig. 64. If much of bone overgrowth is observed over the cover screw, a cover screw mill (*arrow*) in used.

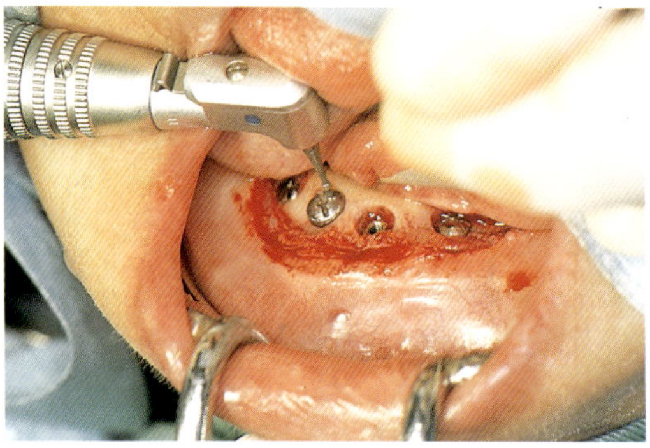

Fig. 65. Instead of the cover-screw mill a small round bur can also be used to remove bone overgrowth of the cover screw.

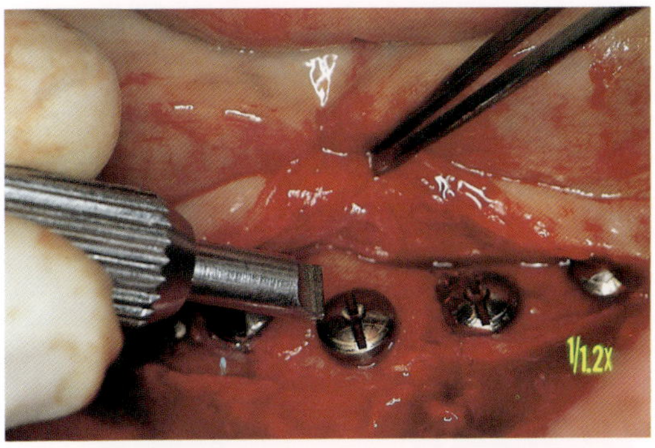

Fig. 66. The cover screw is removed with a short manual screwdriver.

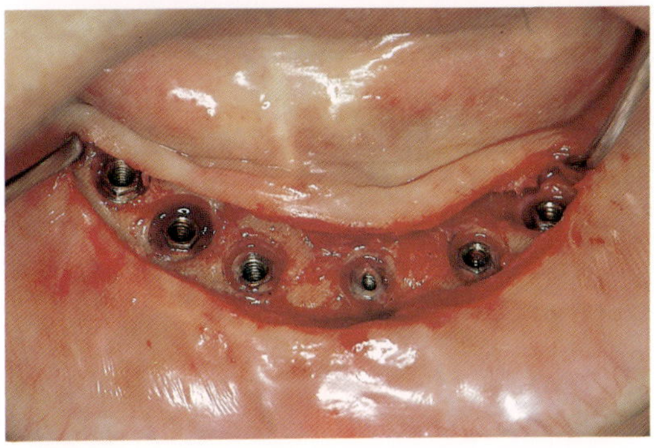

Fig. 67. After screw removal, the horizontal plates around the hex of the fixture is checked for presence of connective tissue or bone. If these are found, they should be removed completely with the punch blade to make subsequent connection of the abutment tight.

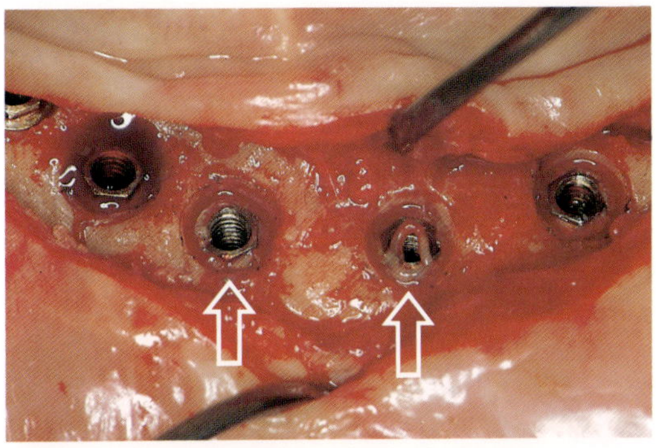

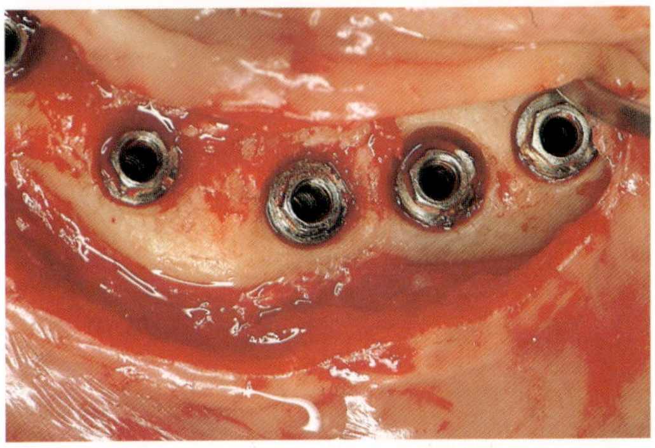

Figs. 68&69.

Remark: Bone overgrowth over the fixture (*arrows*) can easily be removed with a punch blade without damaging the fixture. The cover-screw mill must not be used after cover-screw removal, because it can damage the fixture head.

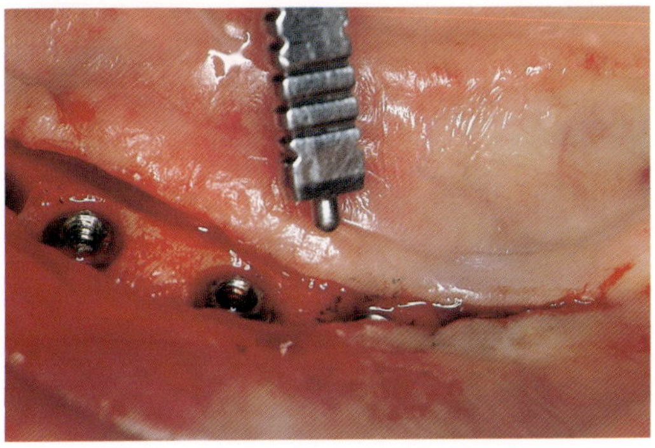

Fig. 70. Select an abutment with an appropriate length. The upper edge of the cylinder should be placed about 2 mm above the gingival margin when applied in lower jaws. A gauge is used for the selection.

Remark: For the upper jaw, an abutment with the top edge of the cylinder at the same level as or about 1 mm above the gingival margin is selected to avoid problem with the phonetics.

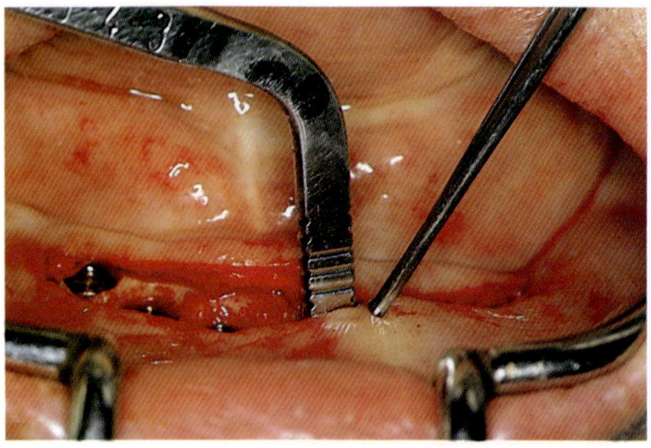

Fig. 71. For measurements, insert the small guide peg of the gauge into the central hole of the fixture.

Remark: An abutment of suitable length is chosen from the 3.0, 4.0, 5.5, 7.0, 8.5, and 10.0 mm abutments available.

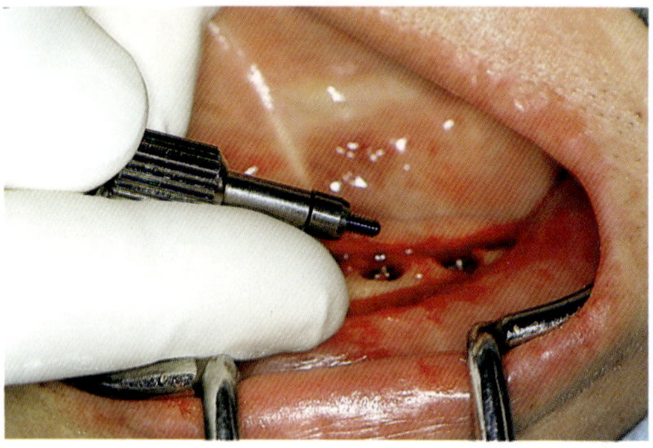

Fig. 72. After inserting the abutment screw into the cylinder, use a short hexagonal screwdriver. Hold the driver between the thumb and middle finger, compressing the abutment with the index finger.

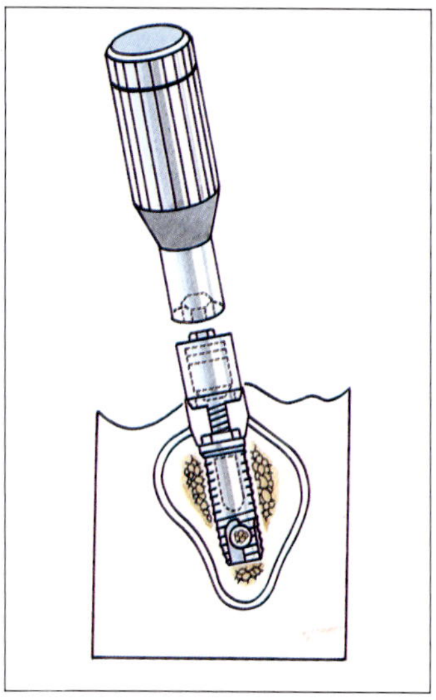

Fig. 73. Insert the abutment screw into the central hole of the fixture and tighten it slightly.

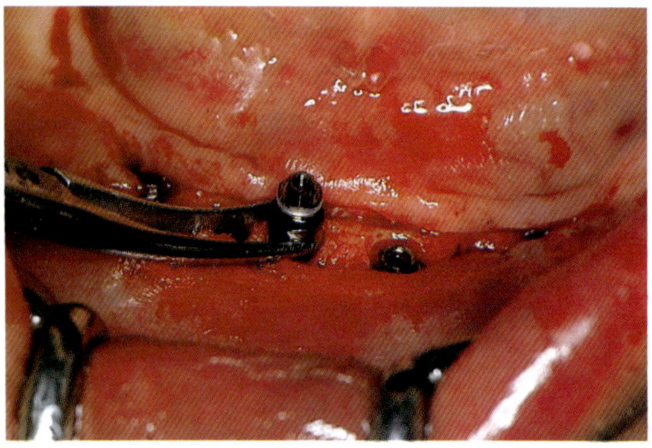

Fig. 74. Hold the abutment cylinder with a small abutment clamp. Press the cylinder in the direction of the fixture while rotating, so that the inhex of the abutment fits the outhex of the fixture head. An abutment holder is very useful for this step (see Figs. 366 and 367).

Remark: This is the most important step in the stage II operation.

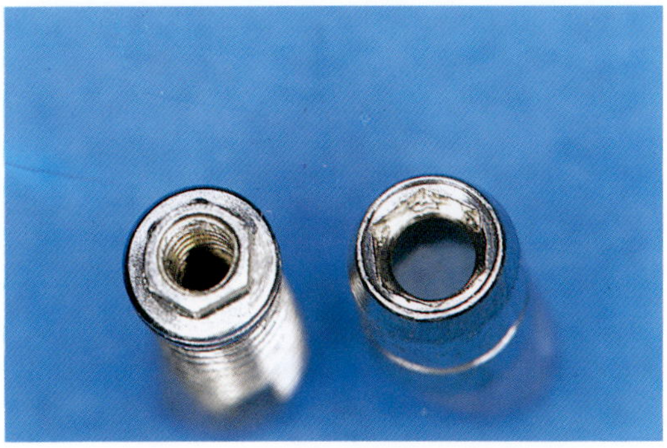

Fig. 75. *Left*: The outhex of the fixture head.
Right: The inhex of the abutment.

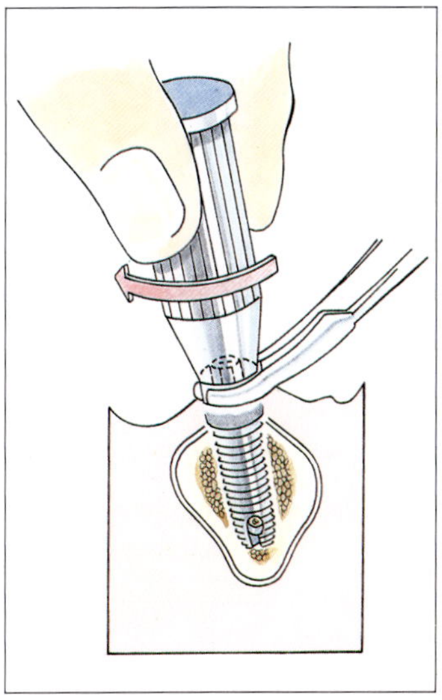

Fig. 76. When the abutment is in good position on the fixture head, hold the cylinder with a large abutment clamp and tighten the abutment screw firmly.

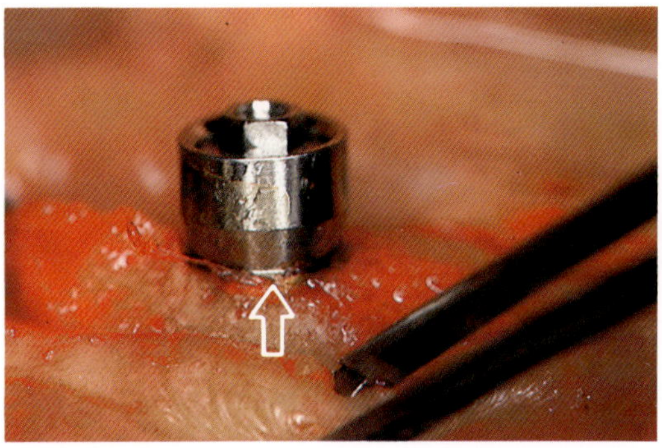

Fig. 77.

Remark: If the abutment has been properly connected to the fixture, a white line (*arrow*) will be detected when light is applied. If not, remove the abutment and eliminate bone tissue or other material preventing complete abutment-fixture connection.

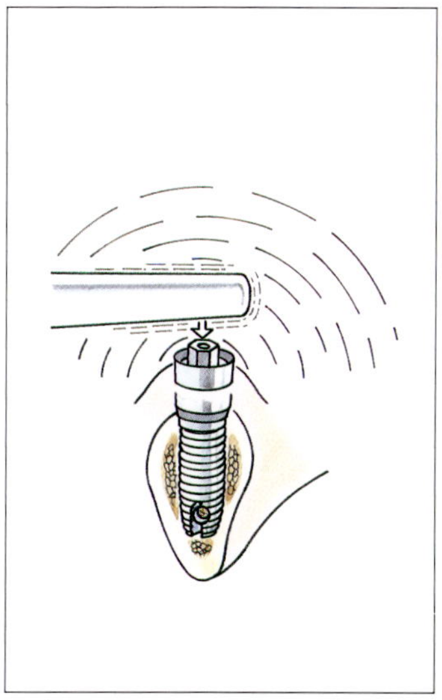

Fig. 78. If the abutment is tapped with a dissector from a height of about 3 cm, a high-pitched metallic sound can be heard, if osseointegration has been established.

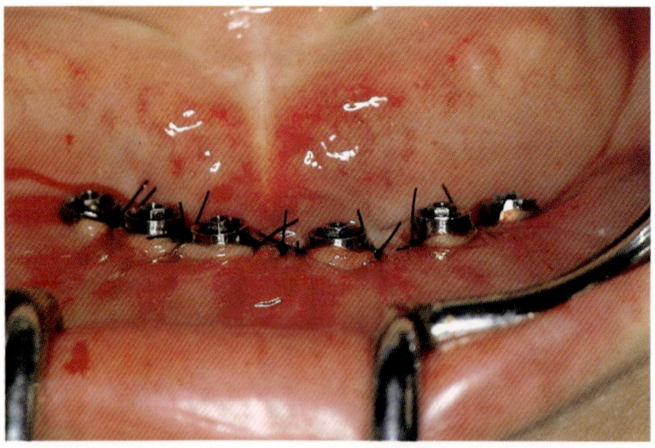

Fig. 79. The gingiva adjacent to the abutments is sutured with 4-0 nylon sutures.

Remark: If the gingiva shows excessive elevation, it should be trimmed before sutured.

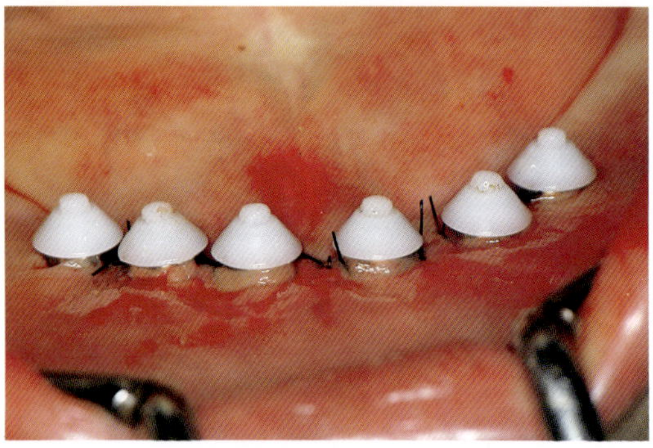

Fig. 80. Healing caps are applied with a short hexagonal screwdriver onto the abutments.

Remark: The healing cap is used to preserve the *COE-PAK* ®, and to protect the top edge of the cylinder.

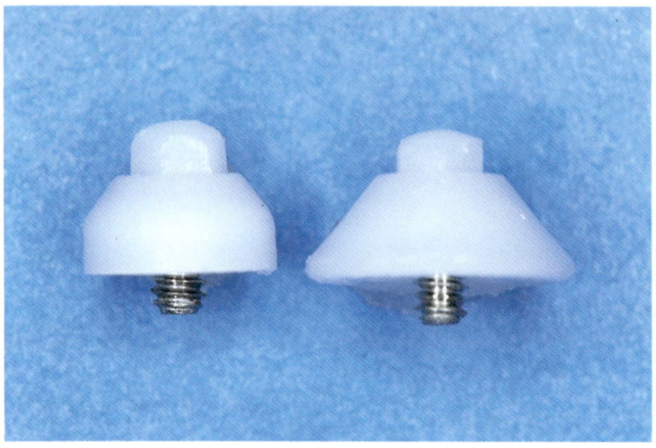

Fig. 81. Two types of healing caps (large and small) are available. The small one (*left*) is used to prevent ulcer formation in the lip and tongue, or when the abutments are placed too close to use the large healing cap. The small type cannot preserve the *COE-PAK* ®.

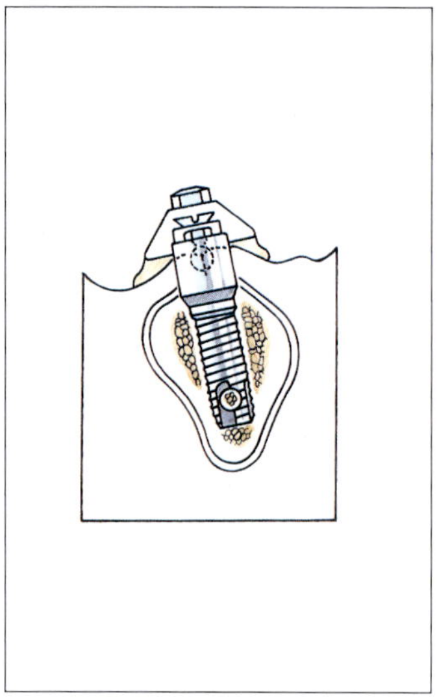

Fig. 82. Hard mixed *COE-PAK* ® is applied between the gingiva and the healing caps and over these.

Remark: This step is easier if the *COE-PAK*®, in a rod-like shape, is pushed in between the gingiva and the healing caps, starting from the lingual side.

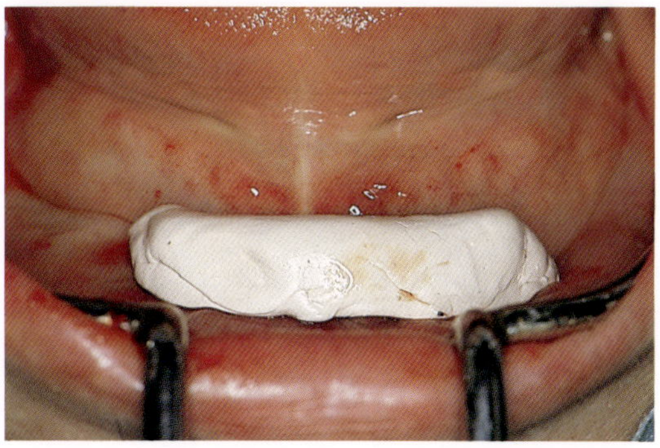

Fig. 83. Completion of the secondary operation.

Precautions after Stage II Operation

1. Immediately after the stage II operation, the fit between the abutment and the fixture has to be checked by radiography. During the interval between the stage I operation and abutment connection, radiography should be avoided unless urgently required. In postoperative radiographic assessment of the abutment, the degree of osseointegration and the linkage between fixture and abutment are particularly important. Periapical radiographs using the paralleling method, are essential for this purpose and are performed in a way similar to that used for the main examination before operation. Rotational panoramic radiography is only employed if the deepest region of the fixtures need to be assessed.

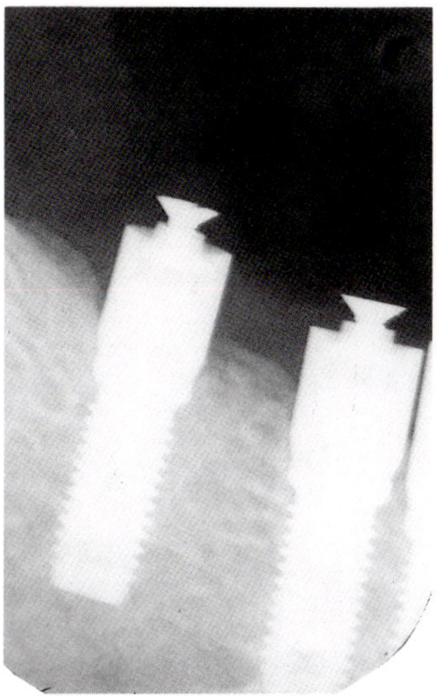

Fig. 84. Postoperative periapical radiograph is aimed at assessing the tightness of the connection between the abutment and the fixture, and to check the degree of osseointegration. Such an observation is possible if a parallel view of the area around the alveolar crest can be obtained.

Remark: If the connection between the abutment and the fixture is not tight, the abutment installation must be repeated immediately, in order to check the reason for the bad fit of the components.

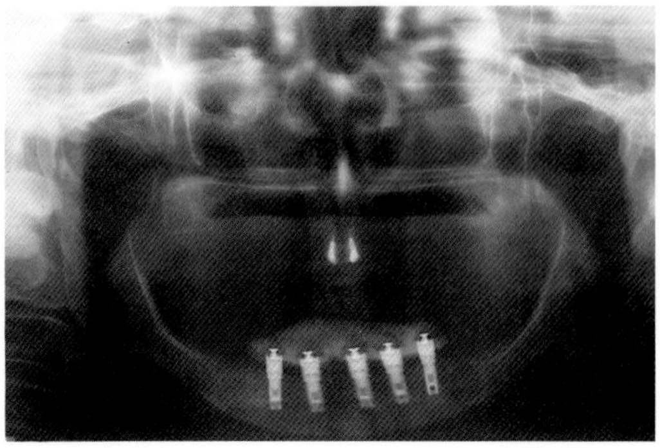

Fig. 85. Rotational panoramic radiography can also be used to assess the abutment-fixture contacts. This technique requires focusing on the fixture. Because the insertion of the fixtures usually is about 10 mm lingual to the teeth positions, the patient has to be positioned about 10 mm forward during radiography (compare with Fig. 4.).

2. An analgesic [e.g., *Diclofenac* sodium, (Voltaren®), 2 tablets×2] is prescribed. Antibiotics (e.g., Lenampicillin, 750 mg / day for 3 days) and gargles [saline or, e.g. *Azulene* sulfonate sodium (*Azulene Granules*®), 3 pack / day for 14 days] are also prescribed.
3. One week post operatively, the *COE-PAK*® and healing caps are removed, together with the sutures. If gingival healing is delayed, healing caps and *COE-PAK*® are applied again for a second week.
4. If the gingival conditions are good 2 weeks after the operation, the *COE-PAK*® is removed, and the prosthetic procedures may begin.

CHAPTER III

SYSTEMIC MANAGEMENT AND ANESTHESIA

Pain Control

Pain control can be divided into the categories of general anesthesia (total removal of pain by suppression of the central nervous system accompanied by loss of consciousness), analgesia (mainly to relieve pain) and psycho-sedation (mainly via sedation). *Analgesia* means temporary suppression or blockage of the sensory center (cerebral cortex) or the pathway of pain from the peripheral nerves to the center, using methods which do not cause loss of consciousness. Analgesia involving the central nervous system is called *general analgesia,* and analgesia involving peripheral nerves is called *local analgesia* or called *local anesthesia*. If a local anesthetic agent infiltrates the nerve fibers in a given region, impulse conduction to the center is blocked.

On the other hand, fear, anxiety and tension based on actual or imaginary experience is stored in the limbic system and retrieved when a similar situation is encountered again, stimulating the sympathetic nerves. This is followed by reactive stimulation of the parasympathetic nerves, leading to neurogenic shock. It is psycho-sedation that eliminates such things as mental pain.

For good patient management, it should be sufficient to use psycho-sedation and efficient local anesthesia for safe and reliable implant surgery.

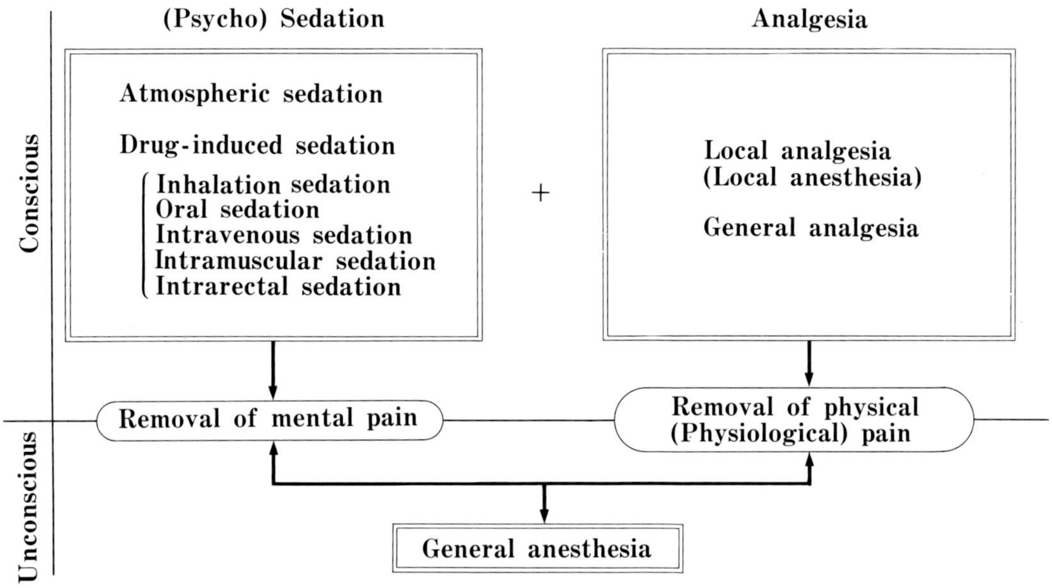

Fig. 86.

Methods of Sedation

(1) Inhalation sedation

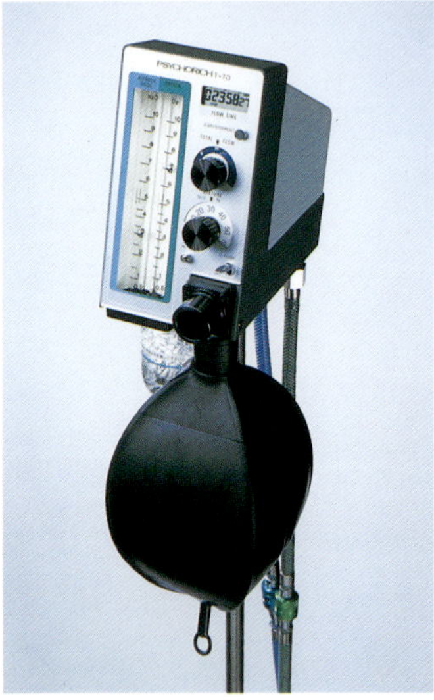

Inhalator for sedation

Fig. 87. Select an instrument which can be used as a respirator and which also is safe and easy to manipulate. This is the *Psychorich T70* ® (Sekimura).

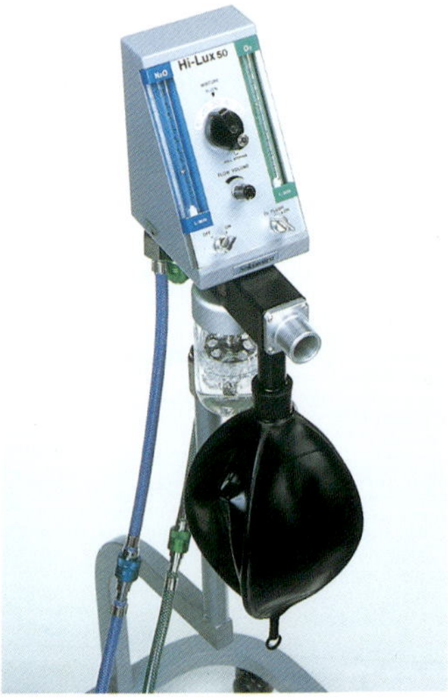

Fig. 88. The *Hilux 50* ® (Sekimura).

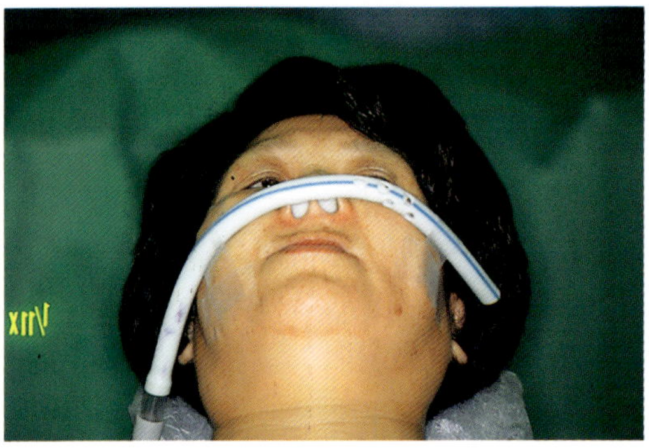

Tools for inhalation

Fig. 89. For Stage II Operation, an ordinary nasal mask can be used. For the primary operation, a nasal cannula or special nasal tube (The Nippon Dental University type) offers smooth operation.

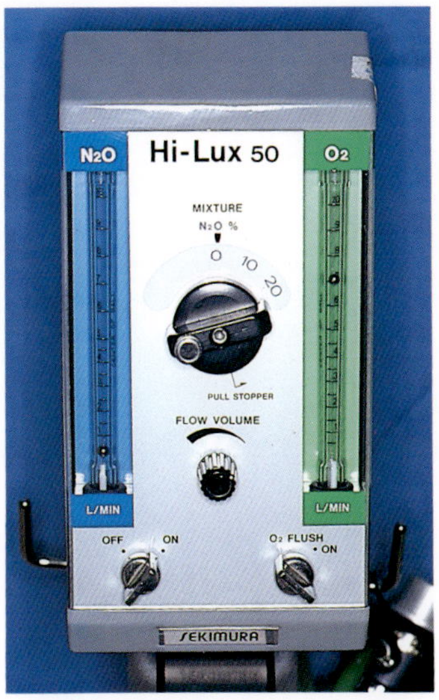

Procedure for inhalation sedation

Fig. 90. A minute amount is initially designated. To minimize air pollution with nitrous oxide, the minimum necessary volume of nitrous oxide (just enough to keep the volume in the reserve bag constant) is applied.

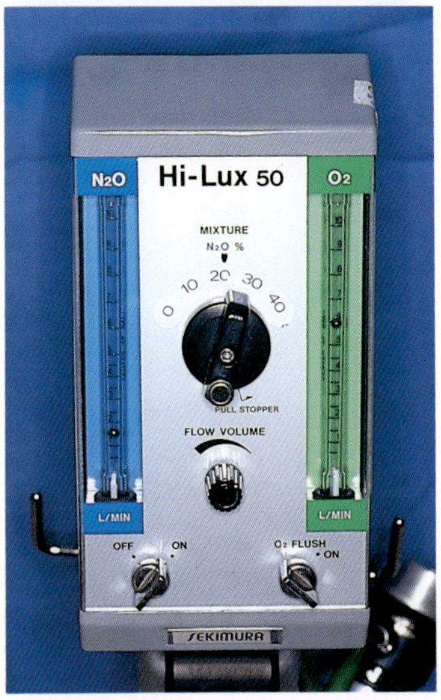

Fig. 91. Inhalation is started, setting the nitrous oxide concentration at 20%. This concentration is maintained throughout the operation.

(2) Intravenous sedation

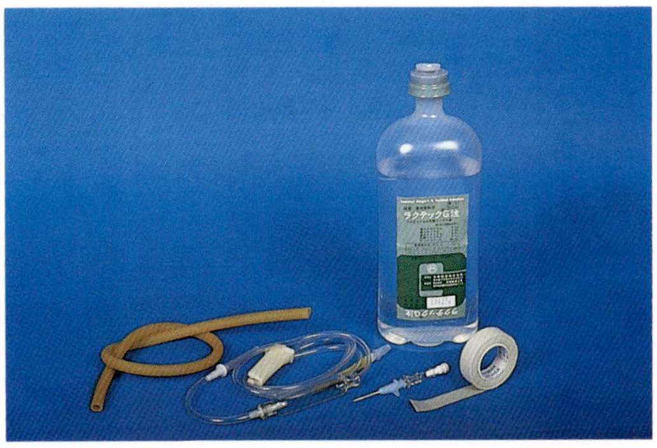

Materials for intravenous sedation

Fig. 92. A needle and an injector are needed. To secure the venous route during surgery, a needle is inserted into the vein and connected to the drip-infusion circuit. Lactated Ringer's solution (to replenish extracellular fluid) or a maintenance solution is infused.

Drugs

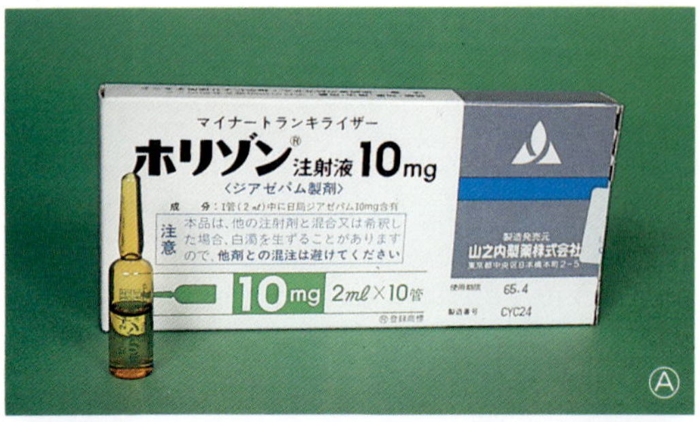

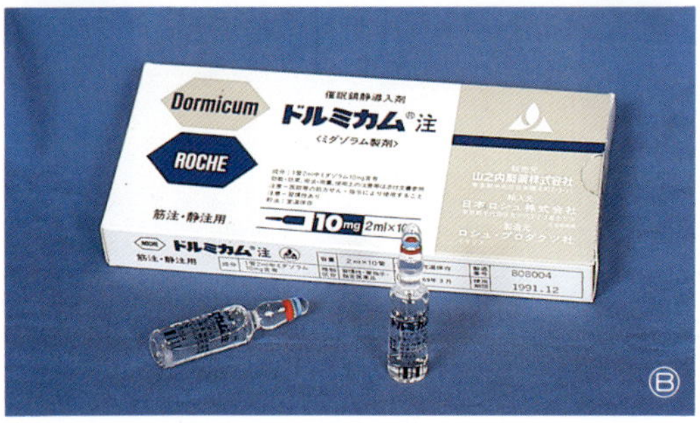

Fig. 93. Diazepam (*Horizon*®) 〈A〉 and Midazolam (*Dormicum*®) 〈B〉 are suitable.

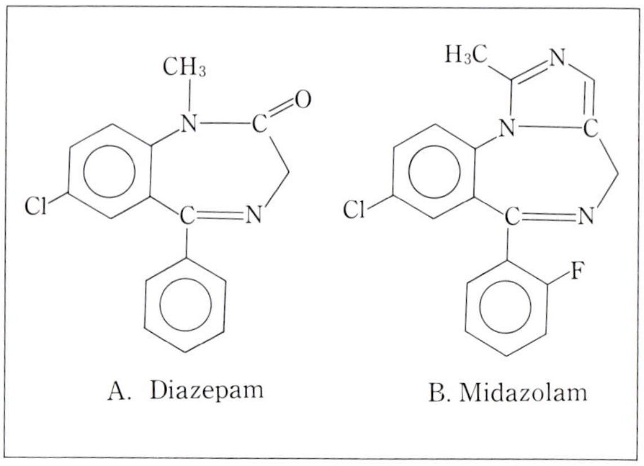

Securing the venous route

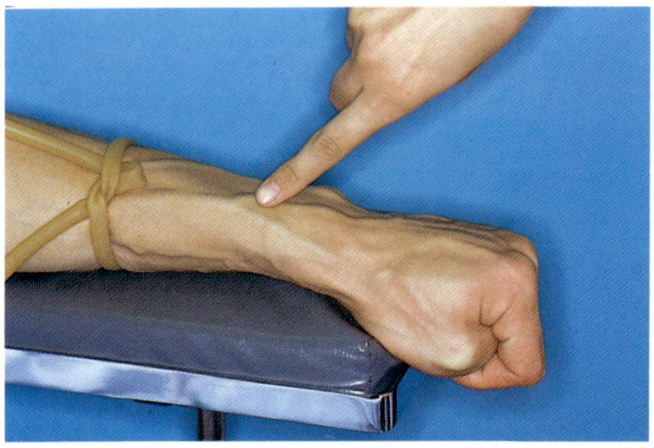

Fig. 94. The vein to be selected must be as large as possible. Avoid curved areas. The median cubital vein, median cephalic vein or dorsal metacarpal vein are suitable.

Procedure for intravenous sedation

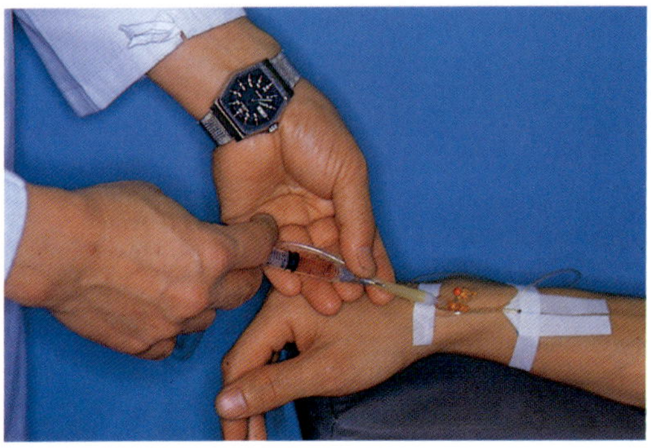

Fig. 95. 2.5 mg (1/4 ampoule) of diazepam and midazolam are administered at intervals of 30 seconds to a total dose of the following.

Ordinary dose per body weight :

Diazepam : 0.2 mg/kg

Midazolam : 0.075 mg/kg

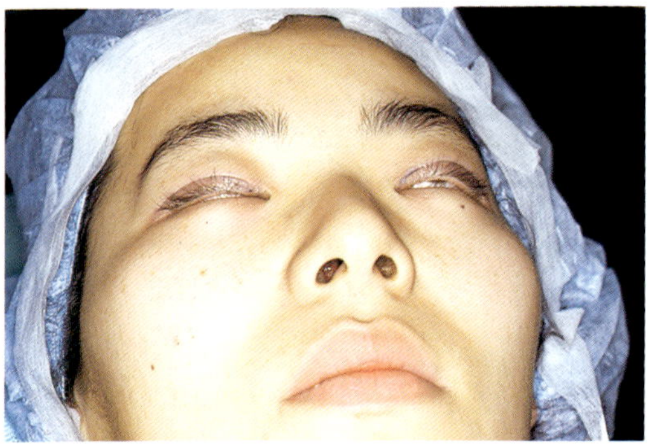

Fig. 96. Optimum sedation is determined, using Verrill's sign as an index. The dose level should be kept within a range in which the patient responds well when called.

(3) Respiratory and circulatory monitoring

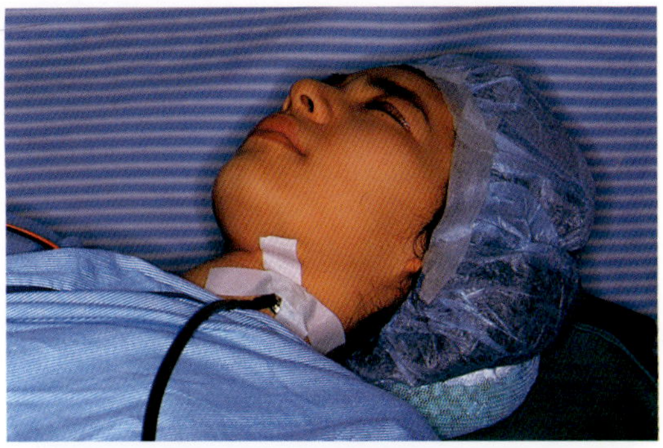

Fig. 97. A staff member is designated as being chiefly responsible for respiratory and circulatory monitoring during the operation. This person auscultates respiration with a stethoscope. If experienced, the person can distinguish the sound of the cervical artery from other sounds and can simultaneously assess hemodynamics.

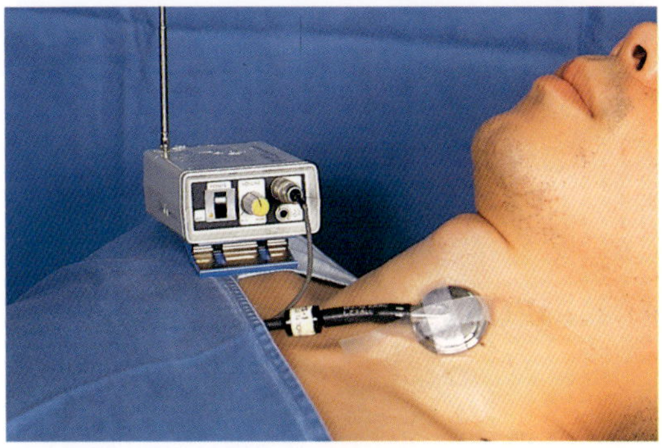

Fig. 98. If an electronic stethoscope (*KMS-1FM* ®, Kimura) is used, monitoring by several persons is possible.

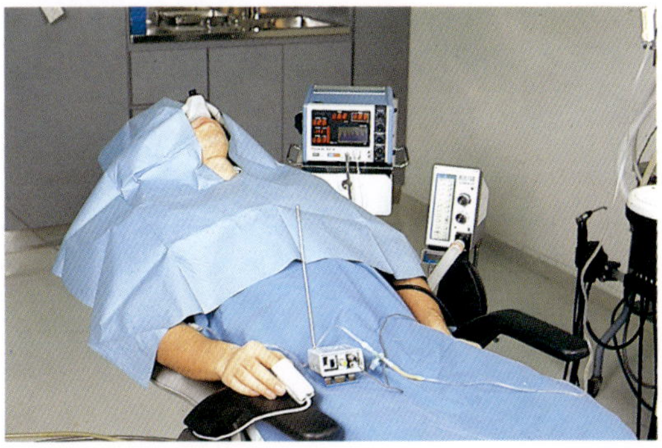

Fig. 99. Intraoperative blood pressure and heart rate must be monitored.

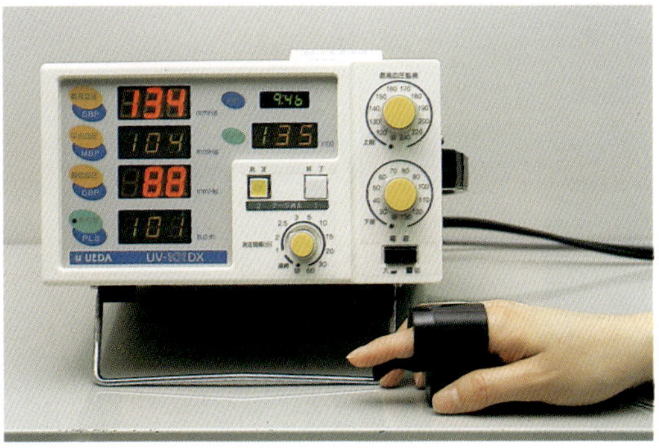

Fig. 100. A reliable automated hemodynamometer is selected.

U-Vision 101DX ® (Ueda).

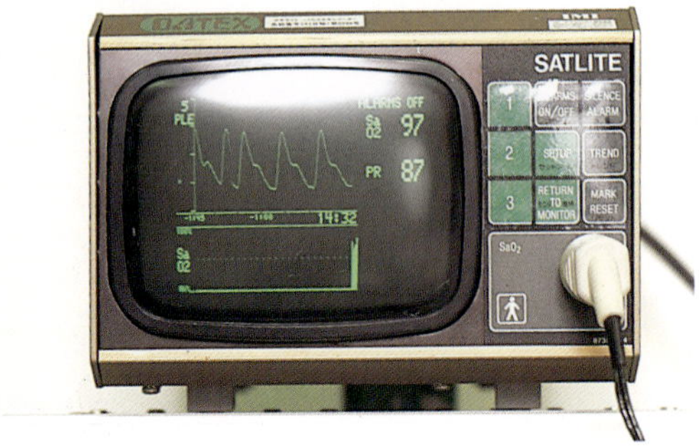

Fig. 101. A pulse oximeter is useful and desirable for respiratory and circulatory monitoring.

Local Anesthesia

(1) Instruments, materials and drugs

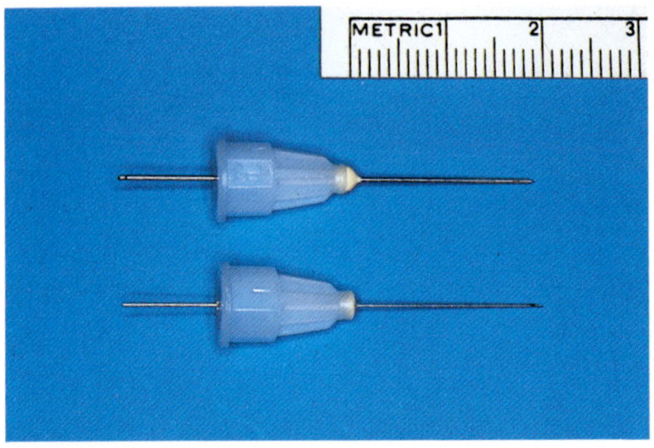

Injection needle

Fig. 102. Disposable needles, which can be fixed on an injector and cause little resistance during puncture, should be used. *Terumo*® *needles* for dental use :

For conduction and infiltration anesthesia	Outer diameter : 0.50 mm (25G) Length : 21 mm
For infiltration anesthesia	Outer diameter : 0.30 mm (30G) Length : 21 mm

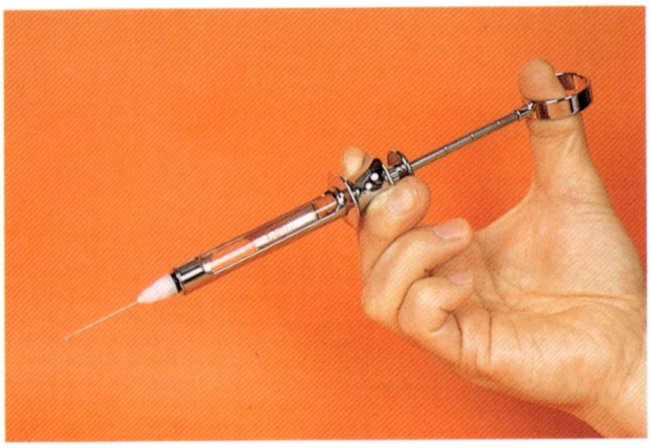

Injector

Fig. 103. To prevent direct injection of the drug into the blood vessels, an injector that proves reliable in aspiration tests should be selected.

Self-aspirating syringe® (Astra, USA)

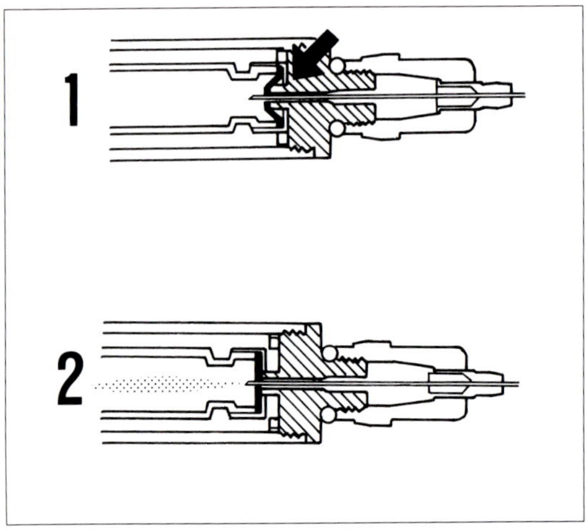

Fig. 104. Mechanism :

1. The small convex part within the syringe compresses the rubber, resulting in elevation of pressure within the cartridge.
2. If the plunger is released by the fingers, the pressure decreases and a sucking force is produced.

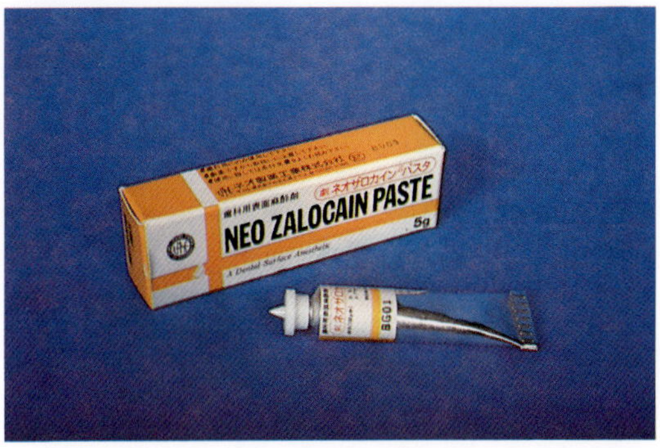

Surface anesthetic

Fig. 105. A drug with a good anesthetic effect, high adaptability to the mucosa, and good taste should be selected.

Neo Zalocain Paste® (Neo)

Composition :

Each gram contains 0.25 gm of ethyl aminobenzoate and 0.05 gm of p-butylaminobenzoic-diethylaminoethyl HCl.

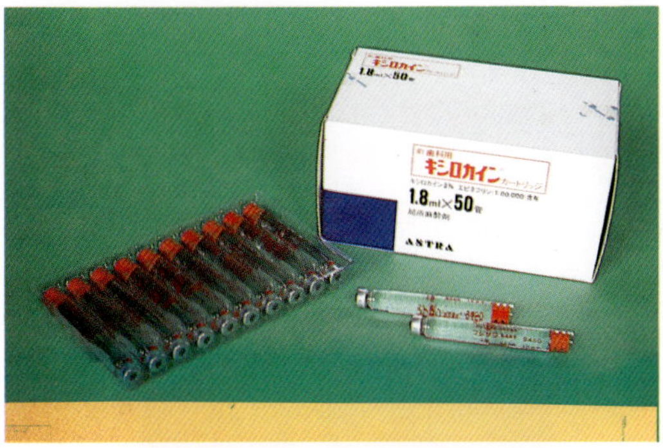

Local anesthetic

Fig. 106. A cartridge drug with high efficacy should be selected. Except in allergic patients, a 2% lidocaine cartridge containing 1/80,000 epinephrine (Astra, Sweden) should be used. The dose level must be adjusted for patients with hypertension or cardiac disease.

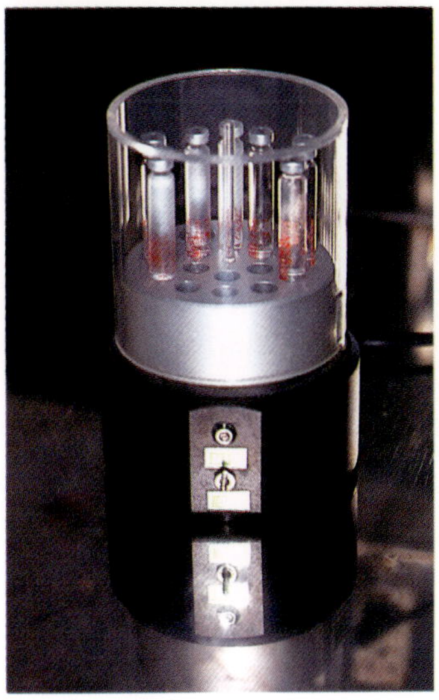

Heater

Fig. 107. To reduce temperature difference between the injectable solution and the body, the drug should be warmed to a temperature near that of the body. This procedure also provides smooth initial movement of the rubber stopper.

(2) **Basic types of local anesthesia**

A good local anesthesia satisfies these three requirements:

(1) It causes no pain,
(2) has a good anesthetic effect,
(3) produces no complication in the patient.

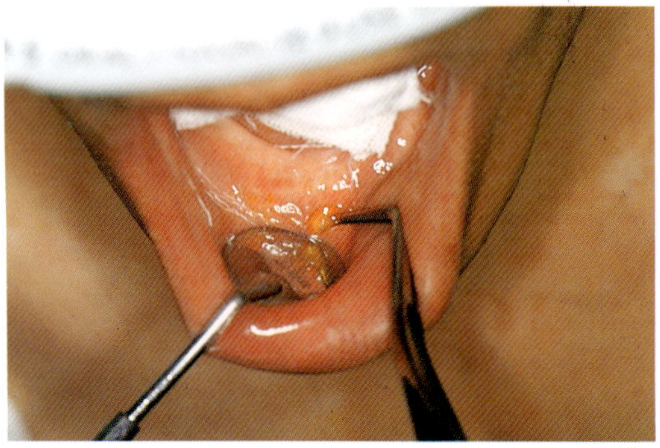

Surface anesthesia

Fig. 108. To ensure that the anesthetic does not act on the non-target region but yet preserves the anesthetic effect on the target area, a dry-field technique is used at the opening of the salivary gland. The anesthetic is applied to a region slightly wider than the outer diameter of the needle.

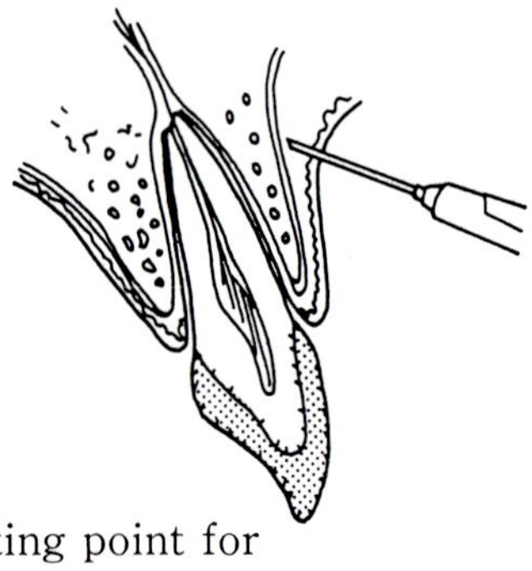

Infiltration anesthesia

Fig. 109. Anesthesia is started on the buccal side of the area. The tip of the needle is kept above the periosteum. The bevel of the needle is inserted parallel to the bone surface, and the needle should not be bended.

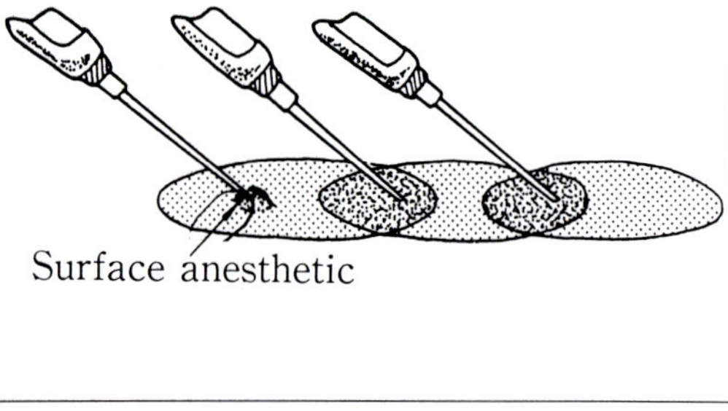

Fig. 110. For cases in which extensive infiltration anesthesia is needed, surface anesthesia is performed at the initial point of puncture. Then areas that show an anesthetic effect are punctured one after another.

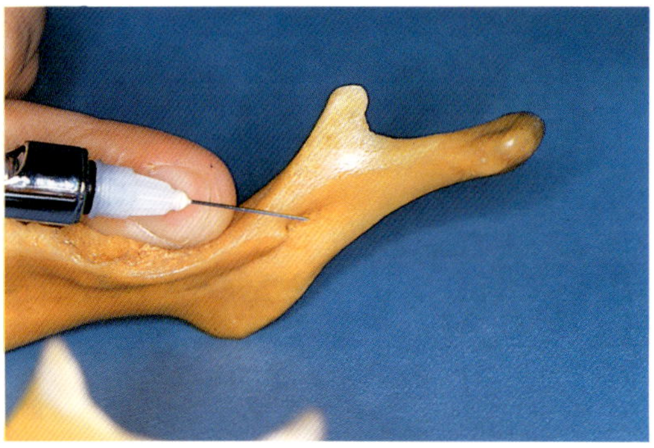

Conduction anesthesia

Fig. 111. In dental conduction anesthesia, the tip of the needle is advanced through the alveolar foramen, the greater palatine foramen, the incisive foramen and the mandibular foramen respectively, where the local anesthetic is injected. Sufficient knowledge of nerve distribution in this region is essential.

(3) Mandibular foramen conduction anesthesia for edentulous jaws

During mandibular implant surgery, an adequate anesthetic effect is difficult to obtain by infiltration anesthesia because the bone is compact and the drug is washed out by the saline solution irrigated during drilling. Mandibular foramen conduction anesthesia is, thus, recommended in such cases. However, the edentulous jaw provides no useful guide in determining the needle puncture point. Therefore, to improve the success rate of this type of anesthesia, the following steps are taken.

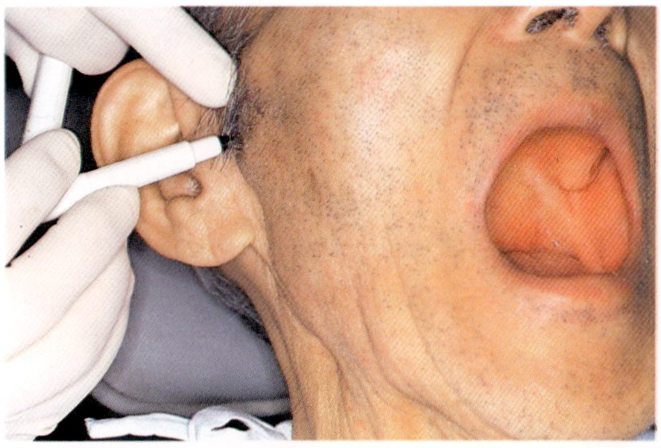

Fig. 112. The lateral edge of the articular process is palpated and marked on the skin during maximum mandibular movement.

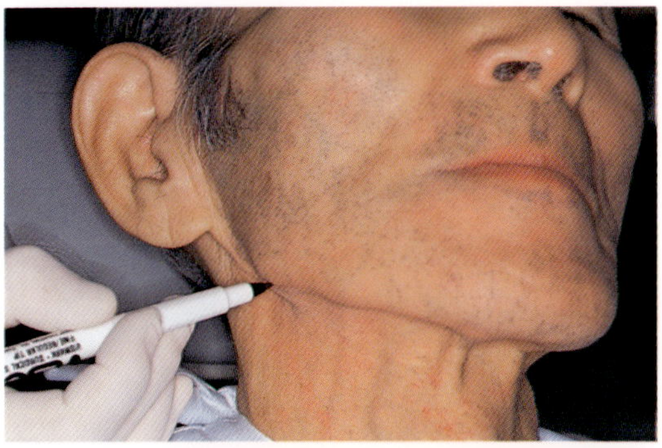

Fig. 113. With the mouth closed, the gonion is marked at the mandibular angle.

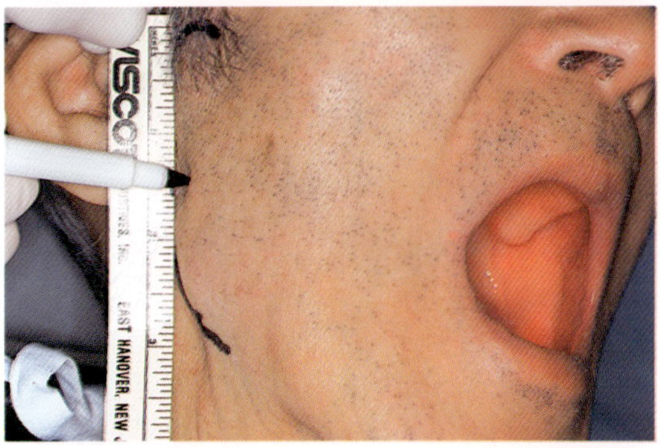

Fig. 114. A line is drawn connecting the lateral edge of the articular process and the gonion. From its center, an extension line is drawn over the skin above the lateral edge of the mandibular ramus. This point serves as a target point for injection.

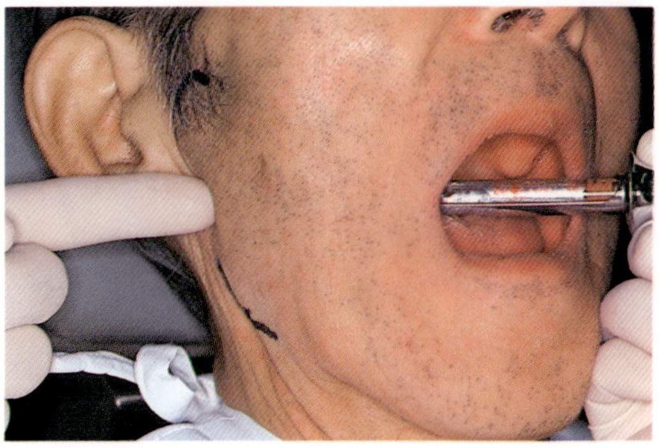

Fig. 115. After palpating the internal oblique line with the left index finger, push the puncture-target point with the left index finger or let an assistant do so. To bring the extension line of the needle to this point, the needle is advanced from a point slightly medial from the internal oblique line. After full insertion of the 21 mm needle, an aspiration test is performed, then the local anesthetic is injected slowly.

(4) Local anesthesia for individual cases

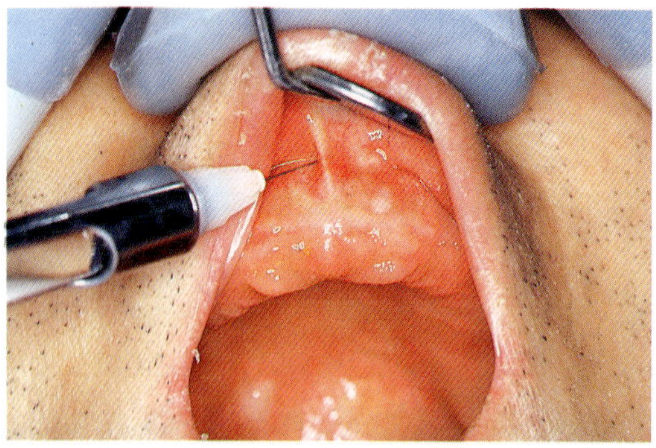

Stage I and Stage II Operations of the upper jaw

Fig. 116. After surface anesthesia, infiltration anesthesia is started in the right labial region. During stage I operation, infraorbital foramen conduction anesthesia is also used. Alveolar foramen conduction anesthesia is sometimes used for the posterior buccal area.

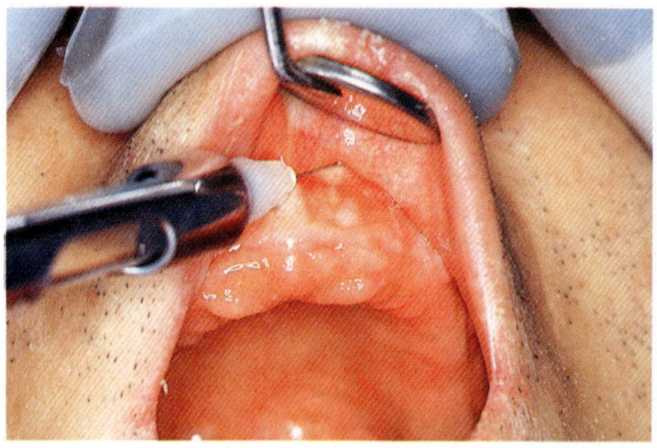

Fig. 117. Infiltration anesthesia is performed for the left labial region. If anesthesia is performed only in the front, one or two cartridges are usually used. To extend the anesthetic effect also to the posterior region, an additional 0.5 cartridge is needed.

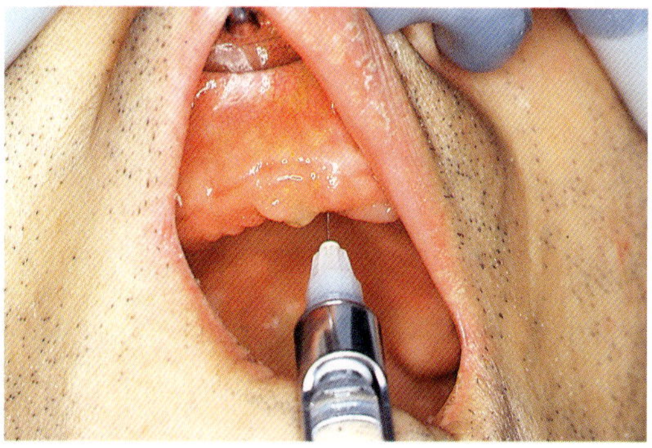

Fig. 118. The nasopalatine nerve can be blocked by injection of 1/3 to 1/2 cartridge into the area near the incisive foramen.

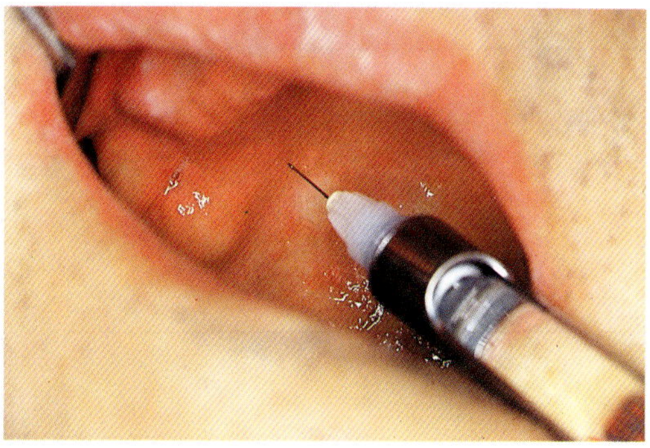

Fig. 119. To anesthetize the area from the posterior to the anterior region of the palate, the mucosa around the greater palatine foramen is punctured to block the greater palatine nerve. From 1/3 to 1/2 cartridge is used for one side. Only three points (the incisive foramen and bilateral palatine foramens) have to be injected in the palatine region.

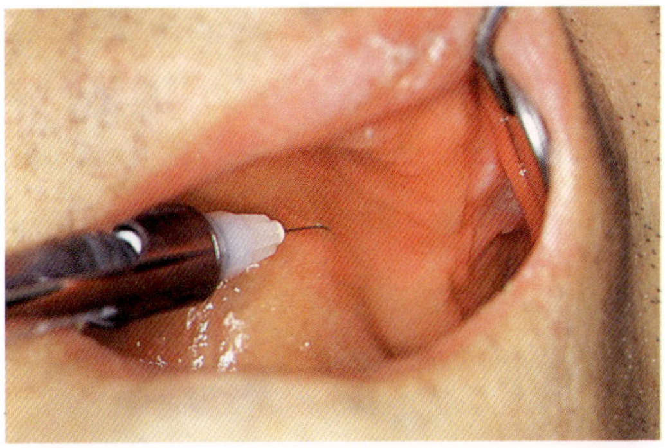

Fig. 120. The left greater palatine nerve is blocked.

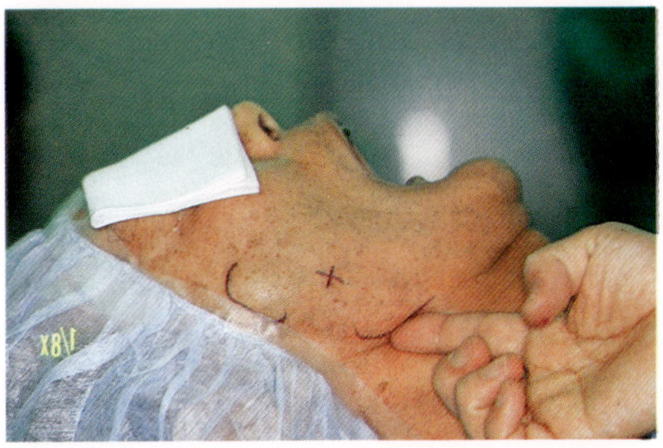

Stage I Operation for the lower jaw

Fig. 121. The injection target point is marked in a manner similar to that described above.

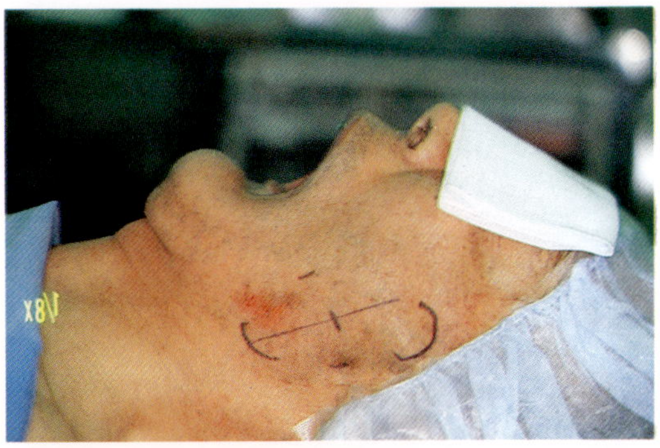

Fig. 122. It is showed that the left side injection target point is marked.

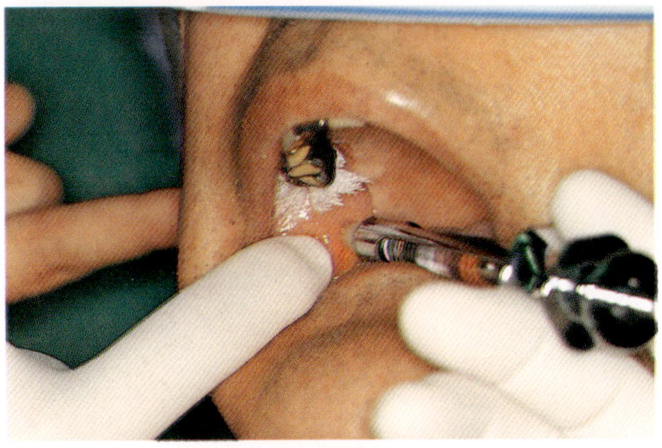

Fig. 123. If fixtures are inserted between the bilateral mental foramina, one cartridge is used for right mandibular foramen conduction anesthesia.

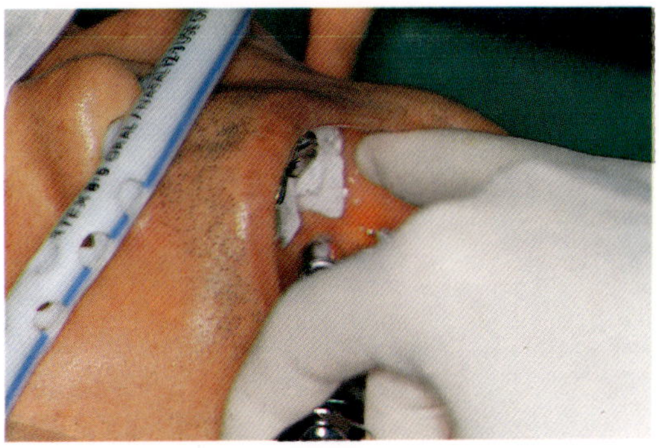

Fig. 124. One cartridge is used for left mandibular foramen conduction anesthesia.

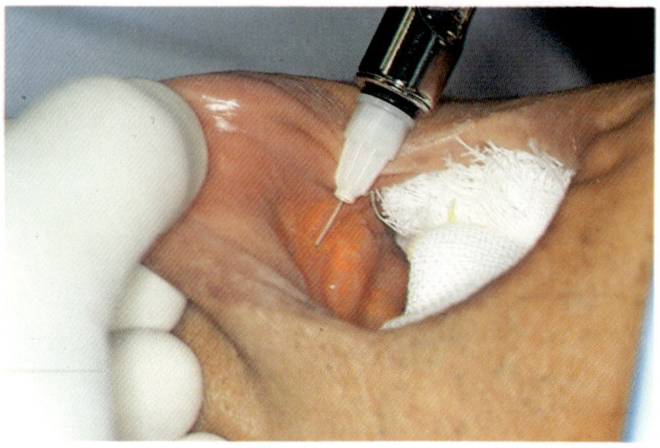

Fig. 125. To achieve anesthesia of the peripheral ramus of the buccal nerve and for hemostasis, 1-2 cartridges are used for labio-lingual infiltration anesthesia. In total, 3-4 cartridges are usually used for the buccal infiltrations, bilaterally.

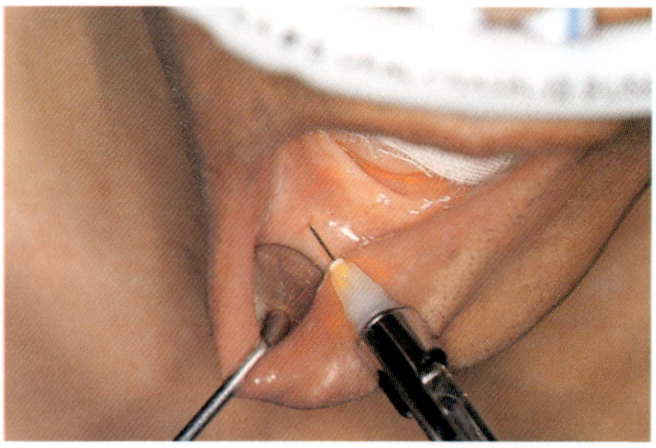

Stage II **Operation for the lower jaw**

Fig. 126. If abutments are connected to fixtures placed between the mental foramina, the needle is inserted towards the mental foramen, avoiding direct puncture of the trunk of the nerve and vessel. Usually, 1/2 to 1 cartridge is needed this region.

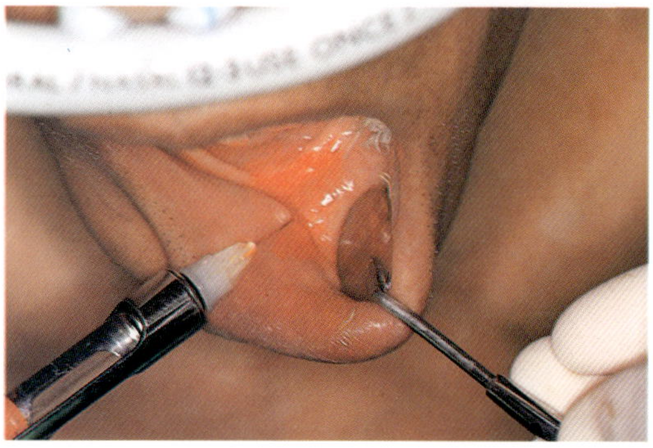

Fig. 127. The process begun in Fig. 126 is continued here.

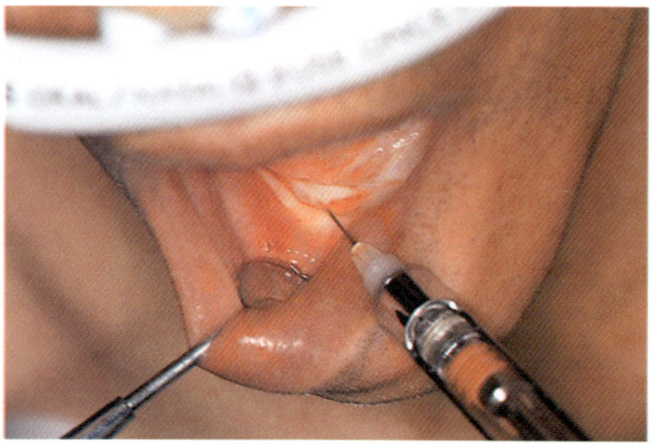

Fig. 128. Next, infiltration anesthesia is injected for the lingual region, using 1/2 cartridge.

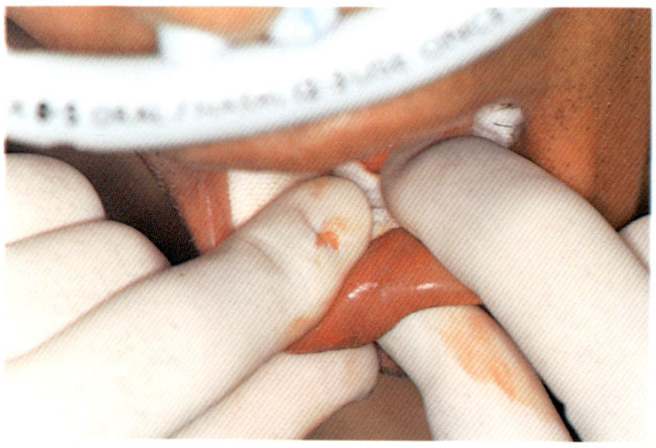

Fig. 129. The injected area is compressed for a while with gauze, soaked with saline solution to better distribute the injection solution within the tissues.

CHAPTER IV

PROSTHETIC PROCEDURES

The procedures for prosthetic treatment will be presented, using a lower jaw case as an example.

Pretreatment

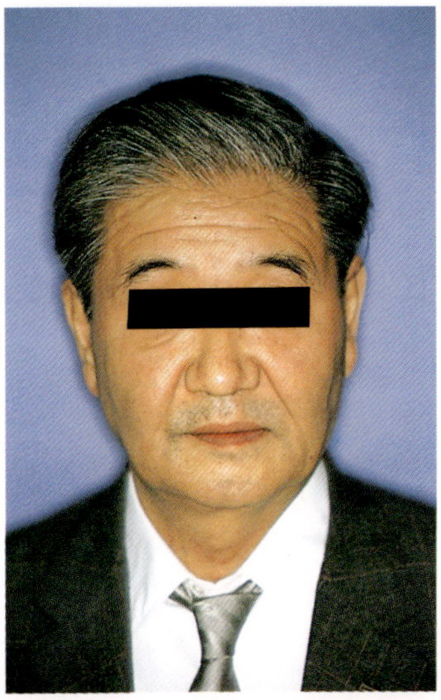

Fig. 130. The patient is a 63-year-old man with severe masticatory problems due to maladaptation of his denture. During habitual occlusion, the face showed at the first examination, wrinkles of about 20 mm on the right and about 7 mm on the left corners of the mouth. In addition, the area of the right half of the lip differed from that of the left half, regarding both the upper and lower lips. These signs indicated a decrease in occlusal vertical dimension.

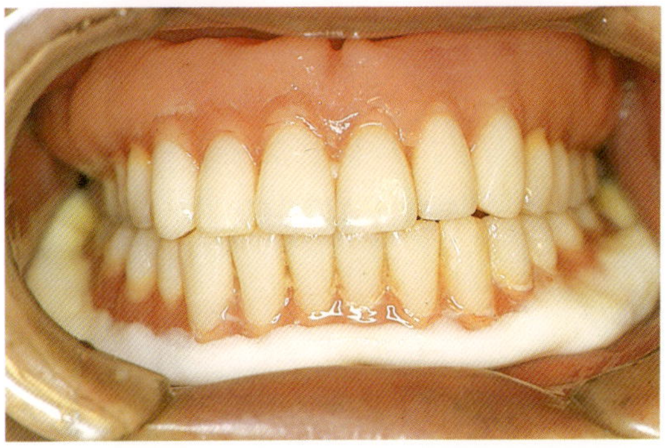

Fig. 131. Existing complete denture, with tissue conditioner in the lower denture.

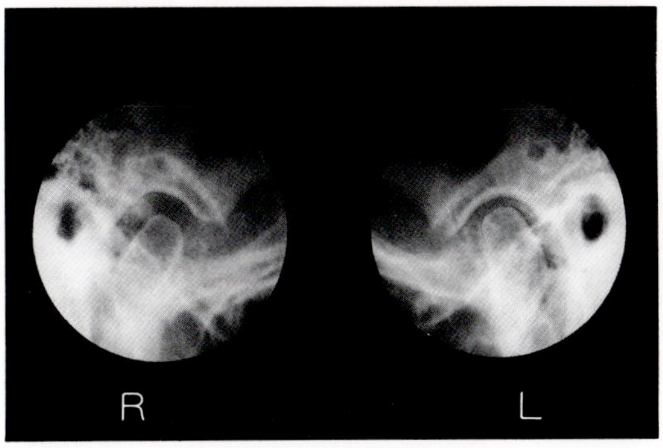

Fig. 132. Transcranial oblique lateral projections of the temporomandibular joints during habitual occlusion with the dentures in place in the mouth. Downward displacement of the right condyle head (*R*) and posterosuperior displacement of the left condyle head (*L*) are visible. This indicates a reduced vertical dimension and forward shift of the occlusion (particularly on the right) due to alveolar ridge resorption.

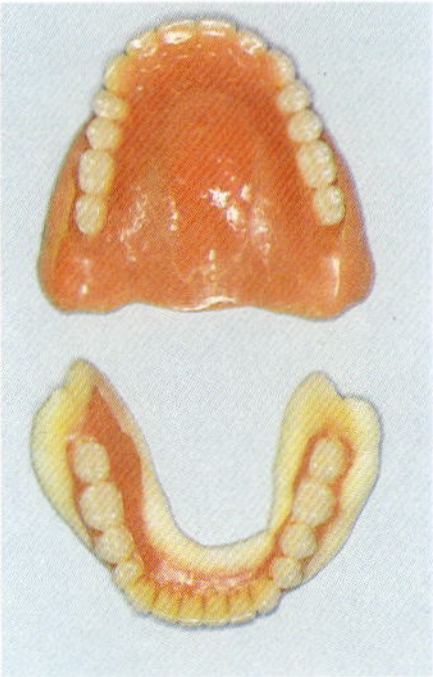

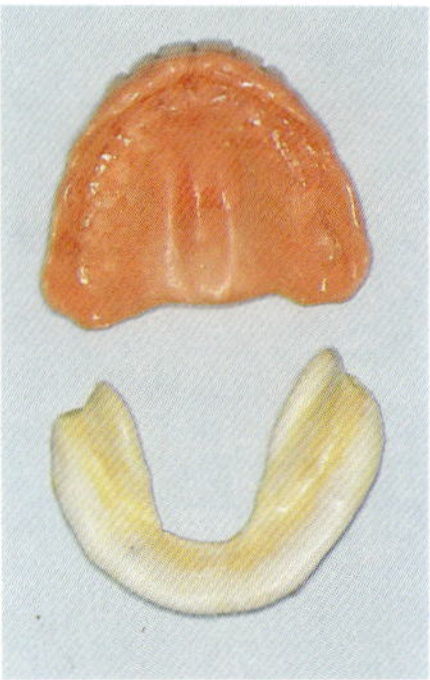

Fig. 133. Existing complete dentures, occlusal surface and mucosal surface.

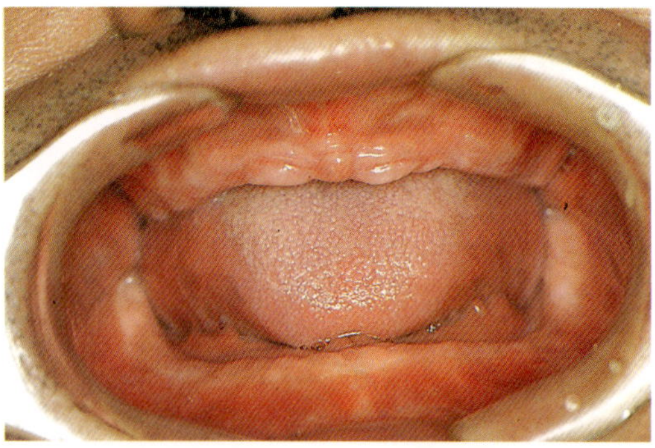

Fig. 134. Examination includes visual inspection, palpation, model assessment and radiography, thereby checking, the oral mucosa, alveolar ridge resorption and position of the mental foramina. Here, resorption of the lower alveolar ridge is marked (especially in the right molar region, which plays a principal role in mastication).

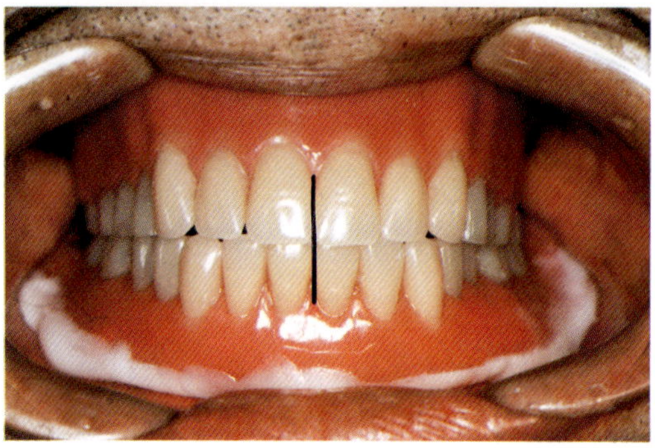

Fig. 135. To condition the alveolar ridge mucosa and correct the mandibular displacement, a treatment denture with cuspless (O°) artificial teeth is used. Occlusal position is arranged as follows: (**1**) centric position is regarded as the horizontal jaw position: (**2**) no difference is seen between the upper and lower lips or between the right and left half of each lip during occlusion: and (**3**) the vertical dimension is set at a level, which produces a wrinkle at the mouth corner of about 1.5 mm (considering the advanced age of the patient). (In this case, it was elevated by 5 mm.) Monoplane occlusion (Hardy's technique) is used. Tissue conditioning is done every 4–5 days. Occlusion is adjusted every 2–3 weeks with a paper strip or sandpaper.

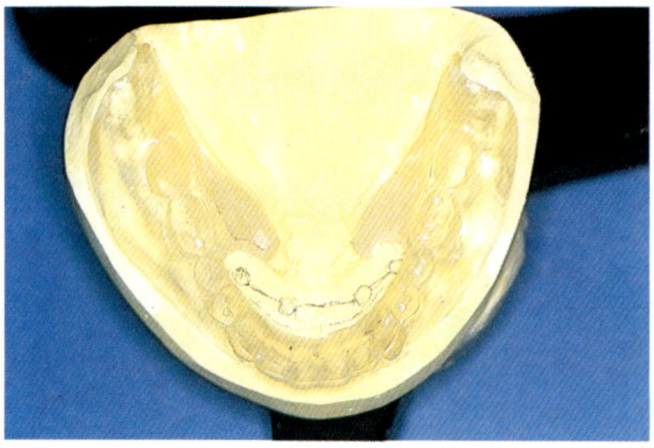

Fig. 136. In the articulator, the relationship between upper and lower jaws is determined, taking into consideration anticipated correction of lower jaw displacement. Referring to the artificial teeth arrangement on the treatment denture, the number, position and direction of fixtures, to be inserted in the stage I operation, are determined on the model. After discussion with the oral surgeon, a surgical stent of transparent resin is prepared to serve as a guide during the operation.

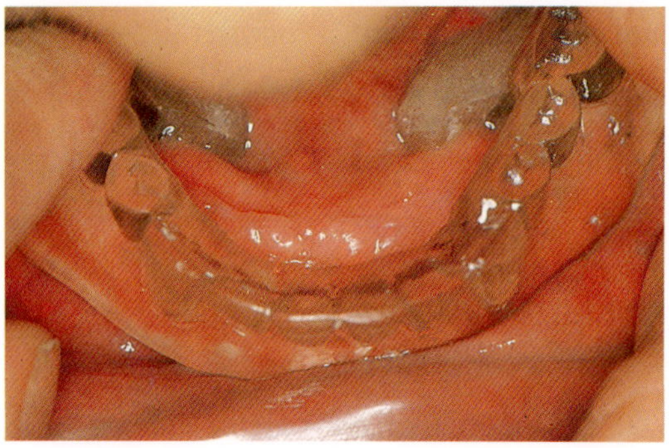

Fig. 137. Try -in placement of the surgical stent.

Prosthetic Procedures after Stage I Operation

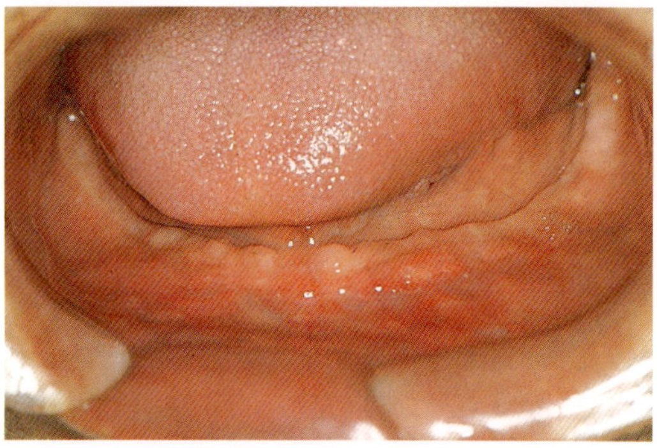

Fig. 138. The oral cavity 2 weeks after the stage I operation. The treatment denture should not be returned until the mucosa has healed properly after fixture insertion. (It takes about 2 weeks.) During this period, the patient may consume only soft and liquid food.

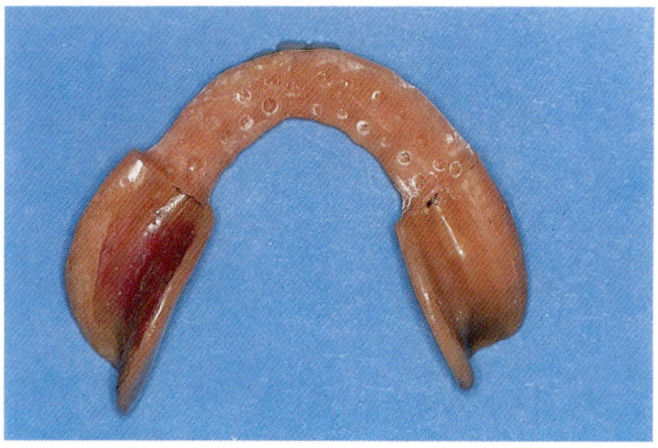

Fig. 139. Two weeks after the stage I operation, the denture base in the area, where the fixtures are inserted, is completely removed to provide a space for lining with a tissue conditioner.

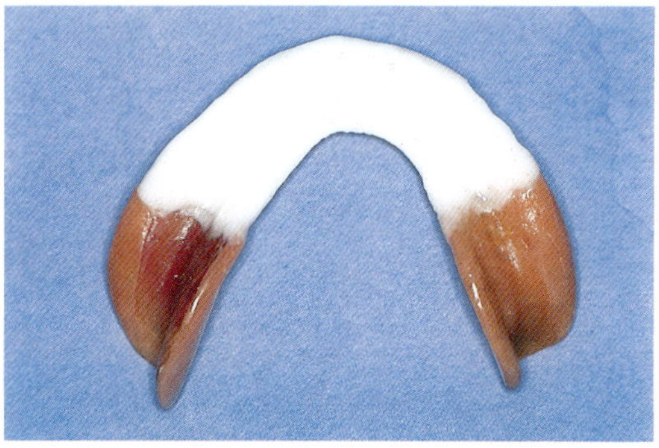

Fig. 140. Mucosal surface of the treatment denture. To achieve sufficient osseointegration, it is essential to keep the inserted fixtures unloaded. For this reason, the conditioner has to be repeatedly replaced at intervals of 5 days to ensure sufficient thickness and flexibility of the denture lining.

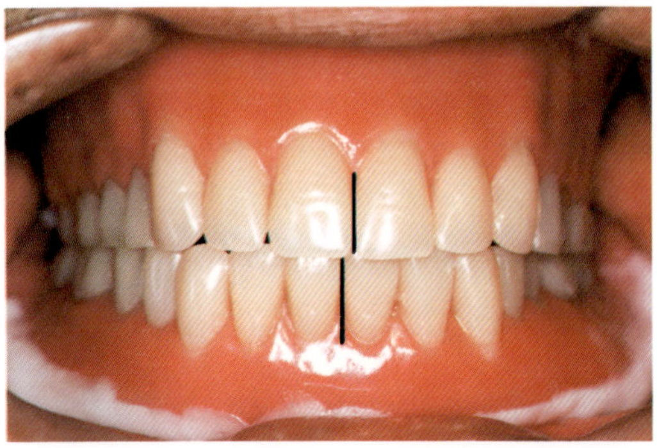

Fig. 141. Habitual occlusion about 3 months after application of the treatment denture. Masticatory function is now excellent, but the median region of the lower arch has shifted to the right by about 1.5 mm.

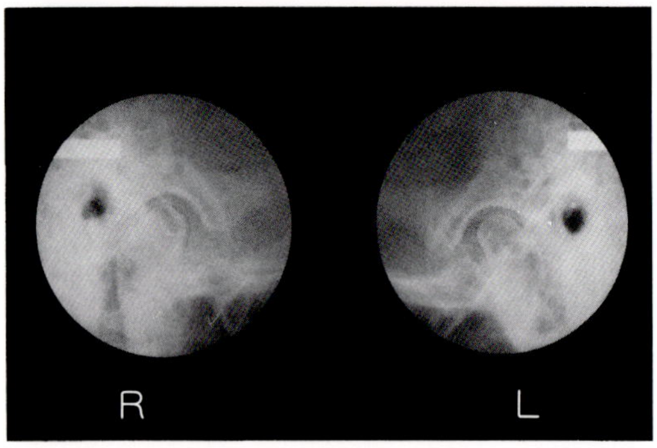

Fig. 142. Transcranial oblique lateral projections during habitual occlusion, about 3 months after application of the treatment denture. The bilateral condyle heads are in the center of the articular cavity, indicating that a correction of the mandibular displacement has taken place.

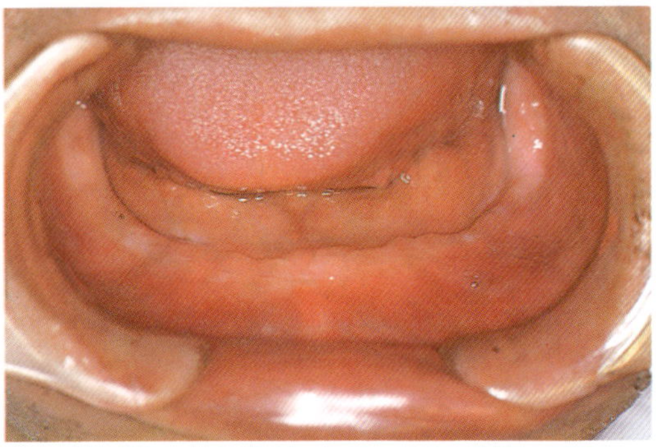

Fig. 143. Oral cavity about 3 months after the stage I operation. A healing period of 3-6 months for the lower jaw and 6-12 months for the upper jaw has to be allowed between the stage I and stage II operations to create sufficient osseointegration before the stage II operation.

Prosthetic Treatment after Stage II Operation

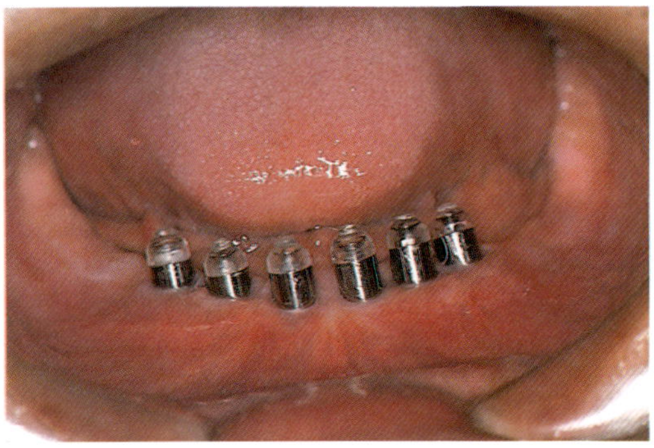

Fig. 144. The oral cavity 2 weeks after the stage II operation. Small healing caps are applied to the abutments. The patient is instructed in plaque control (for details, see the next section on maintenance).

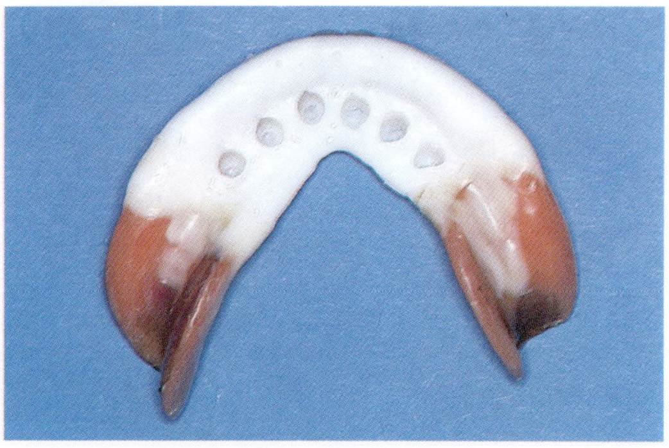

Fig. 145. The resin base has to be completely adjusted, followed by lining with a tissue conditioner, so that the mucosal surface of the treatment denture does not directly touch the small healing caps.

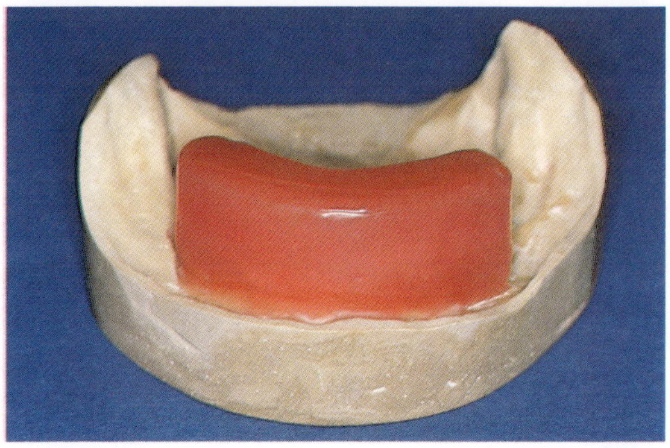

Fig. 146. In order to prepare a custom tray after fabrication of a study model, a wax rim is formed and connected to the model in the area, where the squared impression copings are to be linked to the abutments.

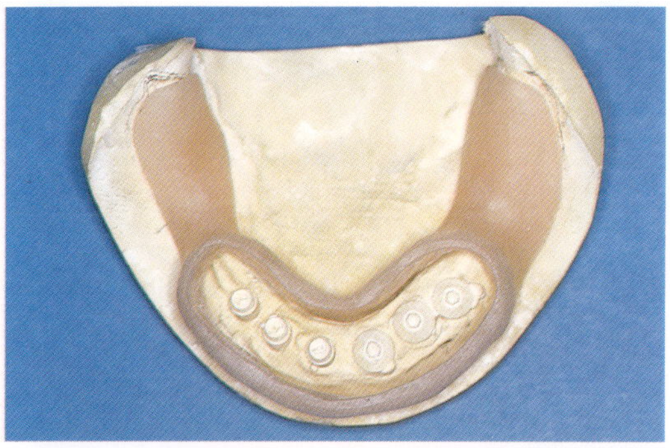

Fig. 147. Preparation of a custom tray, similar to that used for a routine distal-extension partial denture, is performed. In the implant region, the height is adjusted to a level where the guide pins used for impression taking can pass through. The upper region of the tray is kept open, and the retromolar pad in the posterior margin is covered.

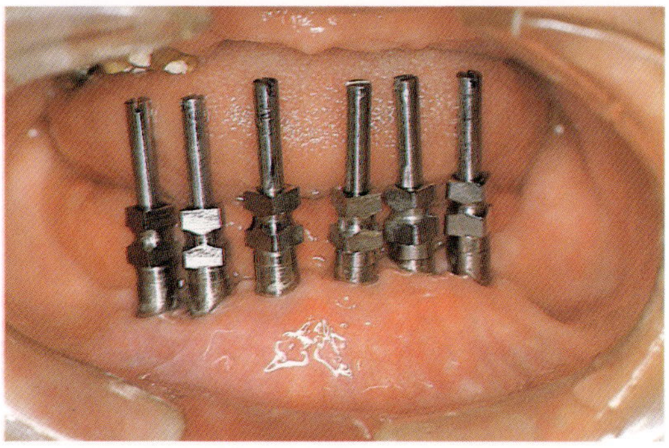

Fig. 148. To take an impression, the squared impression copings are is linked to the abutments, using guide pins. Before manipulation, check that the abutment screws are not loose.

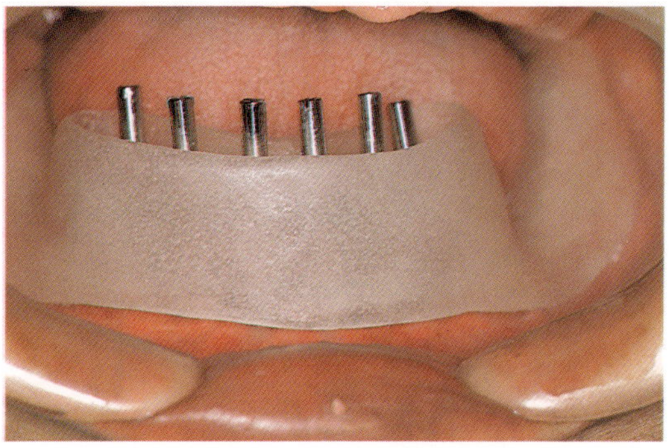

Fig. 149. Try-in of the custom tray. Check that the squared impression copings and guide pins do not touch the tray.

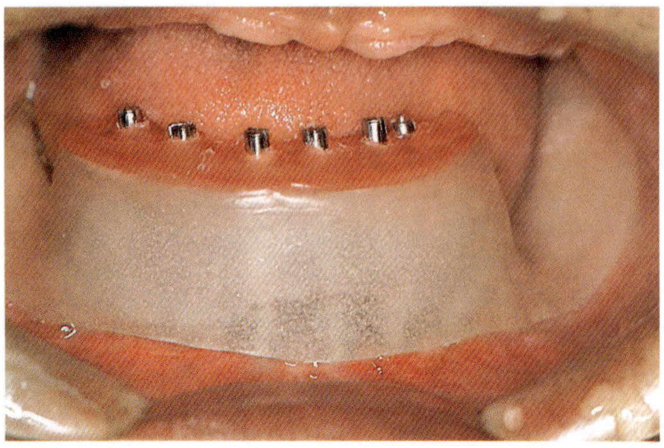

Fig. 150. The window of the custom tray is covered with a layer of wax. When placed in the mouth, the guide pins are allowed to penetrate the wax, marking their positions.

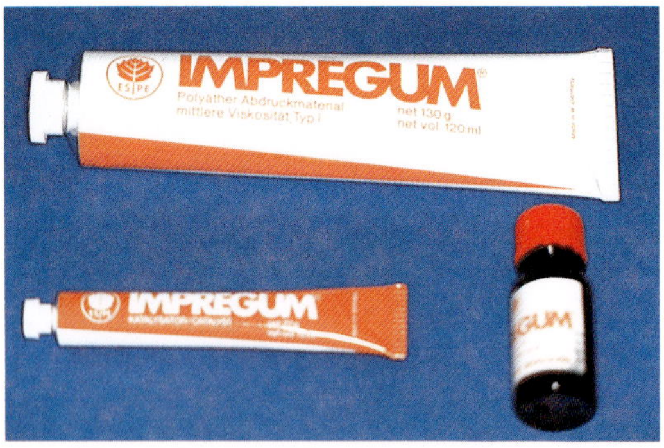

Fig. 151. An impression material, with good size accuracy and morphological stability, is selected. In this case, we selected *Impregum*® (a polyether rubber impression material).

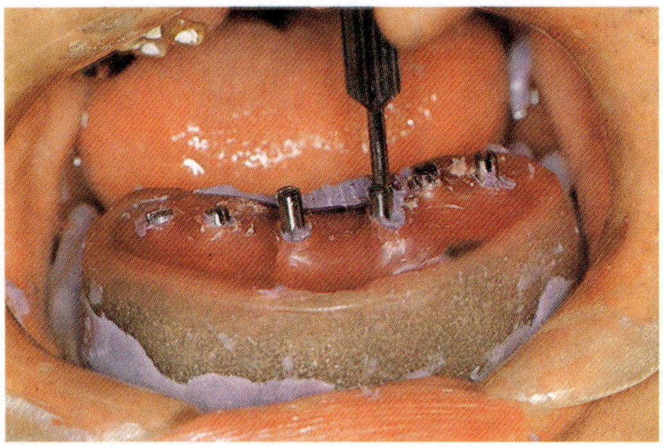

Fig. 152. The impression material is first applied around the abutments using a syringe. Then, the material is applied in the custom tray, which is inserted into the oral cavity, matching the guide pins. When the material has set, all guide pins are loosened with a screwdriver, so the tray can be removed from the oral cavity.

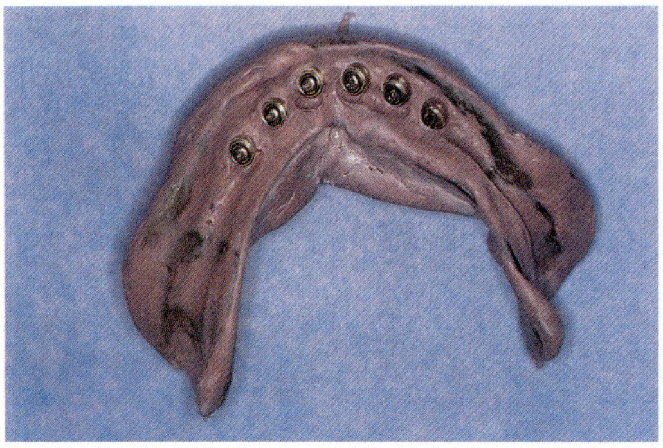

Fig. 153. The impression is carefully studied, and excess impression material (flash, etc.) around the abutments is removed.

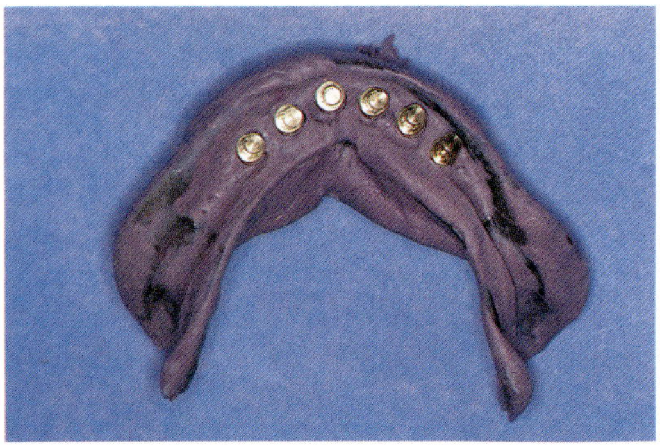

Fig. 154. Abutment replicas are attached to the squared impression copings, using the guide pins.

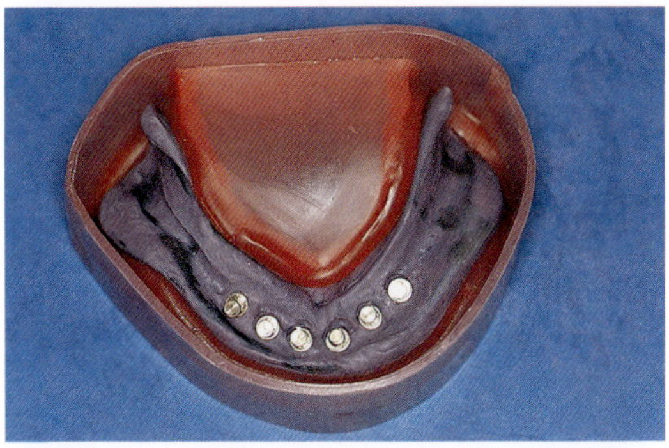

Fig. 155. After routine boxing, plaster (ultrahard plaster) is applied. When the plaster has hardened, the guide pins are loosened and the tray is detached from the model.

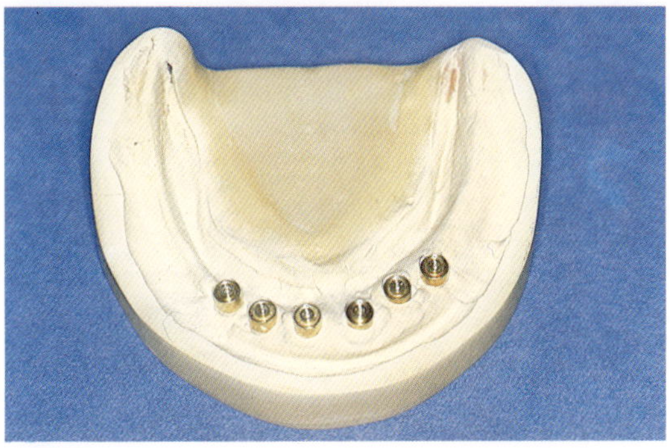

Fig. 156. A complete working model has been fabricated, where the abutment replicas accurately reproduce the abutment positions within the oral cavity.

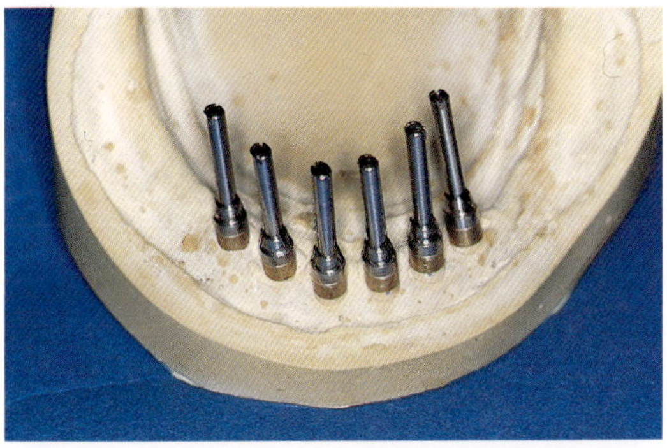

Fig. 157. To fabricate a trial base, gold cylinders are screwed onto the abutment replica with guide pins.

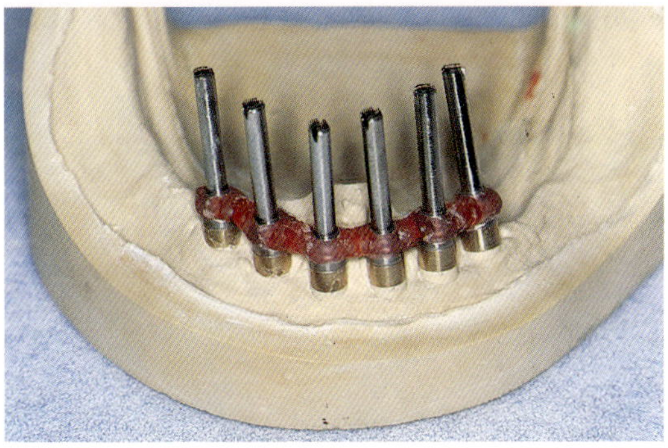

Fig. 158. All gold cylinders are splinted, using *Duralay* ® being applied in a ring-like form around each gold cylinder.

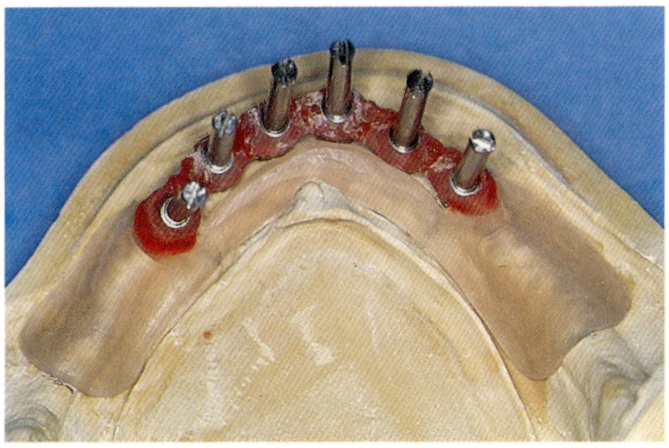

Fig. 159. A trial base is produced, using low-temperature resin, and is linked to the distal end of the *Duralay* ® around the gold cylinders on both sides.

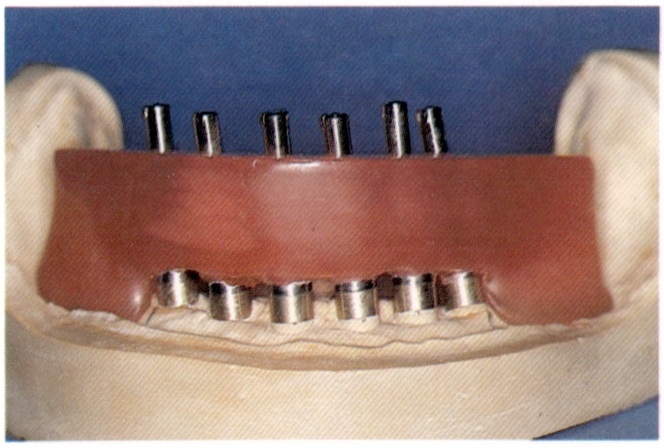

Fig. 160. The wax occlusion rim is stabilized on the acrylic resin trial base. The labial base of the rim is kept open in the area of the gold cylinders, so that the fit of the cylinders and the abutment replicas can be checked.

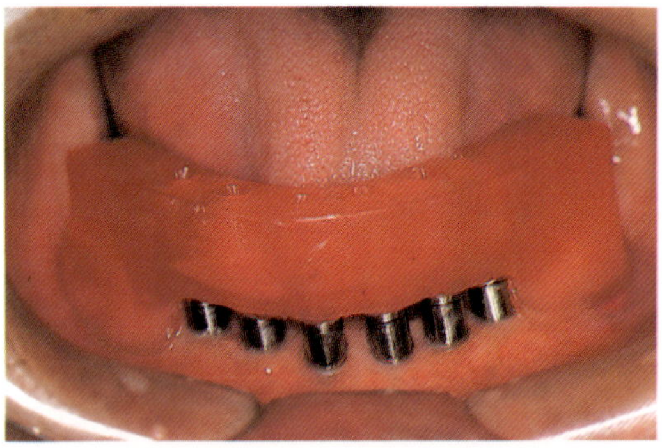

Fig. 161. Using short guide pins, the mandibular trial base is fixed on the abutments in the oral cavity.

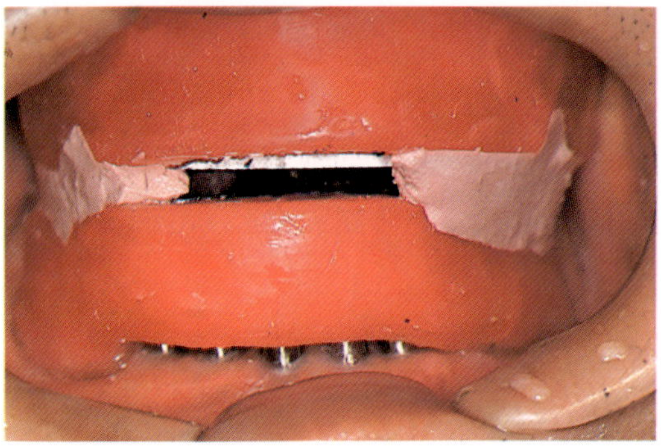

Fig. 162. Gothic archtracer is used for recording centric jaw relation. At the same time, the inclinations of the sagittal and lateral condylar paths are recorded via the check-bite technique.

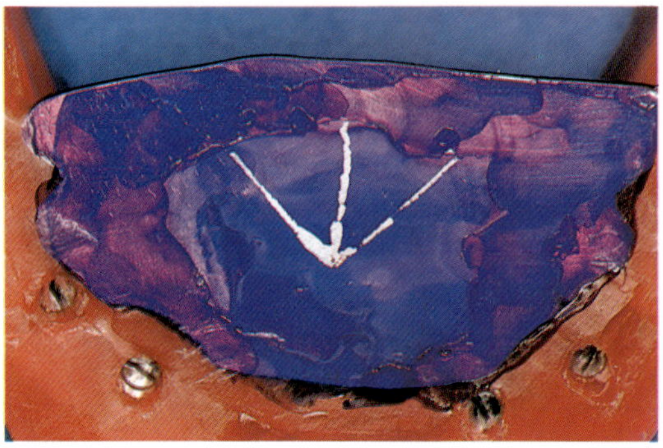

Fig. 163. The horizontal jaw position is the stable position of the condyles (where the Gothic arch apex agrees with the convergence of the 10 tapping points at a frequency of 3/sec) or the so-called muscular position. The occlusal vertical dimension is matched to the facial appearance, as previously corrected with the treatment denture.

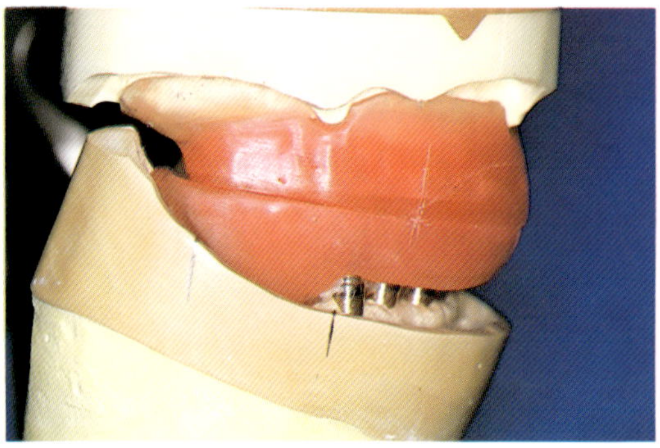

Fig. 164. The jaw casts are mounted in an articulator.

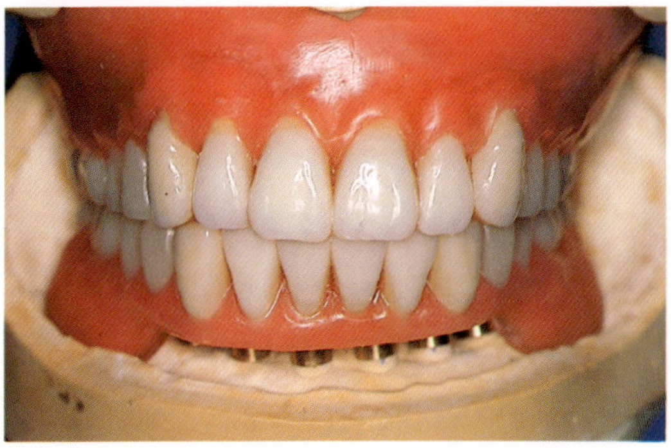

Fig. 165. Arrangement of the artificial teeth is performed, considering resorption of the upper alveolar ridge and the relationship between the upper and lower alveolar ridges. If the implants are used in one jaw, the cusp angle of the artificial teeth has to be minimized. If the resorption of the edentulous alveolar ridge opposite to the implants is moderate or severe, cuspless artificial teeth are indicated. Resin teeth, to absorb the shock of occlusion, are used. Here, we used cuspless artificial teeth.

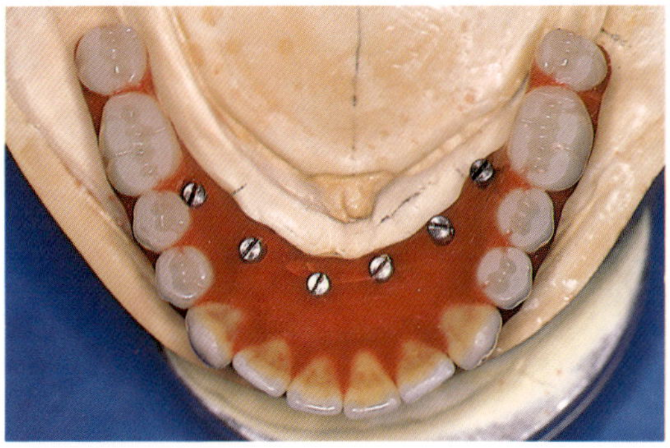

Fig. 166. Relationship between guide pins and artificial teeth.

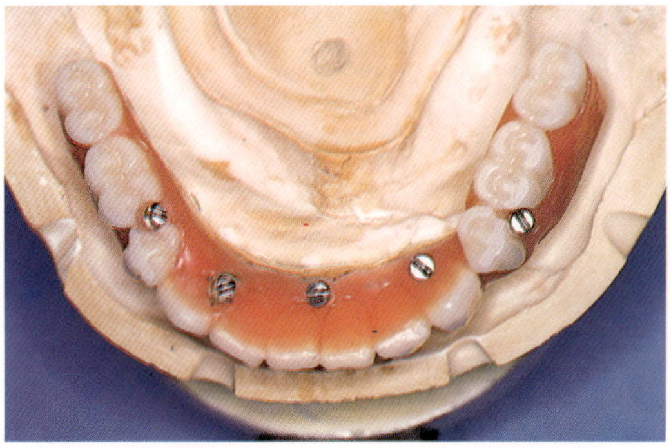

Fig. 167. Depending on the position of the fixtures, the guide pins may occupy the sites for the artificial teeth. In such cases, the artificial teeth are adjusted by trimming. The length of the cantilever distal to the most distal implant should be within 20 mm for the lower jaw and 10 mm for the upper jaw, respectively.

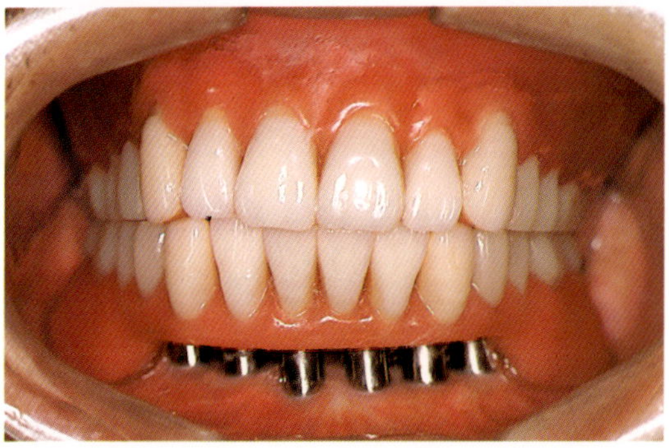

Fig. 168. Acrylic resin teeth are set up in wax on the denture base, which is thereafter tried in the mouth.

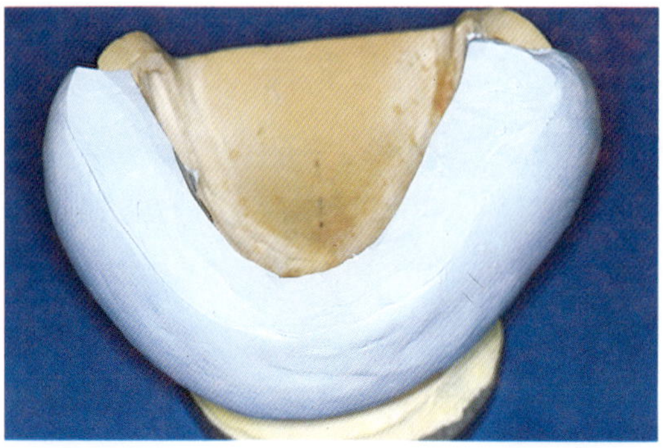

Fig. 169. A labial index of the artificial teeth is prepared, using a silicon (putty) impression material.

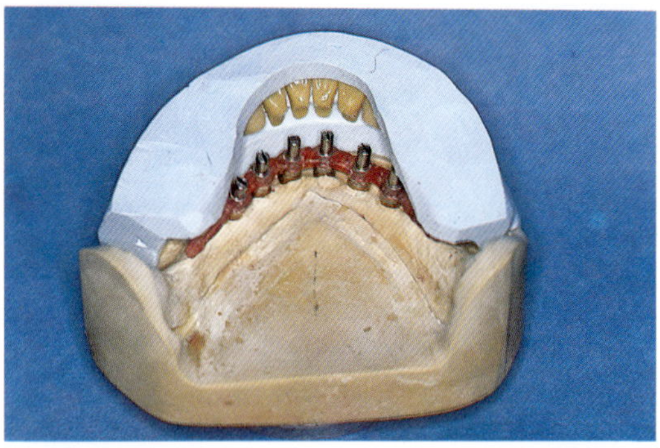

Fig. 170. The try-in denture is separated into the artificial teeth, base plate and wax of the plate. Using the labial index, the artificial teeth alone are returned to the model.

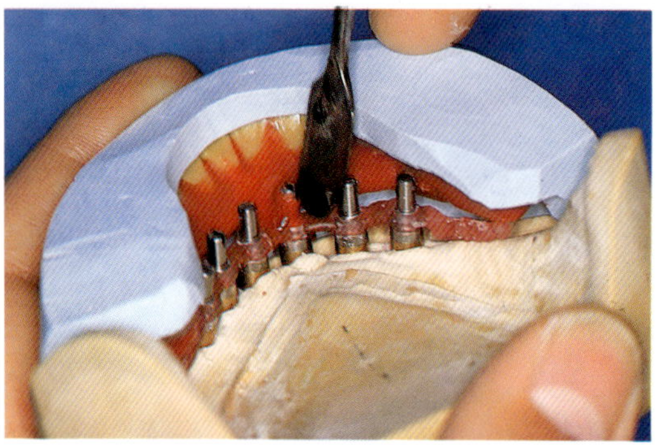

Fig. 171. On the model, loaded with the labial index and the artificial teeth, inlay wax is poured from the lingual side to create a wax form of the framework.

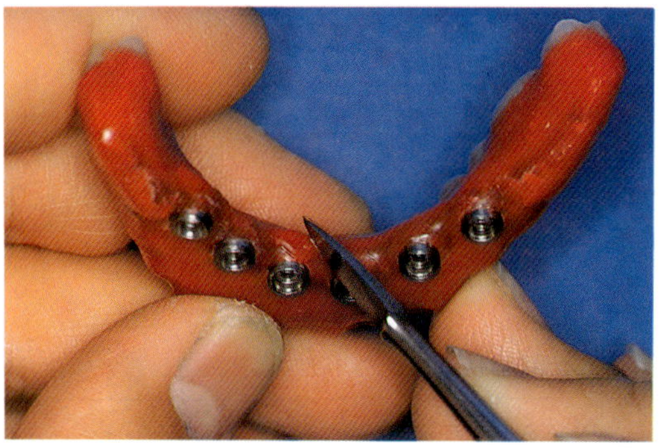

Fig. 172. The bottom of the framework must be Ushaped, with about 1 mm of the gold cylinder exposed.

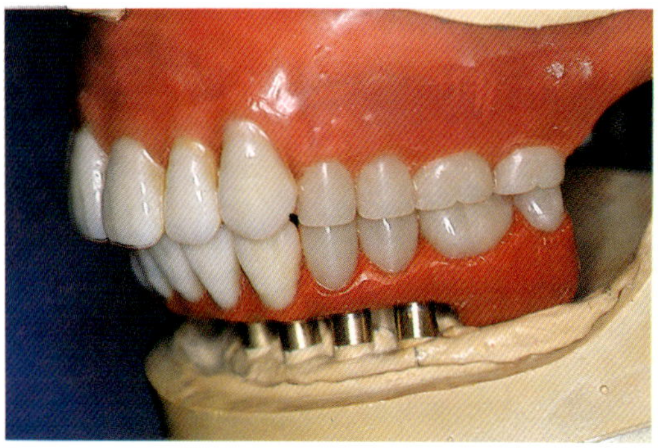

Fig. 173. The peri-abutment form of the framework is determined, with consideration given to allow good cleaning. The base of the structure's free end saddles are formed so that a U-shaped surface towards the alveolar crest is created. The complete denture for the opposite jaw is designed to take a routine form.

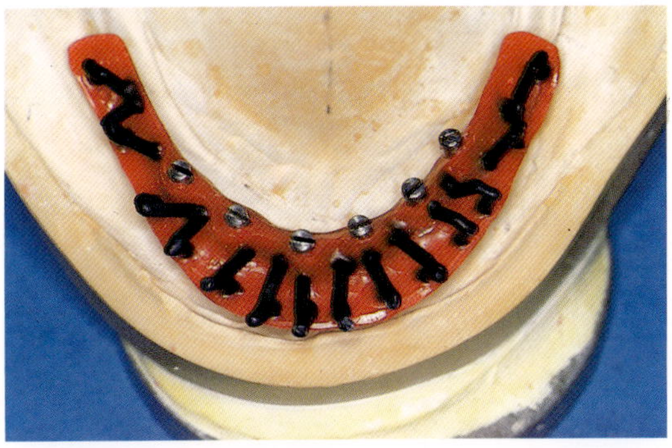

Fig. 174. After removal of the artificial teeth, the framework is adjusted by trimming the wax of the outer surface. To obtain sufficient vertical and horizontal strength, the framework has to be at least 5 mm in width and heigth. A retention loop is attached to each artificial tooth.

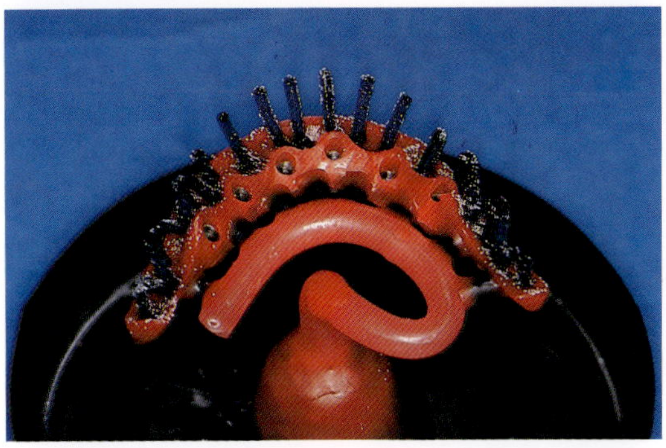

Fig. 175. Investing and casting are performed by routine methods. It is also possible to cast the wax framework in two parts separately and to solder them after casting. Type III or IV gold alloy is usually used as framework material.

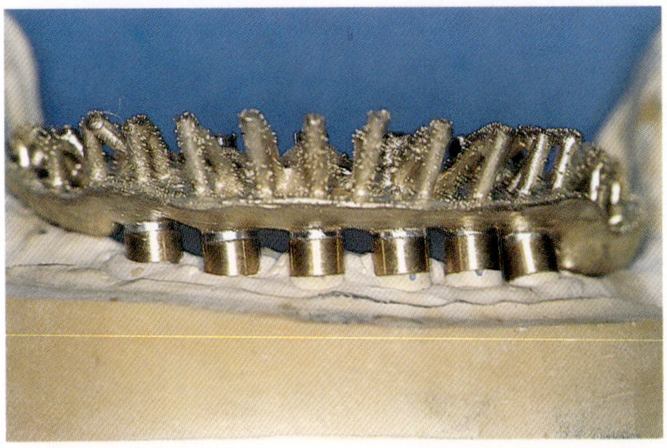

Fig. 176. After casting, the fit of the framework is assessed on the model. If the fit is not good, the framework must be sectioned and resoldered.

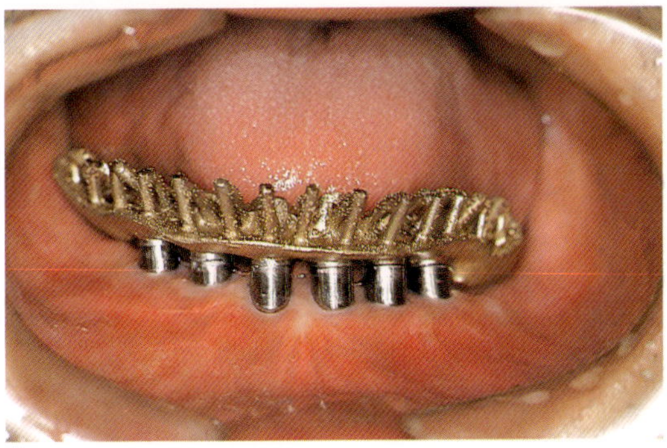

Fig. 177. If the fit was good on the model, the framework is also tested on the abutments intraorally after determing that the abutment screws are tight. First check, without applying pressure, if all the gold cylinders fit the abutments. Then, as the gold screws are gradually tightened, it should also be determined if there is any patient discomfort, due to an ill fit of the framework.

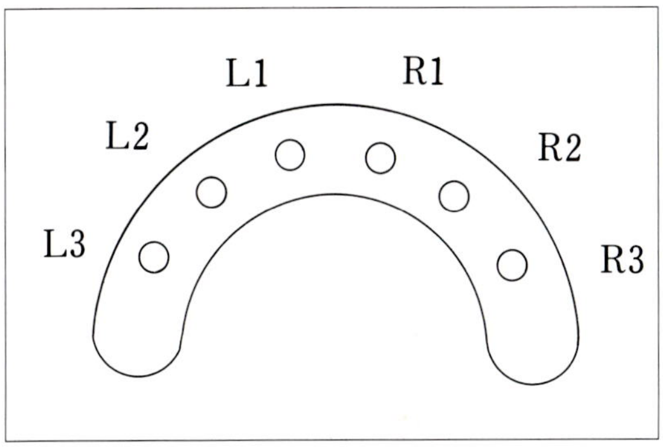

Fig. 178. The gold screws are tightened in the following order: right No. 2, left No. 2, left No. 3, right No. 1, left No. 1 and then right No. 3.

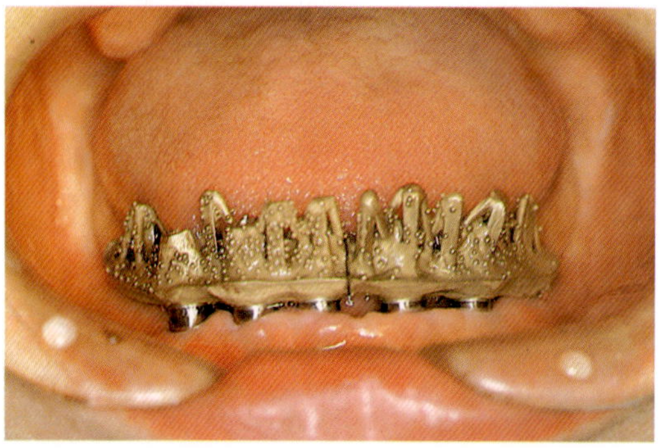

Fig. 179. If the fit between the gold cylinders and the abutments is poor, the framework must be sectioned, and the parts are once again attached to the abutments, where they are fixed to each other and removed from the mouth for corrective soldering.

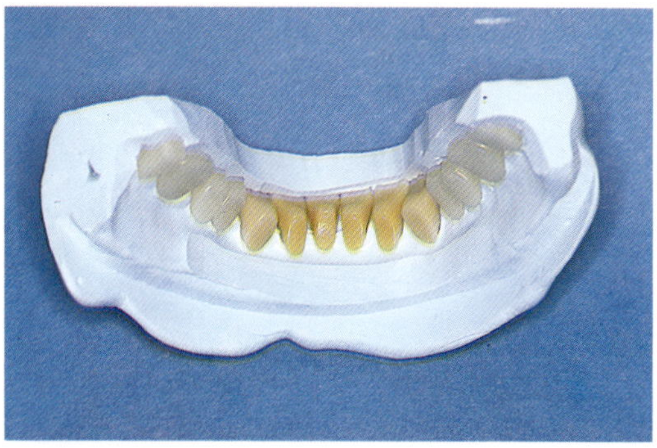

Fig. 180. The artificial teeth are reoriented into the complete framework, using the labial index. Paraffin wax is thereafter poured into the index from the lingual side in order to form the gingiva around the teeth.

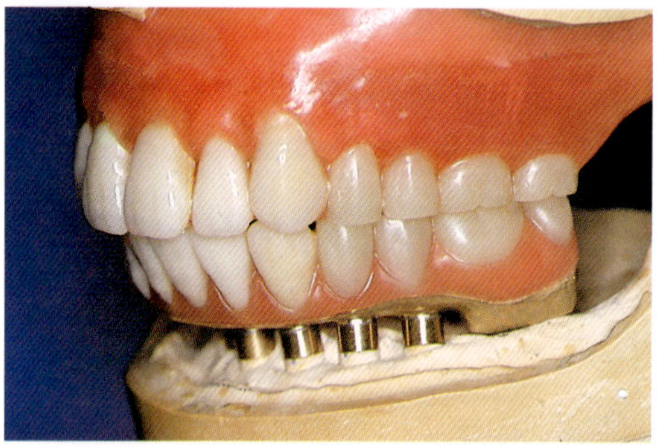

Fig. 181. When the formation of the gingiva is completed, the occlusal relationship is checked on the articulator.

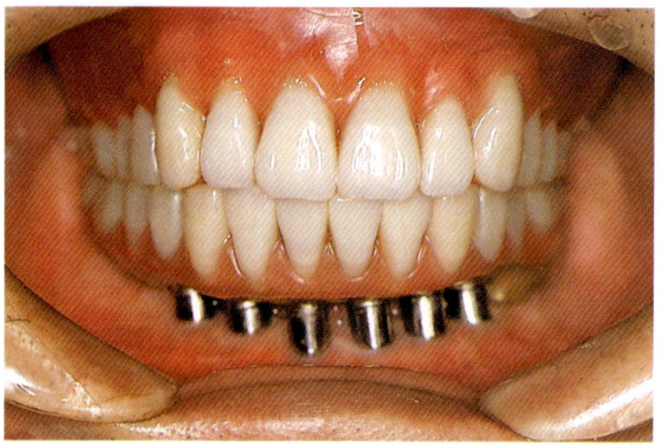

Fig. 182. The construction is tried in the mouth for a final check of occlusion, contacts, phonation and space for the tongue.

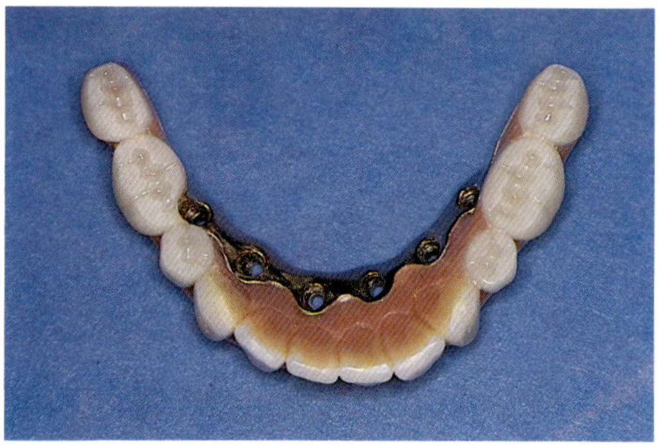

Fig. 183. The wax of the gingiva is replaced with resin to complete the prosthesis.

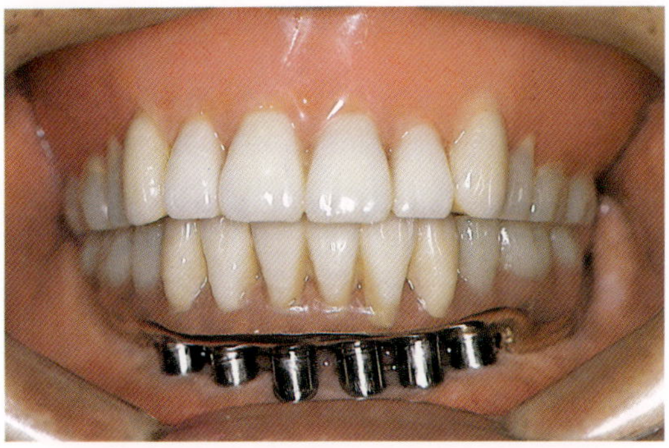

Fig. 184. After determining that the abutment screws are tight, the prosthesis is inserted in the mouth and screwed onto the abutments with the gold screws as described in Fig. 178.

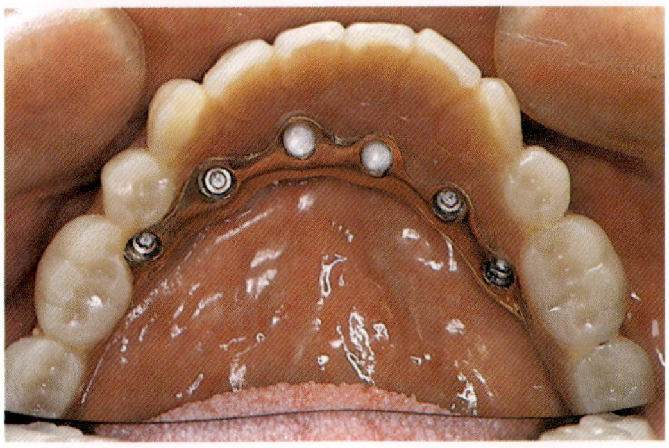

Fig. 185. Small cotton pellets are inserted into the screw holes, which are thereafter filled with a stopping material for temporary sealing.

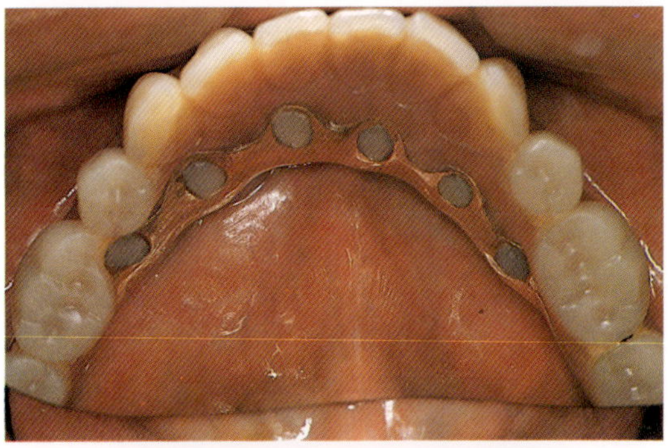

Fig. 186. About one month later, the stability of the gold screws is checked. Thereafter the screw holes are partly filled with a stopping material, sealed with composite resin and polished.

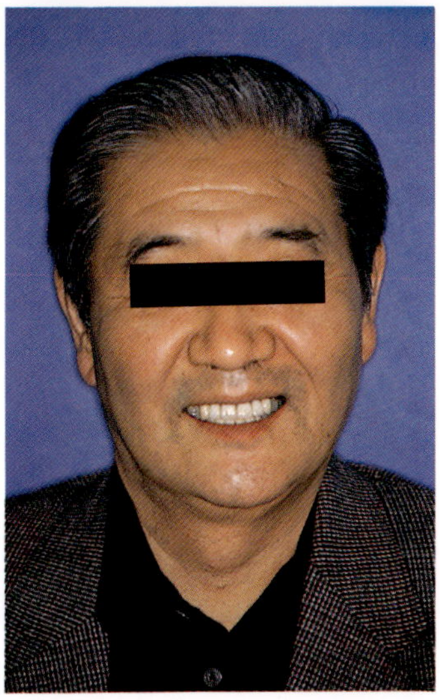

Fig. 187. The prosthesis is checked periodically (1, 3 and 7 months after application) to determine whether occlusal adjustment is needed. Thereafter it is needed to check at least once a year.

Application of Bridges in Partially Edentulous Jaws

After becoming experienced with standard Brånemark implants for edentulous jaws, the system can also be applied to partially edentulous cases. Although the number of partially edentulous patients desiring implants are high, it is not recommended that the practitioner performs his or her first implant operation in a partial case .

In this chapter, prosthetic procedures and problems will be presented for 2 partially edentulous jaws.

(1) Case 1

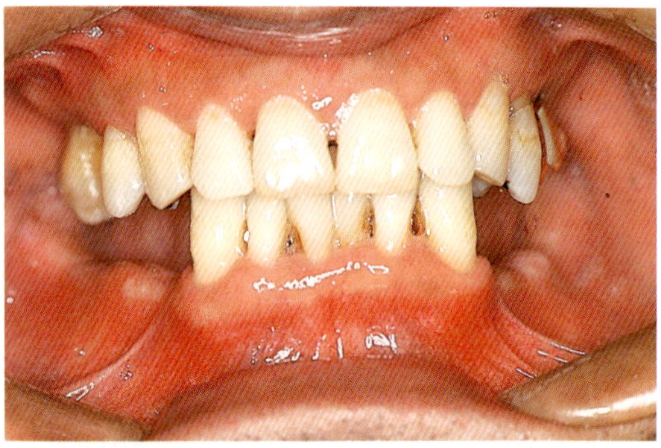

Fig. 188. The first patient is a 50-year-old man, who visited our clinic to receive an implant for a bilateral freeend defect of the lower jaw. He had a partial removable denture but had hardly used it because of an intense sensation of the prosthesis being a foreign body.

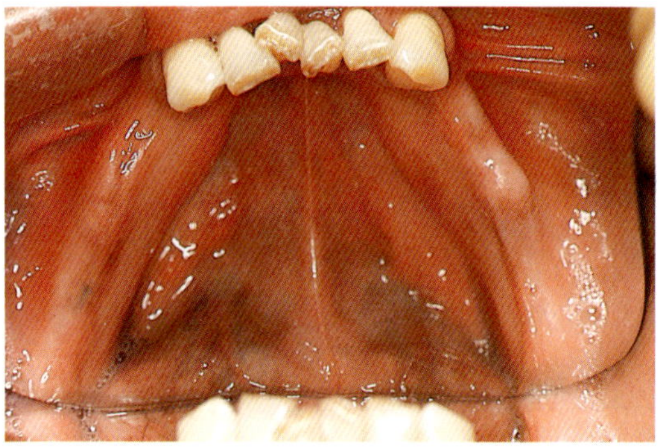

Fig. 189. The oral cavity at the first examination is shown in Figs. 188 and 189. On the alveolar ridge, slight elevation of the left second premolar is visible. No other abnormalities are visible (*mirror image*).

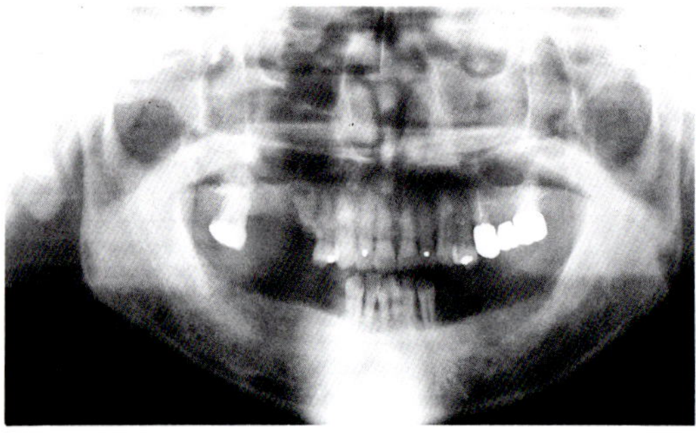

Fig. 190. Radiograph at the first examination.

The upper right second molar showed elongation (because the lower jaw denture had not been applied) and high mobility, and was therefore removed. In lower freeend partial edentulous cases, the position of the mental foramen and mandibular canal have to be elucidated before determining the positions and lengths of possible fixtures.

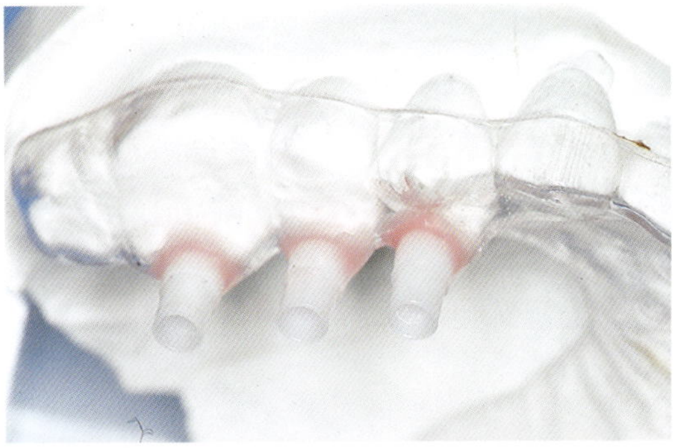

Fig. 191. In addition to the radiographic evaluation, a surgical stent is prepared preoperatively so that the occlusal relationship and esthetic appearance can be checked. The stent in this picture clearly shows the functional cusps of the upper jaw during operation.

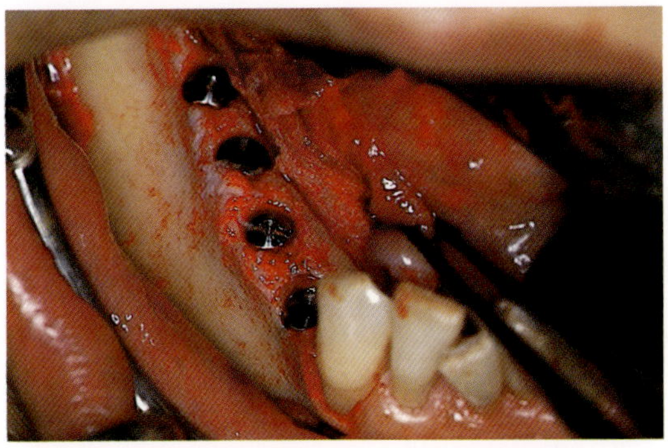

Fig. 192. Stage I operation of right side.

The lengths of the fixtures are as follows:

(distal) 10 mm, 10 mm, 13 mm, 13 mm (mesial)

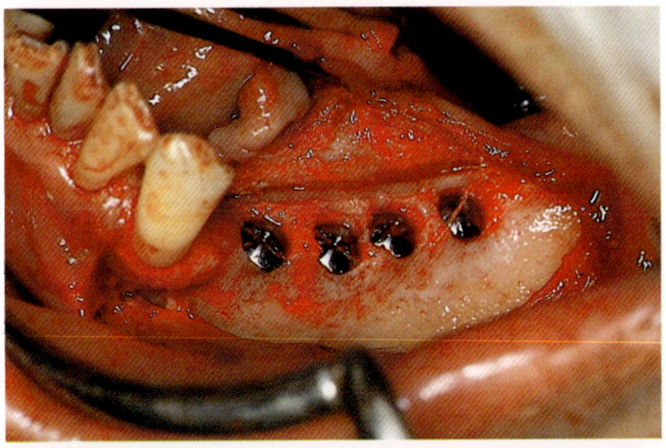

Fig. 193. Stage I operation of left side.

The lengths of the fixtures are as follows:

(mesial) 15 mm, 7 mm, 10 mm, 10 mm (distal)

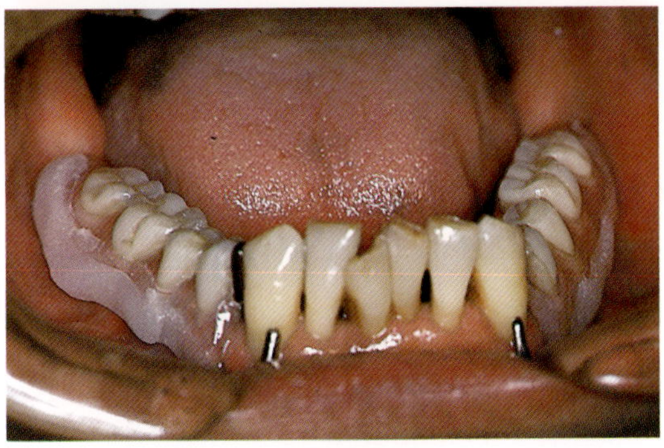

Fig. 194. The operated area cannot be loaded with a denture during the first 2 postoperative weeks, similar to the edentulous jaw. The acrylic resin base of the partial denture used preoperatively is cut so that it will not compress the sutured flaps. The prosthesis is then lined with a tissue conditioner and the material is changed every week for about 2 months.

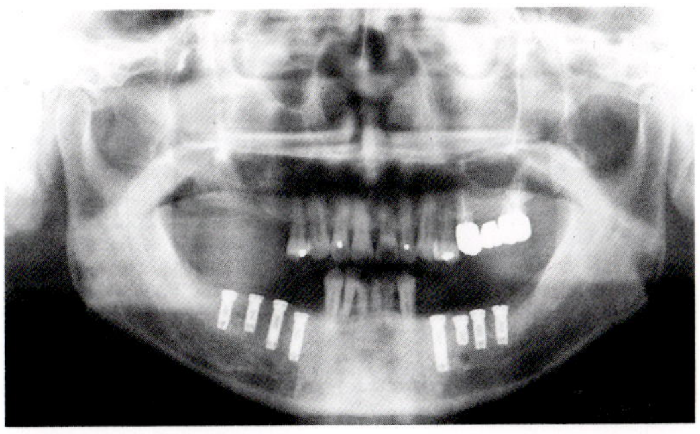

Fig. 195. Rotating panoramic radiograph, taken six months after fixture installation. Because of the lack of abnormalities in the radiograph, and the bone quality observed during the stage I operation, this patient is judged to be ready for Stage II Operation.

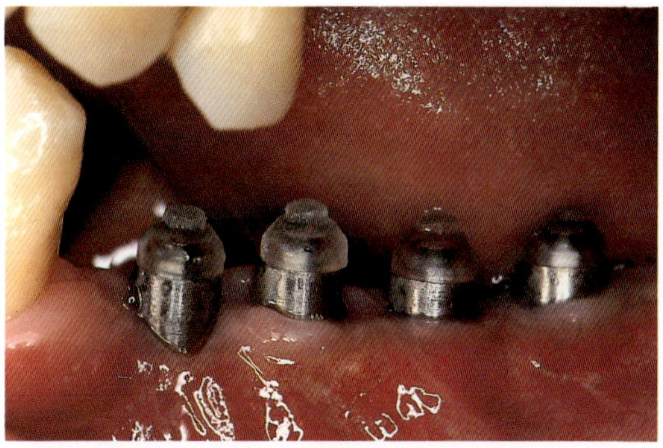

Fig. 196. The right side of the lower jaw after the abutment connection (*mirror image*).

The abutment lengths are as follows:

(distal) 5.5 mm, 4 mm, 5.5 mm, 7 mm (mesial)

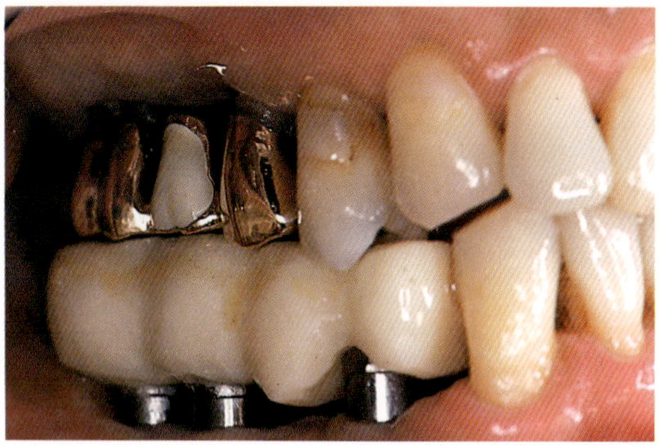

Fig. 197. The left side of the lower jaw after the abutment connection (*mirror image*).

The abutment lengths are as follows:

(mesial) 7 mm, ×, 5.5 mm, 5.5 mm (distal)

The second fixture from the front is not used (i. e., it serves as a "sleeper") because of lack of space to allow smooth preparation of the bridge structure, although the fixture itself shows no problem in osseointegration. What looks like a construction is a temporary bridge.

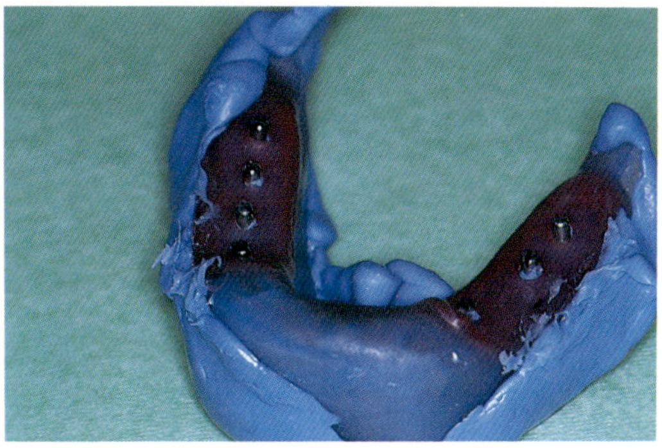

Fig. 198. Impression procedure.

The impression is taken with an custom tray. As in edentulous cases, the upper part of the tray, corresponding to the abutments, is cut so that the guide pins can pass through.

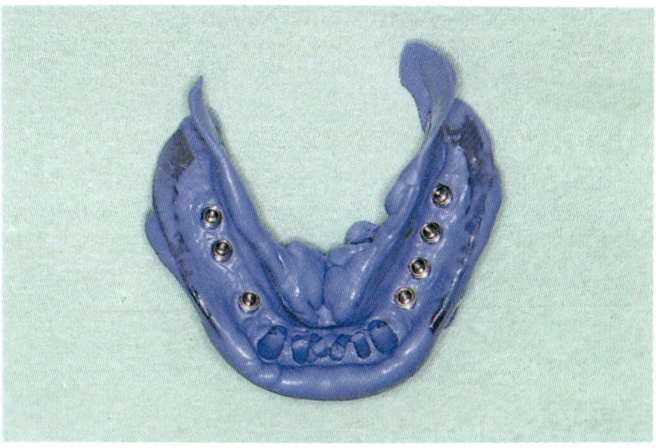

Fig. 199. Connection of the abutment replicas to the squared impression copings within the impression.

The pick-up technique, using a squared impression coping, tends to provide better impressions. In cases where the mouth cannot open sufficiently to allow insertion of the guide pins, the re-seating technique with a tapered impression coping is employed.

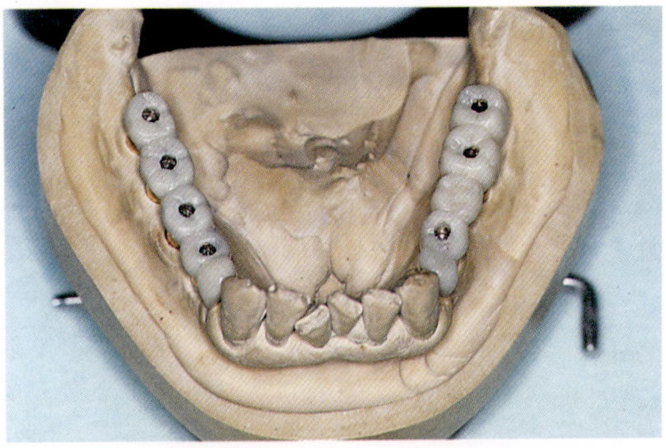

Fig. 200. After taking the impression, a gold framework is manufactured and tried in, and the crown form is built upon the framework with wax so that the patient's comfort (with regard to the tongue), ease of cleaning, and location of the fixtures can be checked. Note that each fixture is located in the central fossa of the crown.

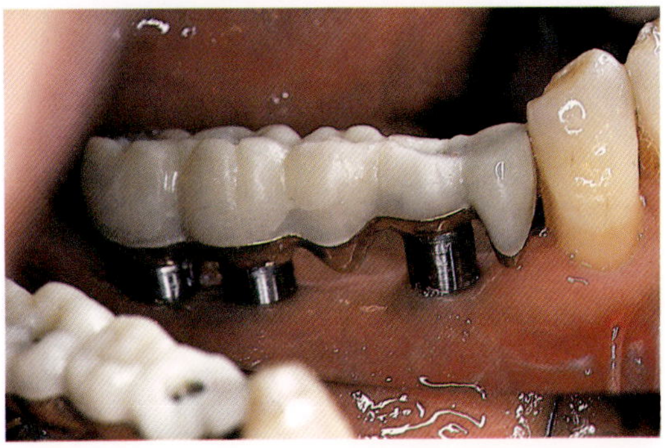

Fig. 201. Application of wax crowns to the left side (*mirror image*).

The same procedure is used for the left and right sides.

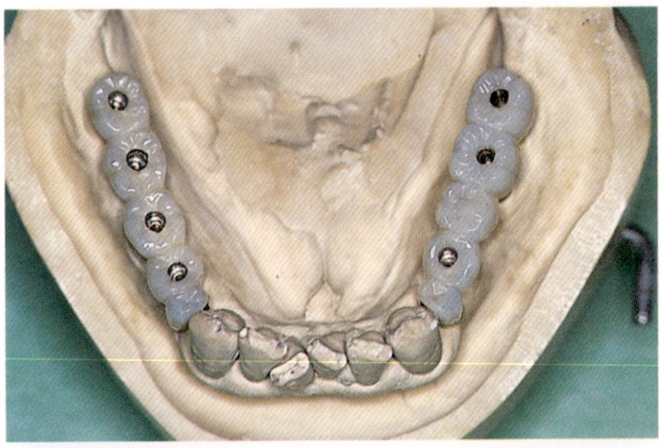

Fig. 202. Preparation of crowns with photopolymerizing hard resin (CESEAD,® Kuraray Co., Ltd.) after taking an impression of the core of the wax crowns.

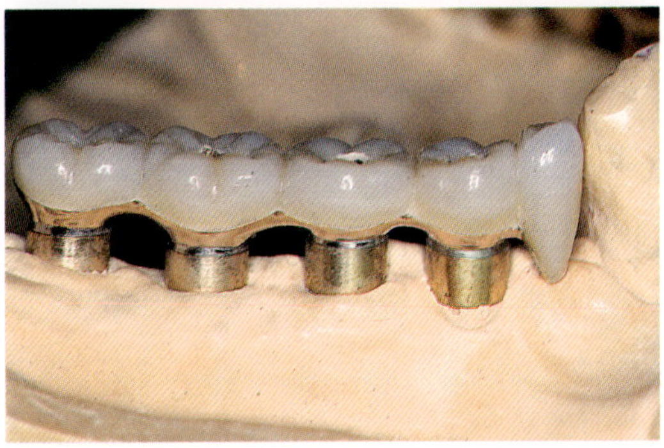

Fig. 203. Complete bridge construction in the right side.

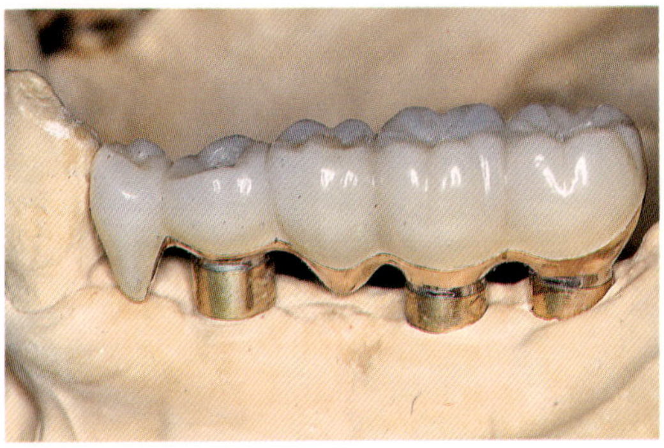

Fig. 204. Complete bridge construction in the left side. In this case, the distance between the canine and first fixture does not seem to be optimal. In partially edentulous cases, the fixture is usually inserted as close to the adjacent tooth as possible. However, if this method seems risky in the light of the bone volume available, it may be esthetically better to place a space of one tooth between the inserted fixture and the adjacent tooth.

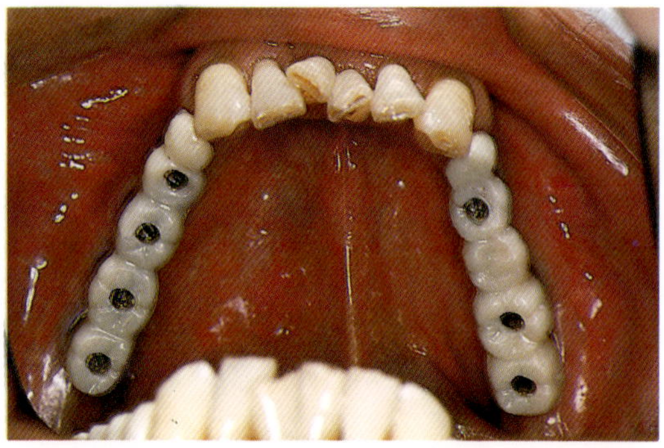

Fig. 205. Bridge constructions placed into the mouth (*mirror image*).

Flat gold screws were used in this case. After the first application of the constructions, the access holes are closed with gutta-percha. About 2 weeks later, it is necessary to check that the bridges' gold screws are not loose.

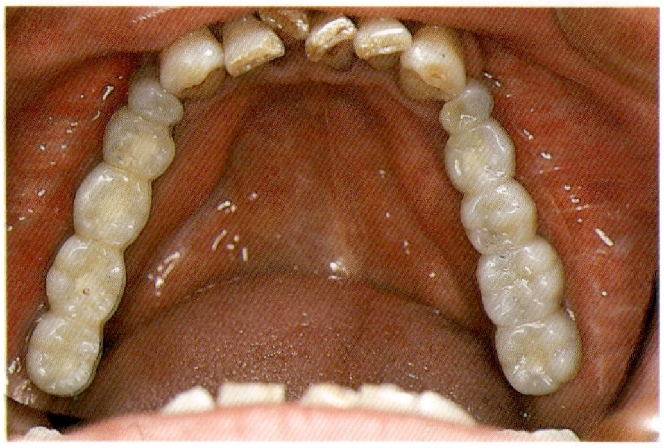

Fig. 206. After checking that the gold screws are not loose, the access holes are closed with a light-curing resin. Thereafter, periodontic maintenance is carried out as mentioned for the edentulous jaws (*mirror image*).

(2) **Case 2**

A 56-year-old woman visited our clinic with a chief complaint of masticatory disturbance due to lack of lower bilateral first and second molars. Although a partial removable denture had been fabricated about one year before, she seldom used it because it caused intense nausea. Based on the patient's desire for implants, and the results of radiography and evaluation of her general condition, indications for implant treatment were judged to be at hand.

The lengths of the fixtures inserted into the lower jaw are as follows:

R 7 mm, 10 mm | 10 mm, 10 mm L

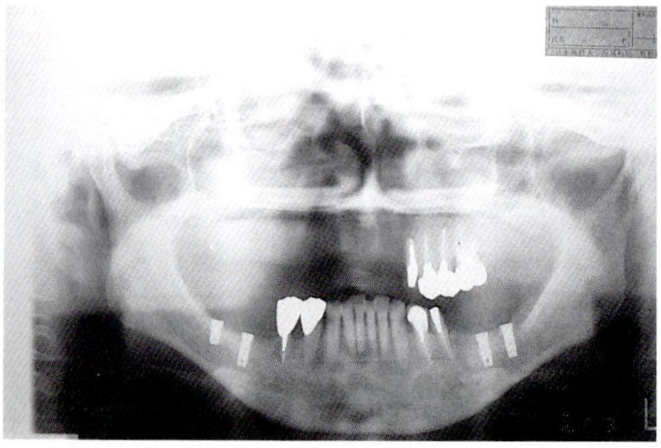

Fig. 207. Panoramic radiograph about seven months after fixture installation. The use of a newly prepared partial denture is planned for the upper jaw, using the preoperative set-up model.

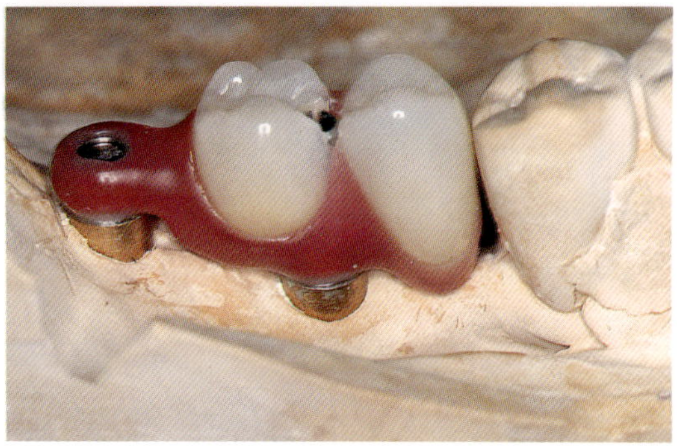

Fig. 208. Abutment connection about eight months after fixture installation.

The lengths of the abutments used are as follows:

R 5.5 mm, 4 mm | 4 mm, 5.5 mm L

The 4 mm abutment on the left side was replaced with a 5.5 mm cylinder, a month later because the original one did not reach above the mucosal level. The picture shows a wax model prepared over the core (including gold cylinders) on the right side.

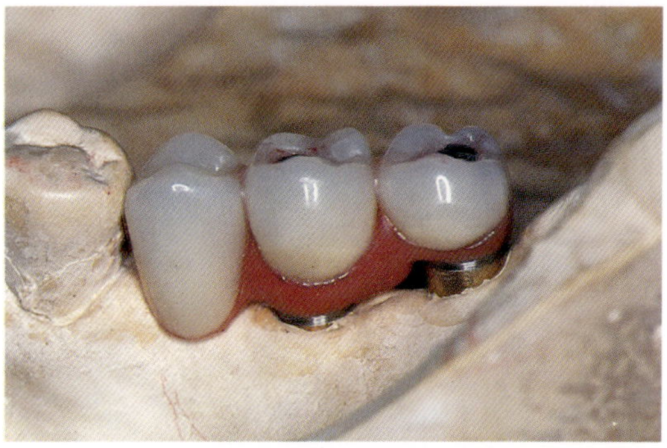

Fig. 209. The same wax model for the left side.

Premolars are used on both sides, because the case was difficult to treat with artificial molars.

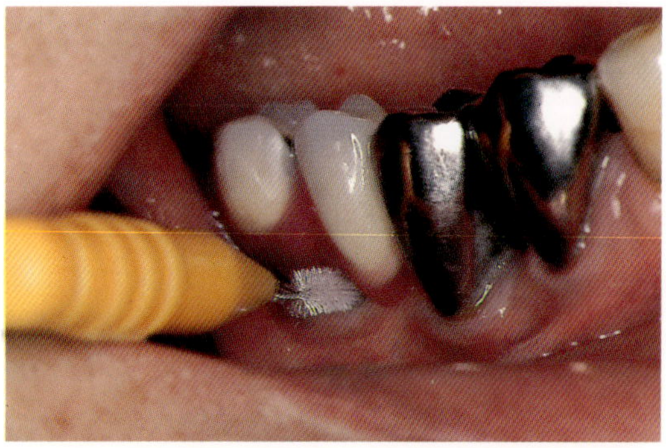

Fig. 210. These wax models are used to determine whether the form of the framework allows for easy cleaning. An interdental brush is used to check the cleaning accessibility.

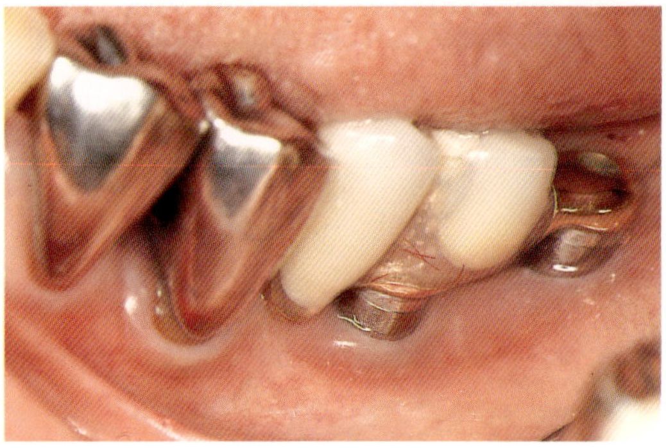

Fig. 211. The completed bridge in the right side (*mirror image*). The last abutment is not loaded with an artificial tooth due to lack of space.

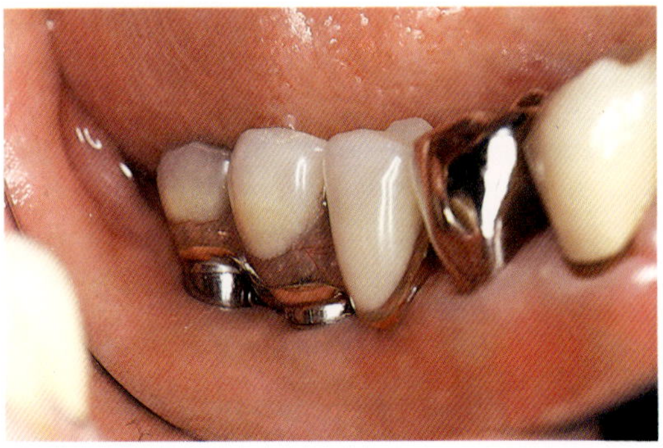

Fig. 212. Completed bridge construction in the left side (*mirror image*).

Three premolars are arranged in a space equivalent to two molars.

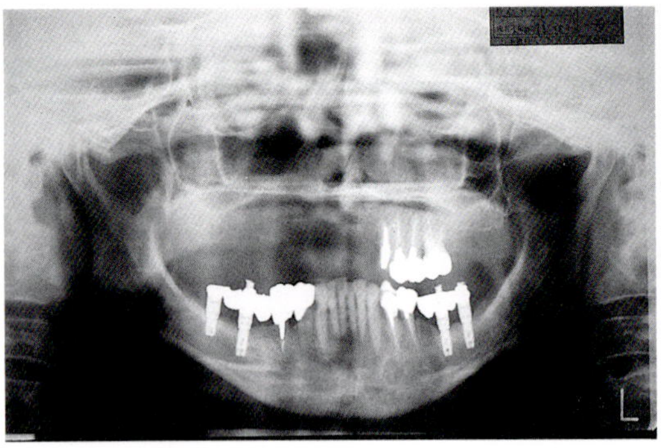

Fig. 213. Panoramic radiograph after application of the partial bridges.

SUPPLEMENT

Radiography upon Completion and During Follow-Up

As a rule, radiography is performed periodically according to a follow-up schedule. Extra radiography is performed if necessary (e.g., with appearance of symptoms). Usually, radiography is performed upon completion of the prosthetic treatment and after 1, 3, 5 and 10 years respectively. Stereoscopic picture pairs, using a parallel technique, are usually taken.

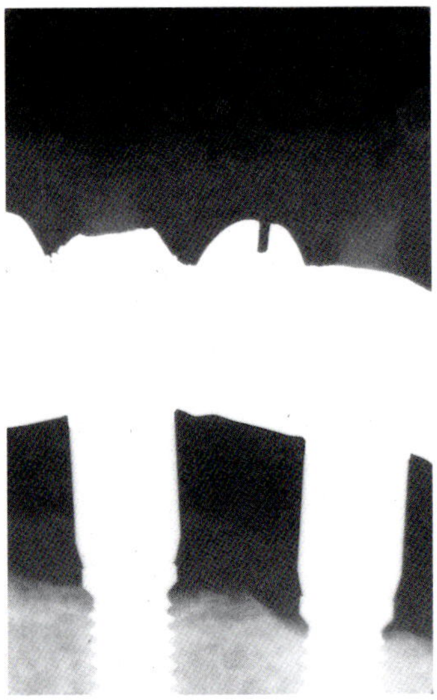

Fig. 214. Bone resorption of the alveolar crest near the implant is particularly important in radiographic followup assessments. At the annual check-up, the condition of the anchorage unit as well as of the osseointegration condition are also examined.

CHAPTER V

MAINTENANCE

Regime in Plaque Control after the Abutment Connection

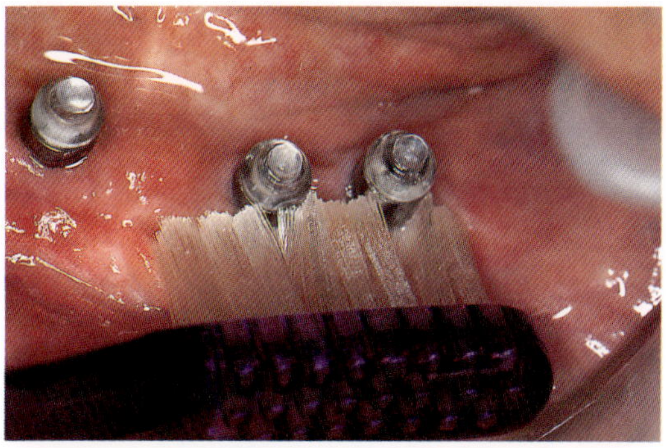

Fig. 215. Poor oral hygiene results in accumulation of plaque and calculus around the abutment cylinders.

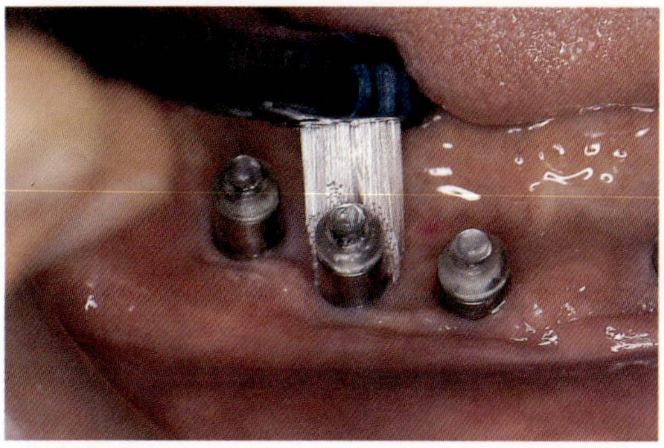

Fig. 216. Cleaning of the abutments is started about 2 weeks after the stage II operation. The buccal and lingual surfaces are brushed by the Bass method using a soft toothbrush.

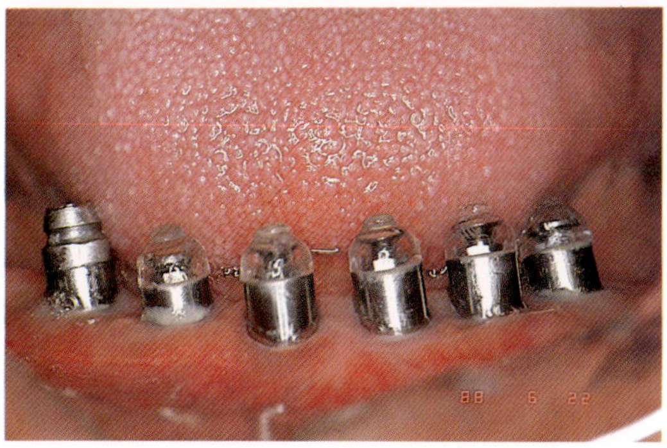

Fig. 217. End-Tuft (Butler® # 307 or # 308) is specifically effective for use on the lingual and proximal surfaces of the abutment cylinders.

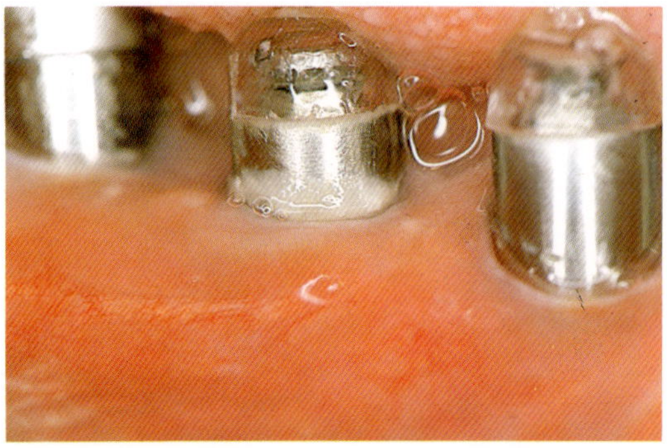

Fig. 218. Accumulation of plaque in the cervical region of the abutments.

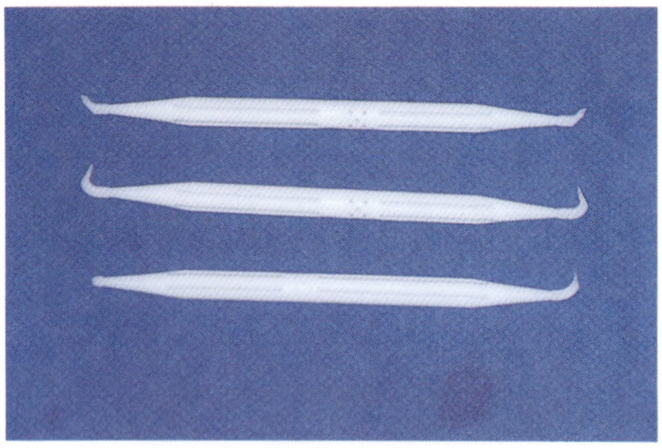

Fig. 219. Plastic scalers have been developed to aid in the removal of debris and calcified deposits, taking care not to damage the surface of the titanium abutment cylinders.

Nobelpharma plastic scalers
Buccal scaler DIA240 (*top*)
Lingual scaler DIA239 (*middle*)
Universal scaler DIA238 (*bottom*)

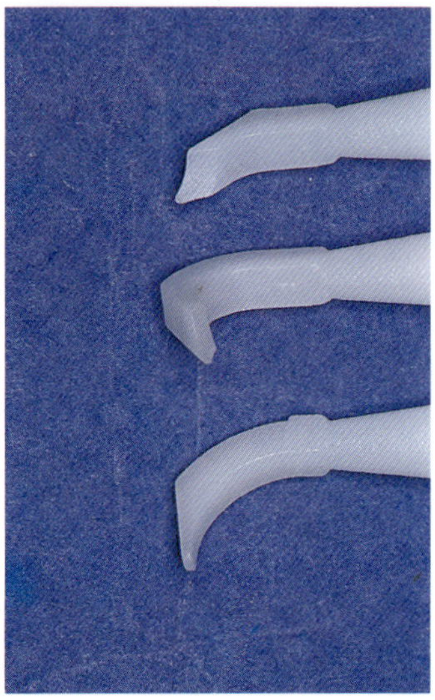

Fig. 220. The working edge of the *Nobelpharma* scalers :

Top : buccal scaler
Middle : lingual scaler
Bottom : universal scaler

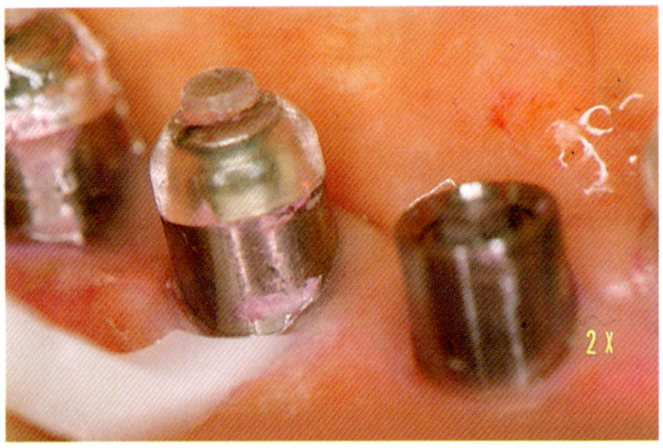

Fig. 221. The working edge of the buccal plastic scaler is designed to fit the buccal surface of the abutment and to remove plaque and calculus.

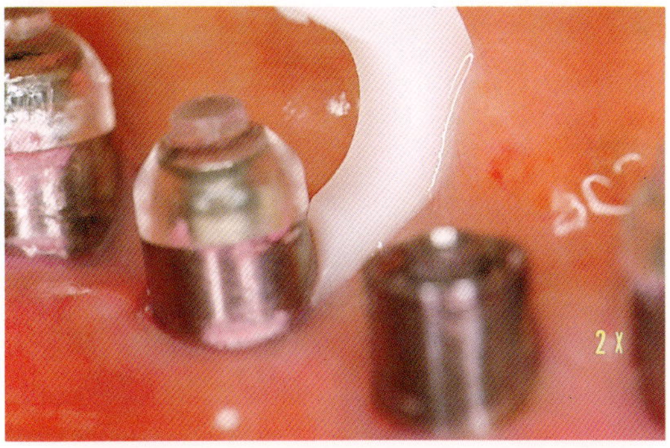

Fig. 222. The working edge of the lingual plastic scaler is designed to fit the lingual surface of the abutment and to remove plaque and calculus.

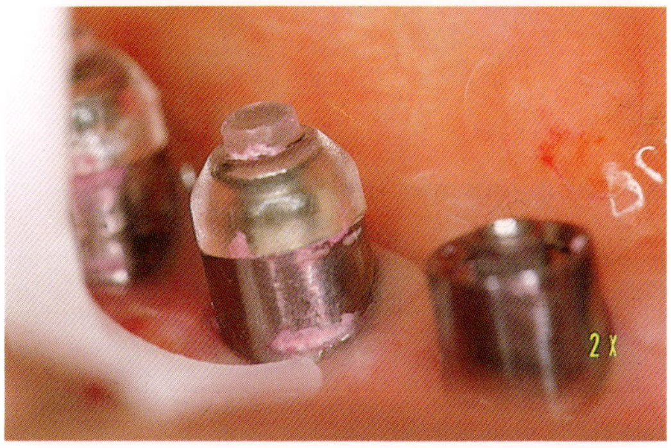

Fig. 223. The universal plastic scaler can be used on the distal surfaces to remove plaque and calculus.

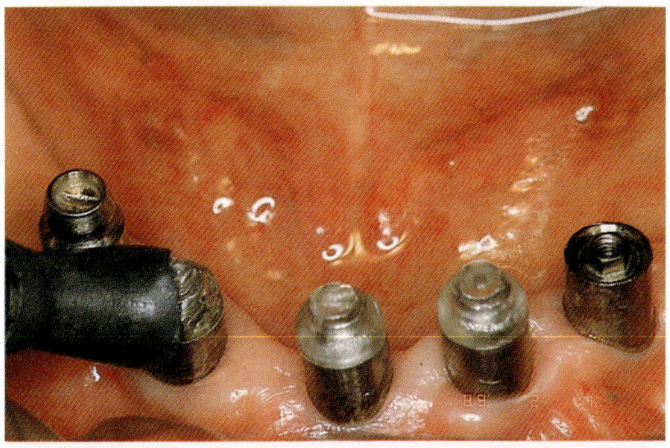

Fig. 224. The abutment surface is polished with a rubber cup.

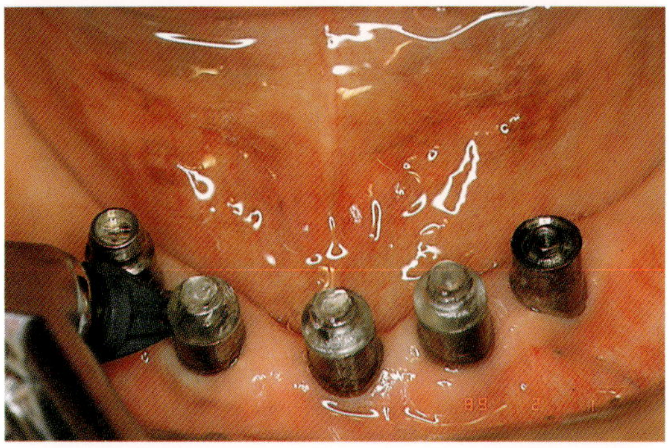

Fig. 225. The abutment surface is polished with a prophy point.

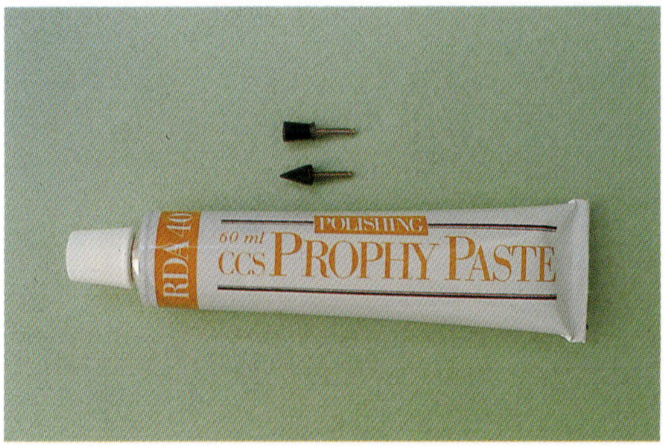

Fig. 226. A fine abrasive paste may be used, such as Prophy Paste (CCS, Sweden).

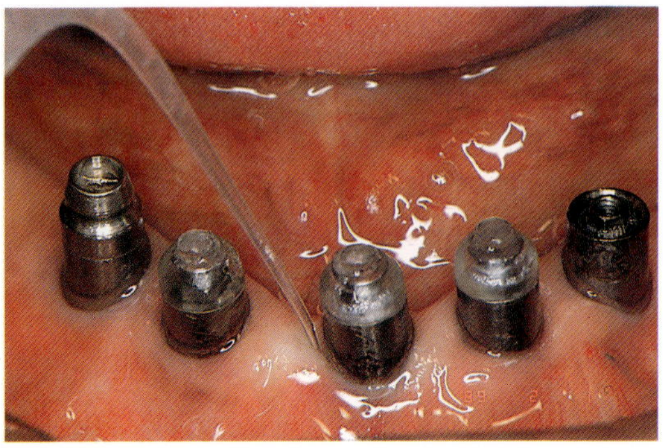

Fig. 227. Antimicrobials are applied with an plastic irrigation syringe, in order to reduce subgingival plaque.

Brushing Method

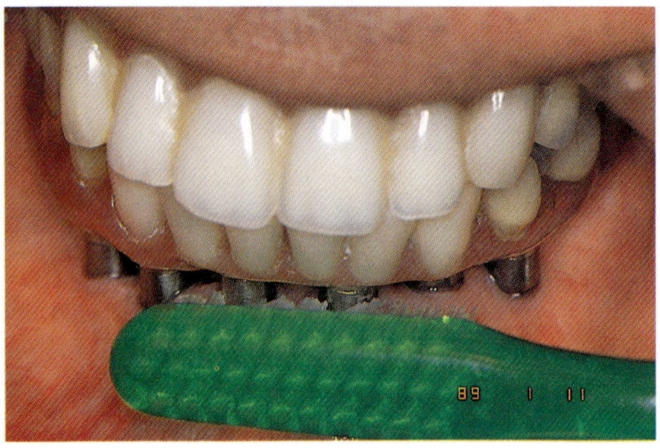

Fig. 228. (1) **Brushing method for buccal surfaces.** Brushing by the Bass method is effective, because the depth of the vestibule is very small and the keratinized mucosa is thin.

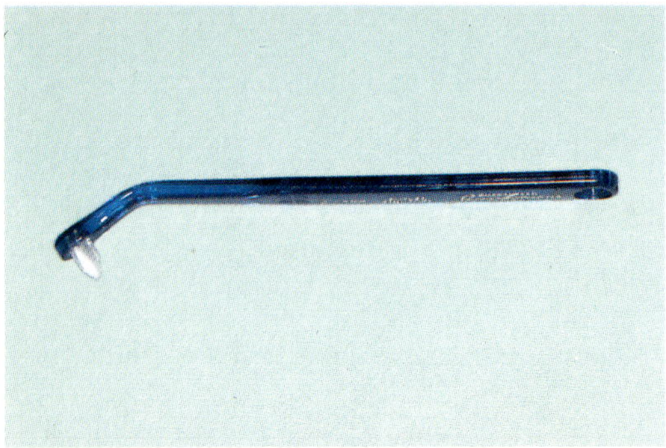

Fig. 229. (2) **Brushing method for palatal and lingual surfaces.**

The shaft of End-Tuft (Butler® #307 or 308) is curved toward the inside, so that it can easily reach the abutment on the lingual surface.

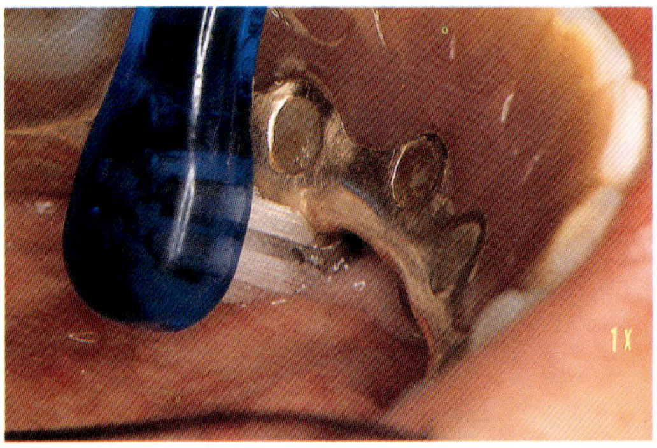

Fig. 230. The lingual surfaces are cleaned with short vertical and horizontal movements.

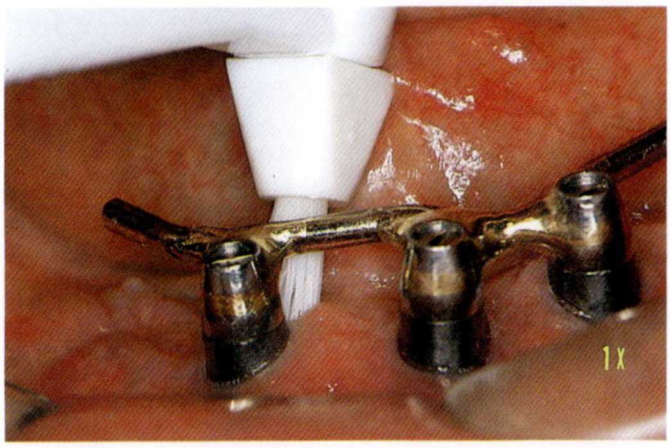

Fig. 231. An inter-space brush allows removal of plaque from "hard-to-reach" areas on the palatal and lingual surfaces.

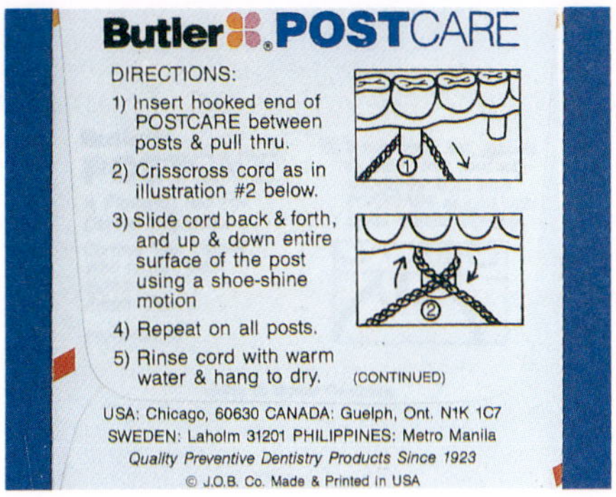

Fig. 232. POST CARE™ (Butler®) is also effective in removing plaque from the abutment on the lingual and mesio-distal surfaces.

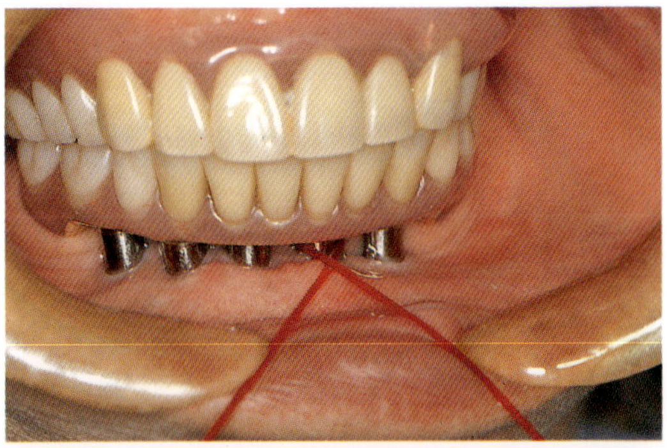

Fig. 233. The bent end of the POST CARE™ (Butler®) is inserted between the abutments and pulled through. The entire surface of the abutment is flossed to remove plaque.

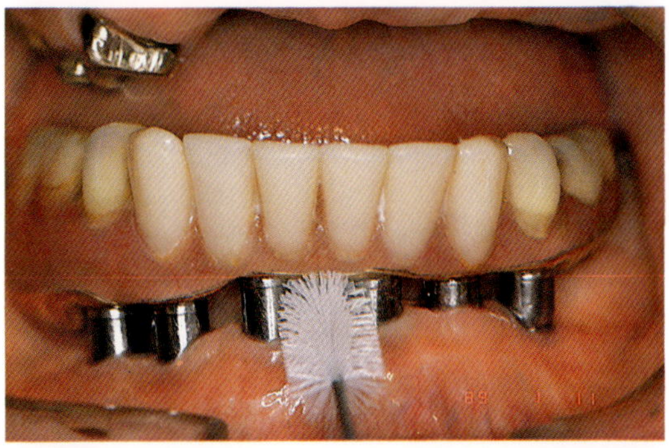

Fig. 234. (3) **Brushing method for the mesio-distal surfaces.**

The interdental brush is carefully inserted through to the lingual side. It must be used with care so as not to scratch the surfaces of the abutments.

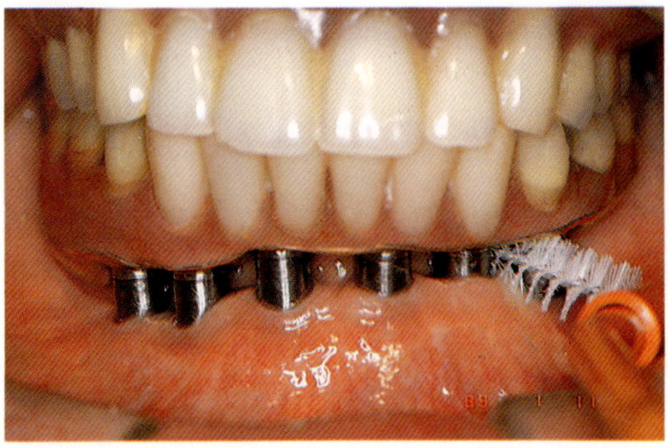

Fig. 235. If a curved interdental brush is used, plaque on the mesio-distal surfaces of the posterior abutments can easily be removed.

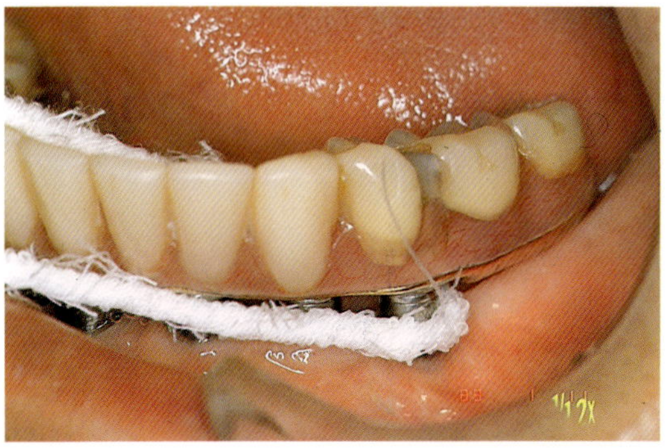

Fig. 236. A gauze strip (or POST CARE™) is pulled under the cantilever towards the distal aspect of the abutment and used to clean the cylinder surface.

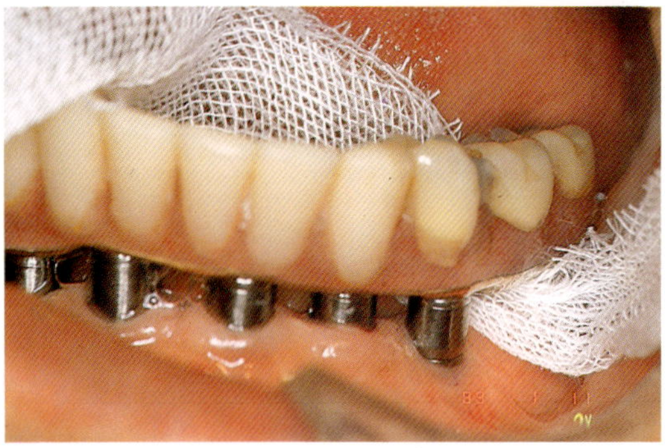

Fig. 237. A gauze strip is inserted under the posterior cantilever and used to clean and polish the pontic area.

Cases in which Plaque Control is Difficult

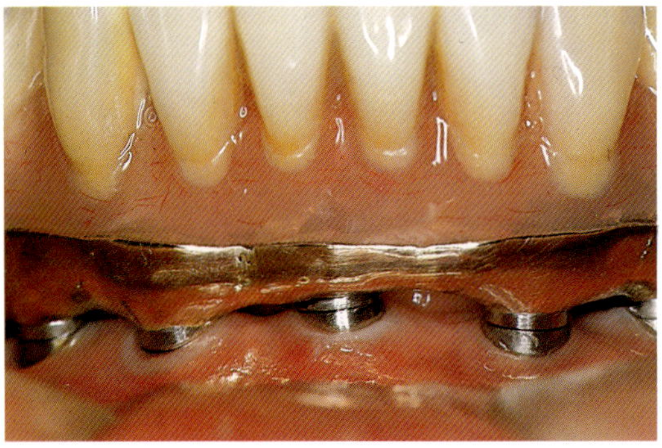

Fig. 238. (1) Situations in which the distance between the margin of the prosthesis and the marginal gingiva is less than 2 mm. In this case, it is difficult for a toothbrush or interdental brush to reach the marginal gingiva, all around the abutment.

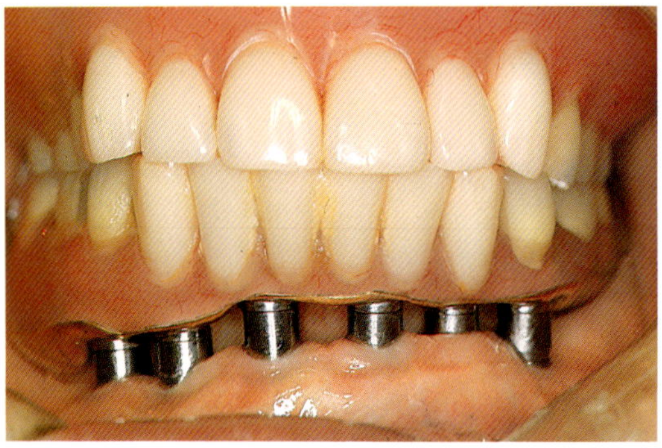

Fig. 239. (2) Situations in which the distance between the margin of the prosthesis and marginal gingiva is not uniform (unnecessary long abutments). In this case, it is difficult to remove plaque on the buccal and lingual sides with a toothbrush.

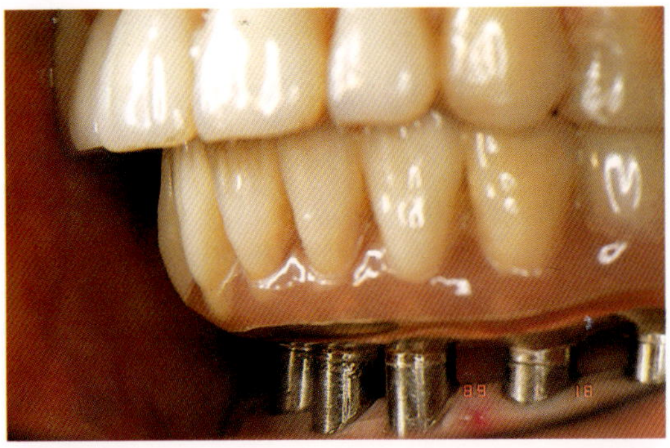

Fig. 240. (3) Situations in which the prosthesis either has a buccal or a lingual overhang due to bad position of the fixtures. In this case, the excessive inclination of the prosthesis makes plaque removal with a toothbrush difficult on both sides of the bridge work.

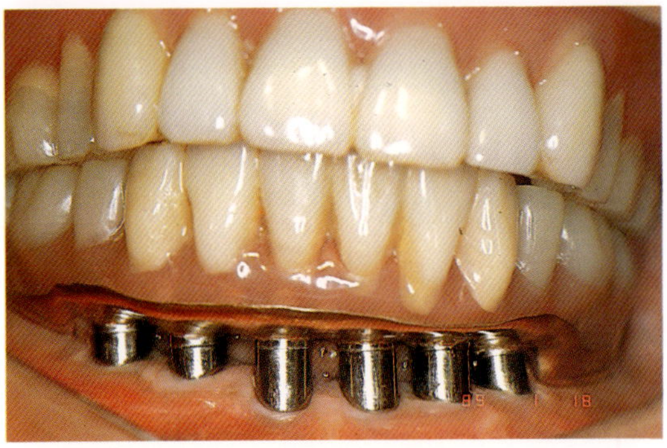

Fig. 241. (4) Situations in which individual implants have been installed outside the arch. In this case, it is difficult for a toothbrush or interdental brush to reach the target point.

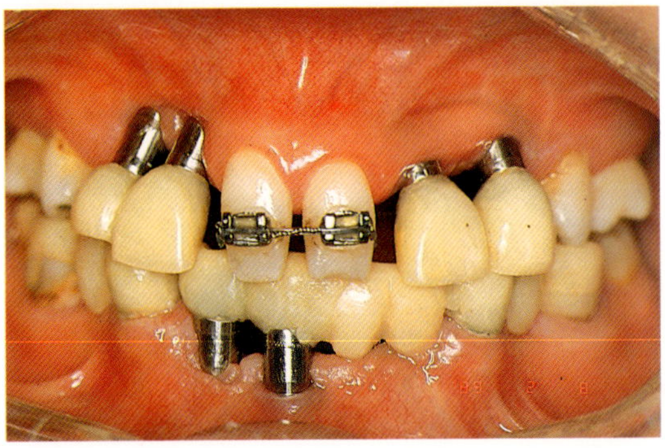

Fig. 242. (5) Situations in which the position of implants is different from that of the natural teeth in the labio-lingual aspect, or in which the implants are excessively angulated. Inclination of implants may lead to malposition of the marginal gingiva around the implants. In such cases, plaque removal on the mesio-distal sides can be difficult.

Maintenance of Peri-Implant Tissue

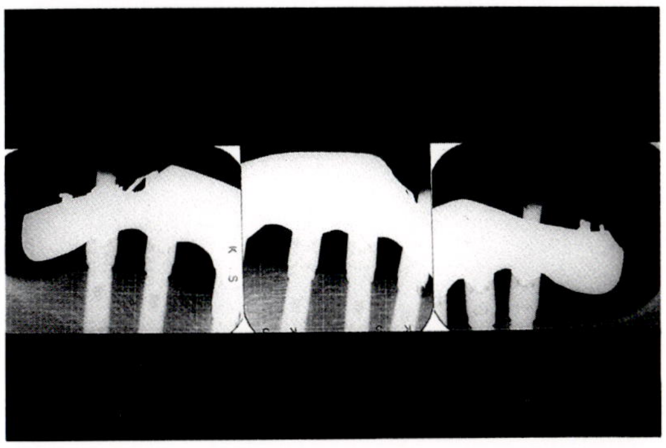

Fig. 243. Condition after the prosthesis has been connected. The level of the marginal crest is uniform, and the bone trabeculae are dense.

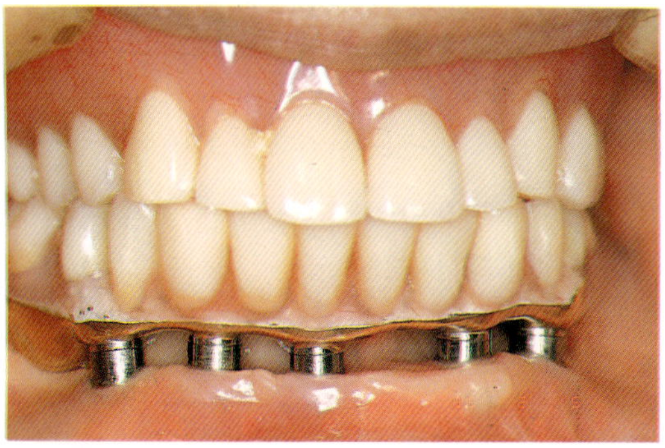

Fig. 244. Frontal view of lower full bridge. Plaque control on the bucco-labial sides is performed by the Bass method. The patient is instructed to use a gauze for plaque control on the lingual and distal sides of the abutments and under the pontics.

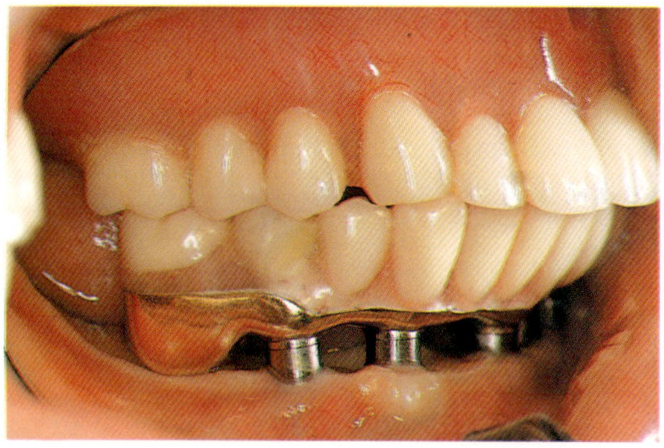

Fig. 245. Lateral view of the full arch bridge, indicating good oral hygiene and healthy gingiva.

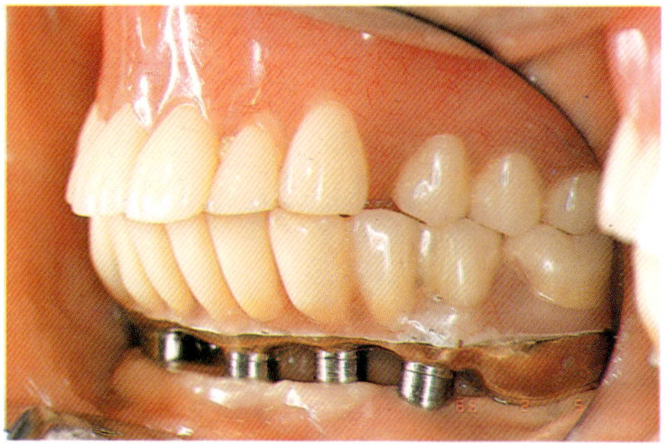

Fig. 246. The opposite side of the case in Fig. 245.

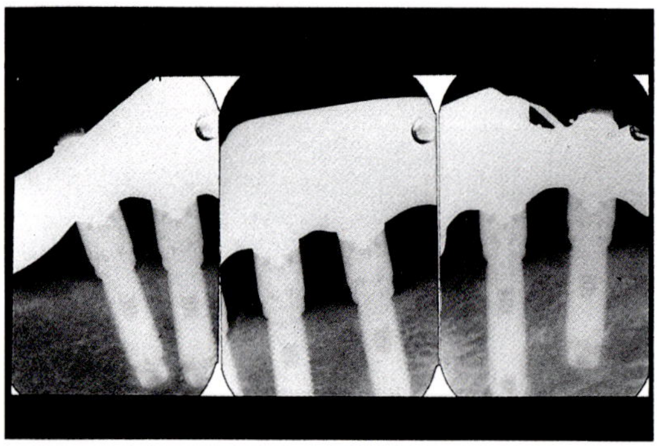

Fig. 247. Radiographs taken three years and two months after the stage II operation. The radiographs show a uniform crest of the marginal bone and also dense bone trabeculae.

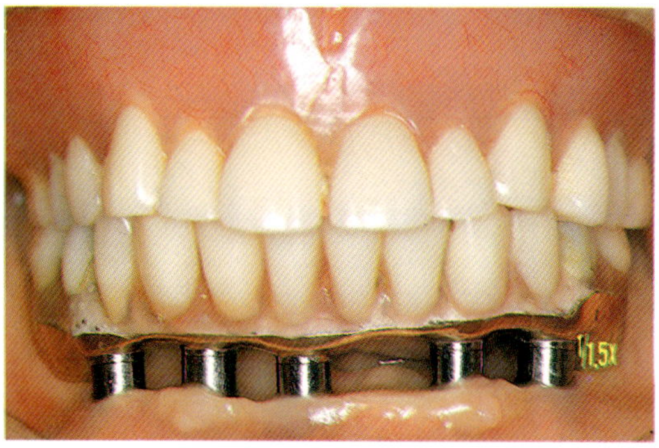

Fig. 248. A frontal view of the situation shown in Fig. 247. Recession of the marginal gingiva is visible as compared with the condition immediately after prosthesis application (cf. Fig. 244). The gingiva tends to sink for about one year after the stage II operation.

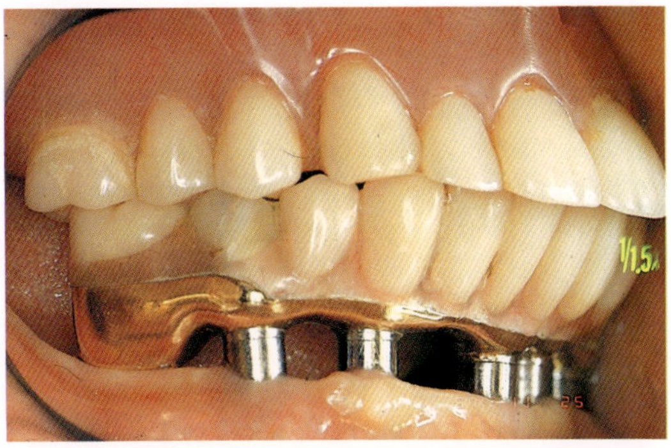

Fig. 249. Lateral view after three years, showing good plaque control.

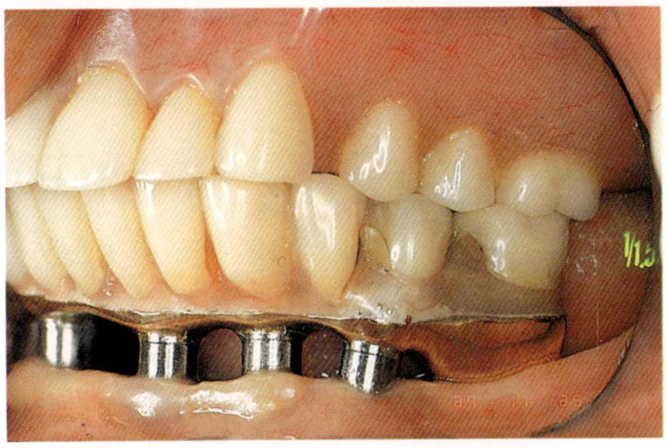

Fig. 250. Lateral view of the left side, showing healthy gingiva.

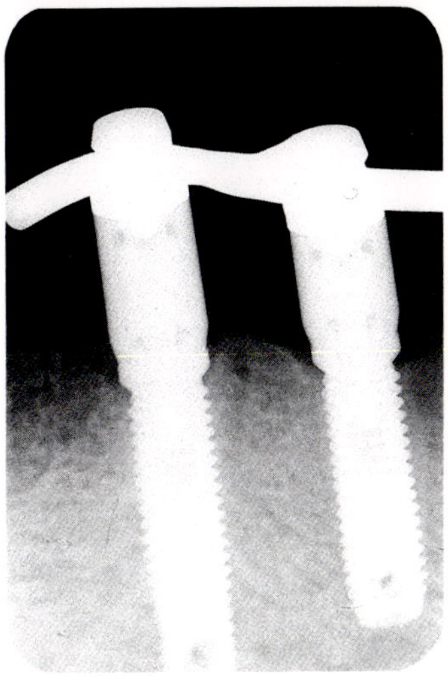

Fig. 251. Radiographs taken after prosthesis application, showing good contacts of the components and a well leveled marginal crest together with dense bone trabeculae.

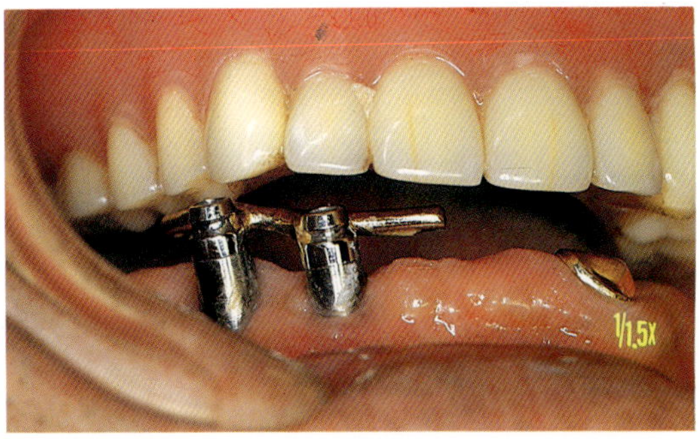

Fig. 252. Frontal view of a bar-construction for an overdenture (cf. Fig. 251). Plaque accumulation on the mesial side of one of the implants (in the region of the lower right second incisor) is visible. The Bass method was used for plaque control on the labial aspect. Brushing with an interdental brush has been used for the mesio-distal and lingual sides.

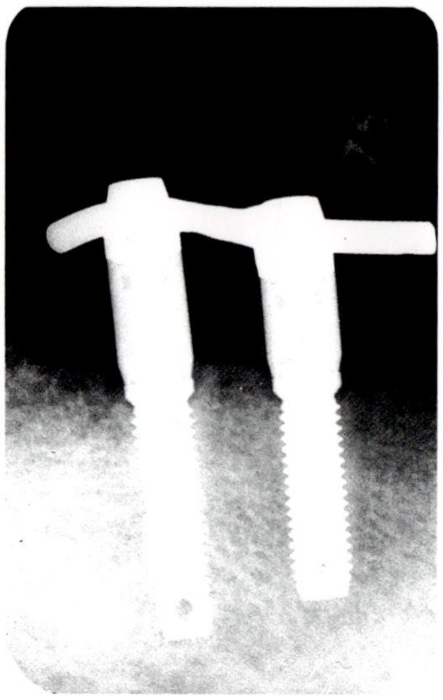

Fig. 253. The overdenture situation three years after the stage II operation. The radiograph shows good marginal bone conditions and dense bone trabeculae.

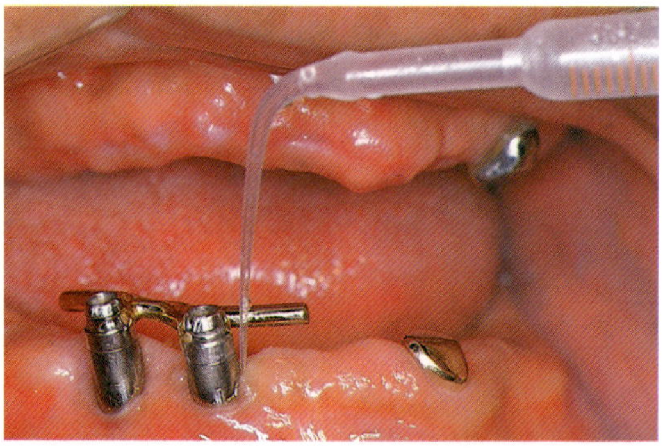

Fig. 254. Sometimes it is difficult to completely remove all of the plaque from the peri-implant sulcus. Antimicrobials like chlorhexidine solution can then be used to irrigate the sulcus.

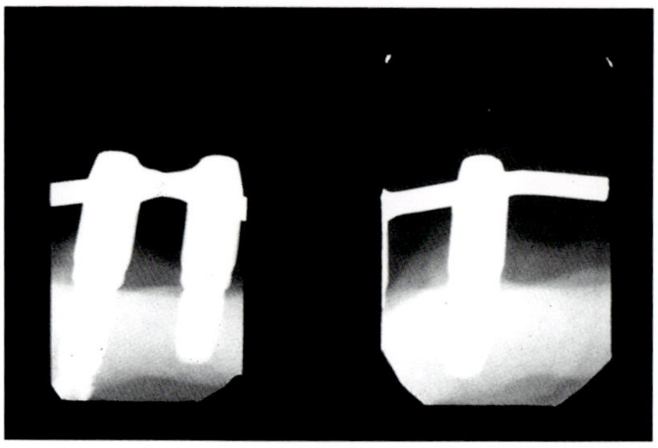

Fig. 255. Radiographs of a bar-construction taken after prosthesis application. The radiographs show that the most posterior fixture on the right side perforates the inferior border of the lower jaw.

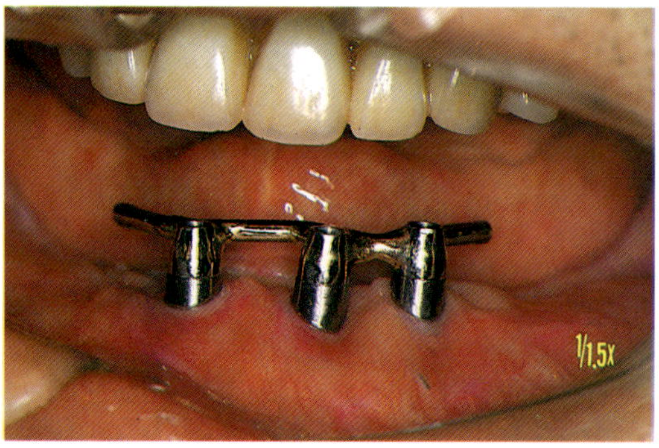

Fig. 256. The clinical situation of Fig. 255 in a frontal view. The Bass method has been used for plaque control on the labial side and interdental brush for the mesio-distal and lingual sides.

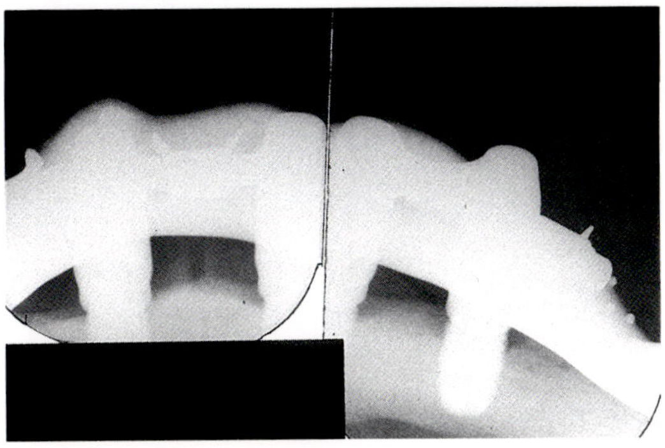

Fig. 257. Radiographs of the overdenture situation two years and six months after the stage II operation.

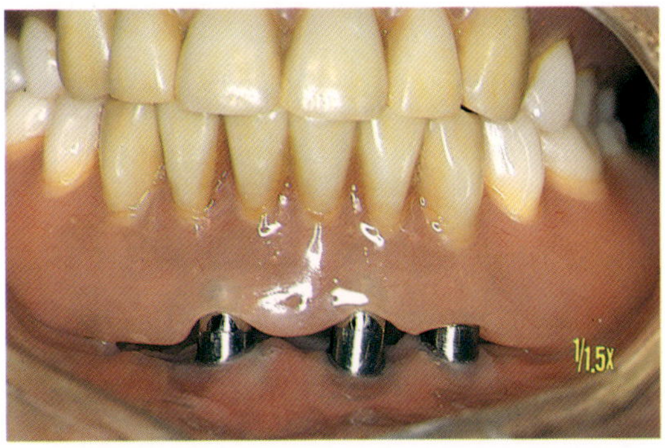

Fig. 258. Frontal view of the case presented in Fig. 256, showing healthy peri-implant tissues.

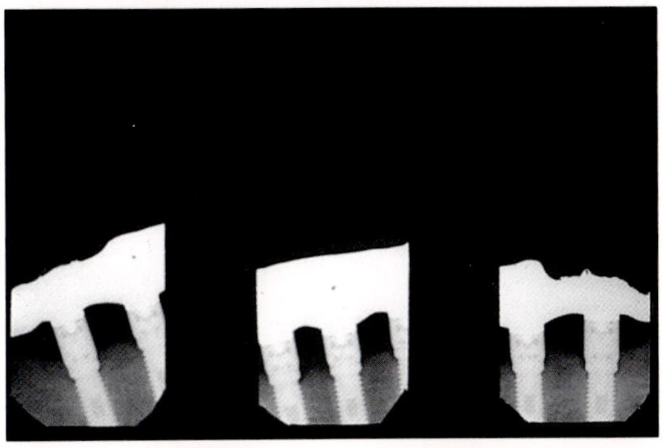

Fig. 259. Radiographs taken after bridge connection. The radiographs show good marginal bone levels and dense trabeculae around the implants.

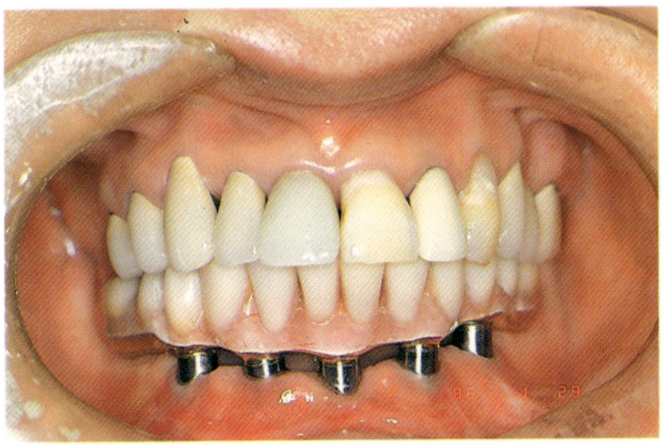

Fig. 260. Frontal view of the case presented in Fig. 259. Plaque has been controlled by the Bass method on the bucco-labial side, brushing with an interdental brush on the mesio-distal sides, and inter-space brush on the lingual side.

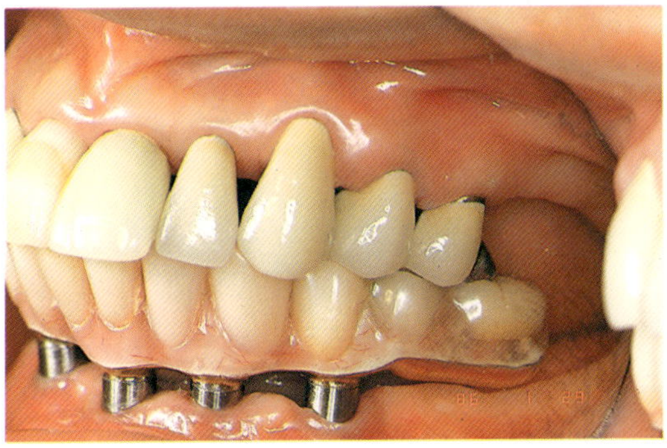

Fig. 261. From the lateral view it is obvious that the gingiva is healthy.

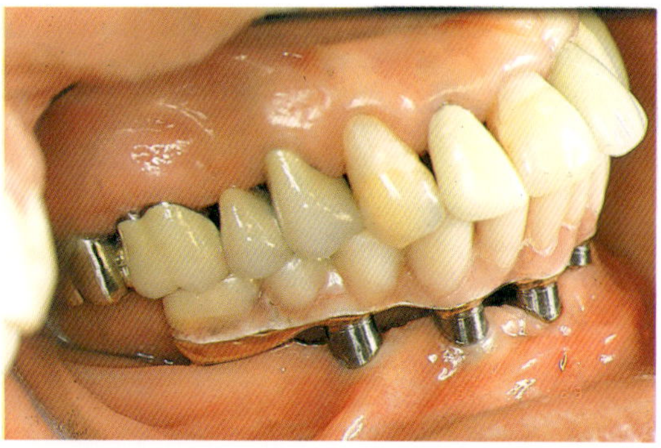

Fig. 262. Also the lateral view of the opposite side (cf. Fig. 261) shows a healthy gingiva. During probing, bleeding was not observed in any site.

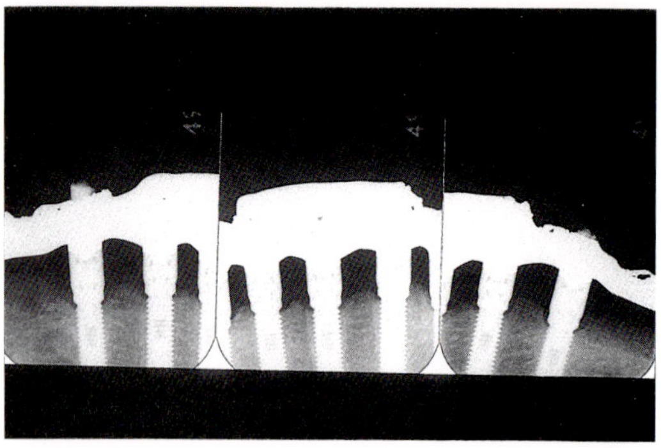

Fig. 263. Radiographs of the bridge three years and two months after the stage II operation, showing good marginal bone conditions around the implants.

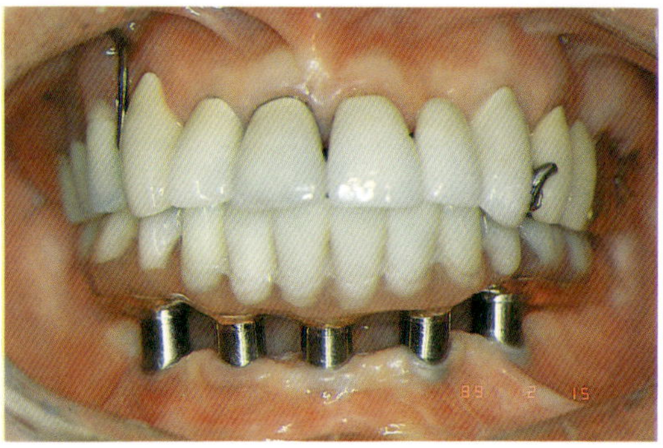

Fig. 264. The situation in Fig.263, showing slight recession of the gingiva.

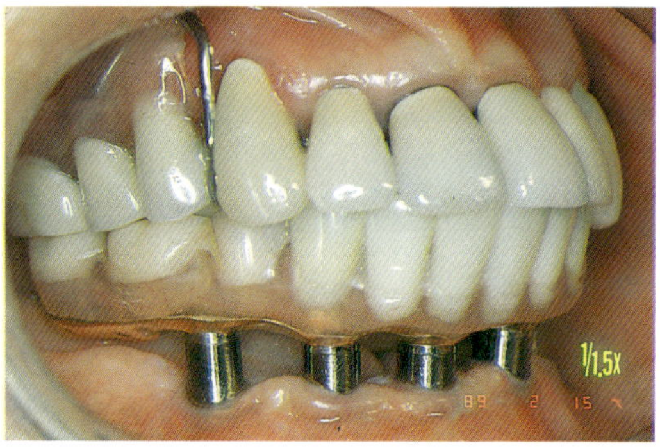

Fig. 265. Also in the lateral view, the gingiva looks healthy due to good plaque control.

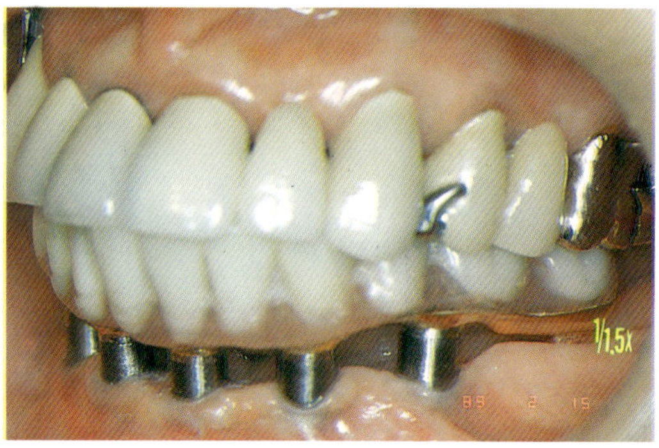

Fig. 266. The lateral view of the opposite side showing healthy gingiva too.

Complications Appearing at Follow-Up Controls

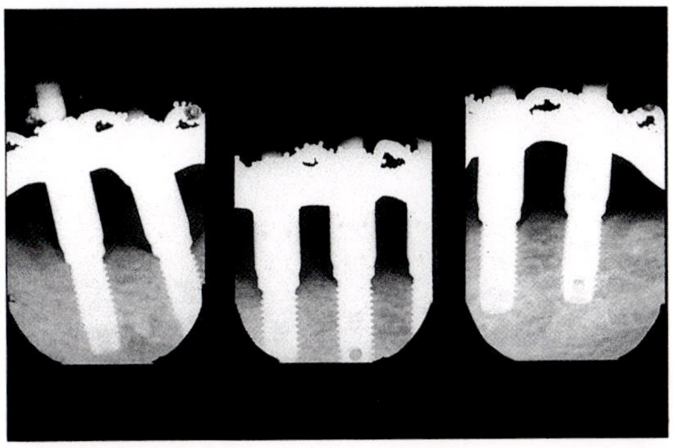

Fig. 267. Radiographs taken immediately after prosthesis application, showing well osseointegrated fixtures and good marginal bone conditions.

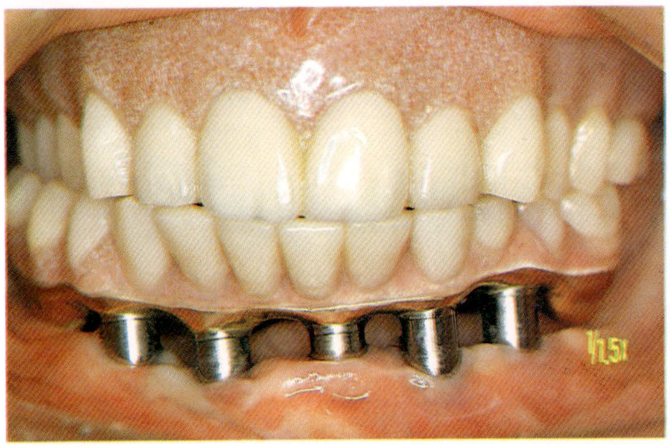

Fig. 268. One month after bridge connection, the gingiva is clinically healthy, but some plaque formation is noted in spite of plaque control.

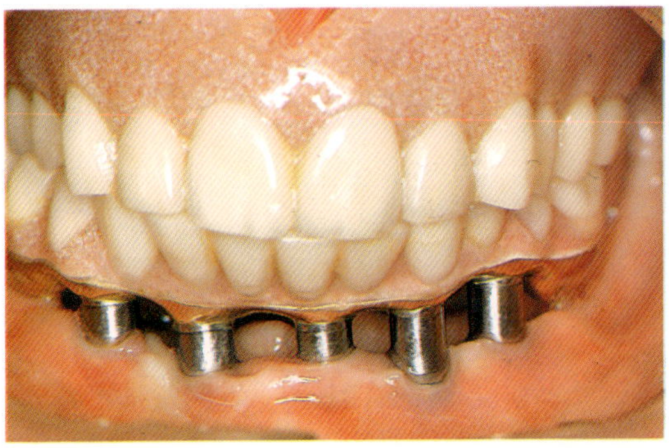

Fig. 269. Six months after bridge connection, showing mild gingivitis around some of the abutments.

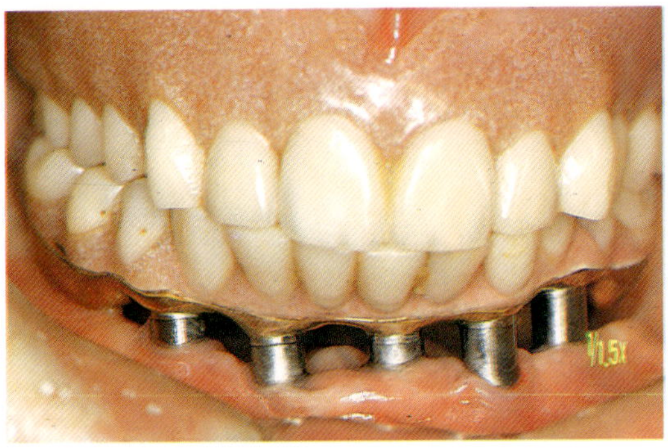

Fig. 270. Twelve months after bridge connection. Moderate to severe gingivitis and plaque formation can be observed at most abutments.

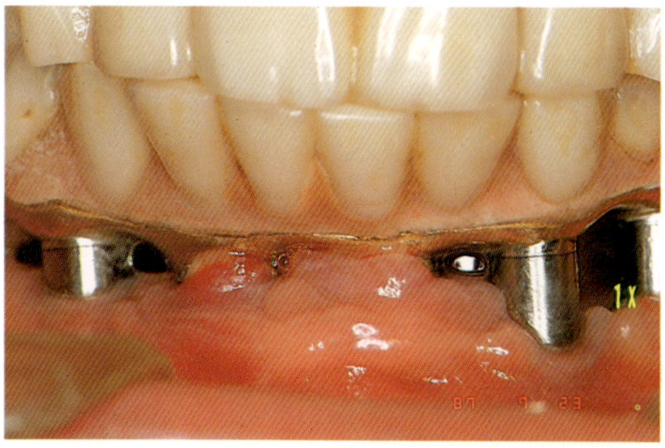

Fig. 271. One year and six months after prosthesis insertion, it is possible to see dark-red gingival hyperplasia formation around the abutments, making mechanical plaque control with a toothbrush impossible.

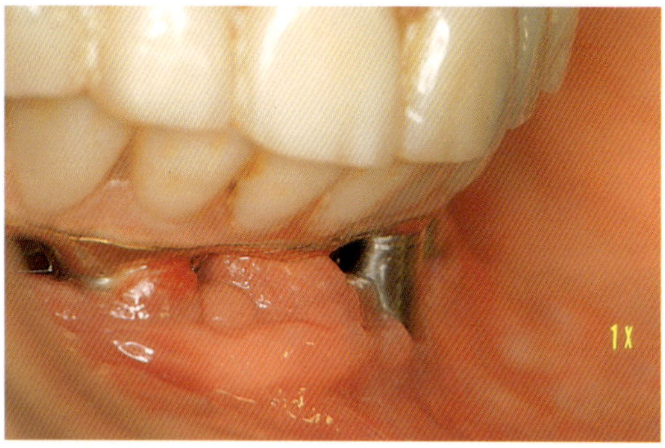

Fig. 272. A lateral view of the gingival proliferation shown in Fig. 271.

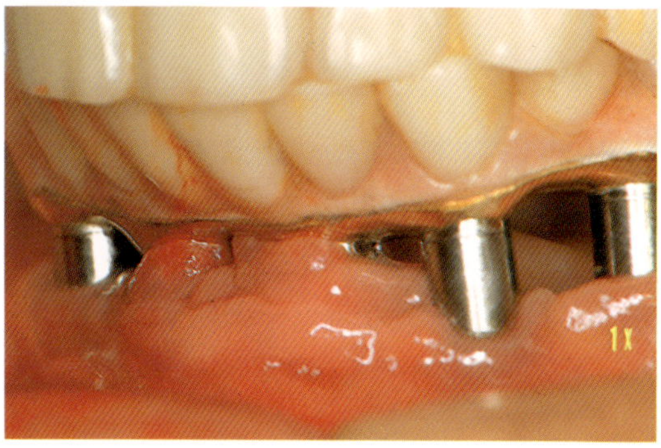

Fig. 273. Treatment of gingival proliferations starts with intensified plaque control combined with the use of an antimicrobial agent applied locally.

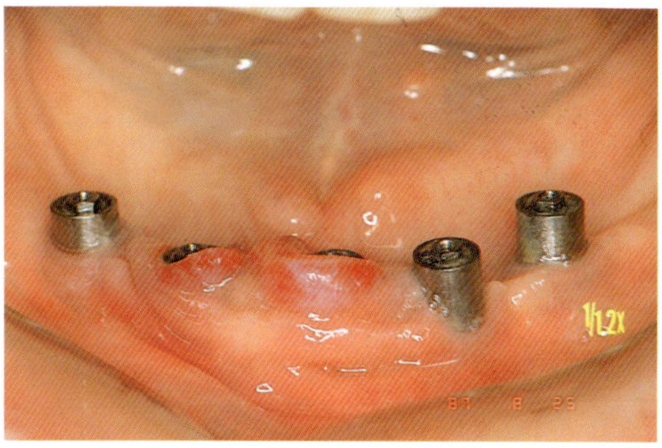

Fig. 274. Frontal view one month after starting the treatment of gingival proliferations. The condition is slightly improved due to the use of local antimicrobial drug therapy and gargling with 0.2% chlorhexidine (CH).

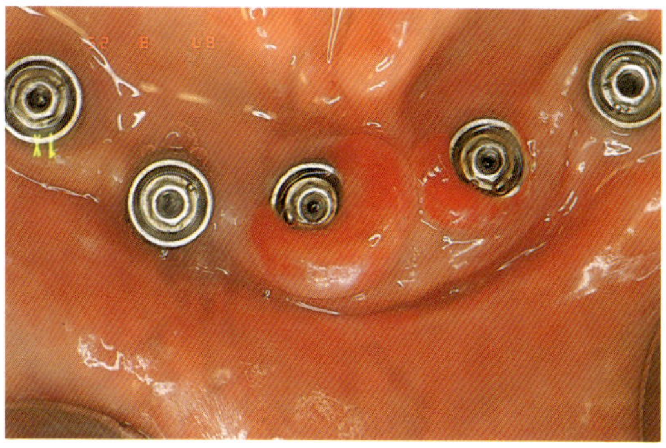

Fig. 275. Occlusal view of the situation shown in Fig. 274. Despite reinforced plaque control, the peri-implant sulcus remains deep, and hence, periodontal surgery is decided to be used.

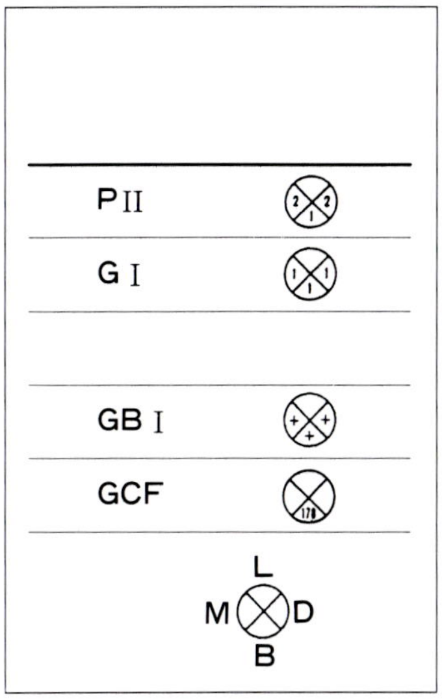

Table 2. Clinical registrations at the time of upon the detection of the gingival proliferations.

The results show a high gingival crevice fluid (GCF) and that the probing depth (PD) was too extensive to allow measurements.

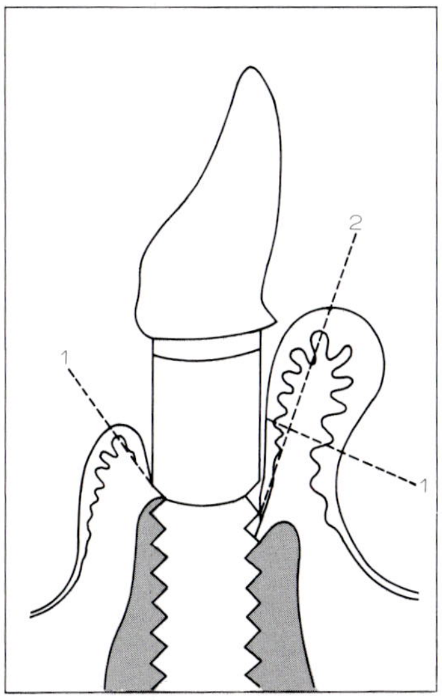

Fig. 276. Schematic presentation of surgical procedures to eliminate gingival proliferation.

1 : primary incision 2 : secondary incision

In this example, the inflamed tissue was removed due to the following reasons: (1) the mouth floor was not sufficiently deep, (2) inflammation had markedly reduced tissue resistance, and (3) the mucoperiosteal flap was expected to become mobile.

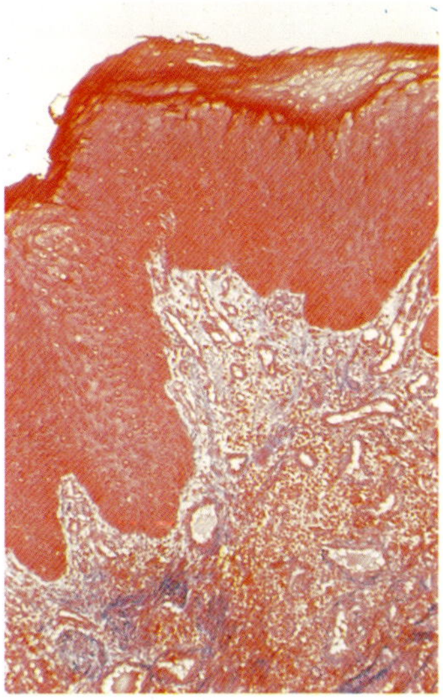

Fig. 277. Histopathological picture of the proliferative gingiva, removed from the case presented Fig. 271. The outmost layer of the gingival epithelium shows parakeratosis, and gingival epithelial cell layer is thick. Irregular epithelial proliferations are visible toward the area of intense infiltration of inflammatory cells (chiefly polymorphonuclear leukocytes).

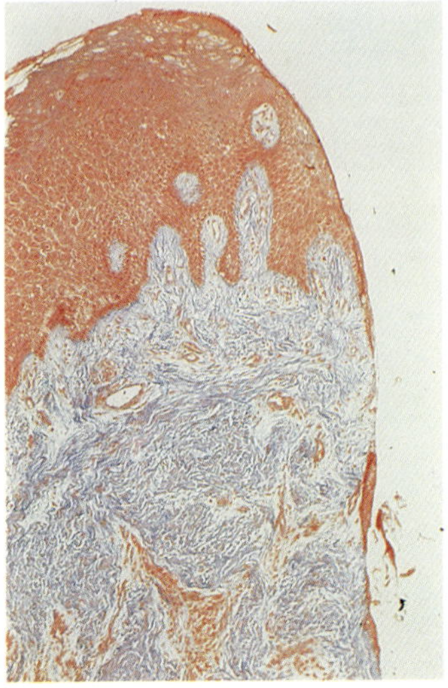

Fig. 278. Histopathological picture of the peri-implant gingiva. The gingival margin at the inner edge, which seems to constitute a part of the peri-implant sulcus, shows parakeratosis and is composed of thick cell layers. The gingiva facing the abutment is thinner (composed of only 1-2 layers) and continues to the lower region. The sub epithelial connective tissue is relatively dense.

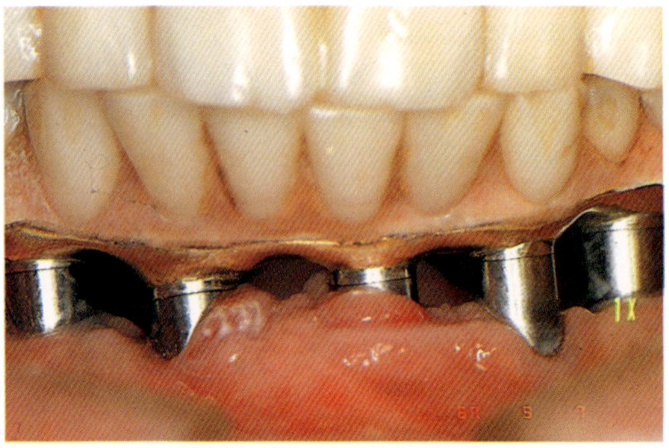

Fig. 279. One month after periodontic surgery the proliferations occurred again, probably because plaque had not been completely removed at the surgical intervention.

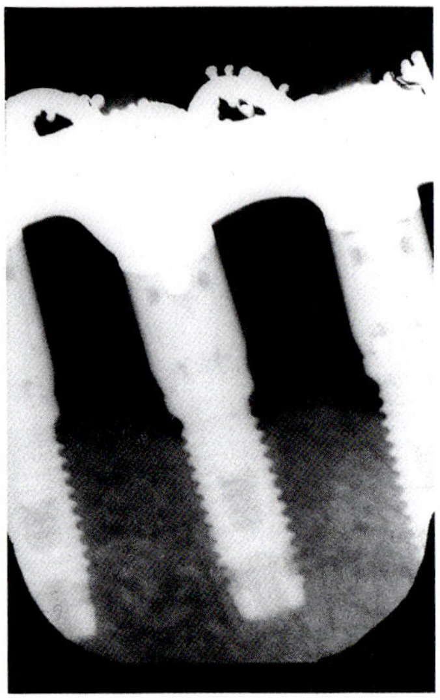

Fig. 280. A radiograph from the time of hyperplasia detection. The density of the bone trabecula is low on the distal side of the central fixture.

P. gingivalis	−
P. intermedia	−
B. melaninogenicus	−
E. corrodens	−
F. nucleatum	−
Capnocytophaga sp.	+
A. actinomycetemcomitans	++

− : 0/4.5m*l*
\+ : $0 < \times < 10^3$/4.5m*l*
++ : $10^3 \leq \times < 10^4$/4.5m*l*

Table 3. Results of the bacteriological test performed at the time when the proliferations, reoccurred *A. actinomycetemcomitans* is predominant. Based on oral condition, radiographic findings and the bacteriological test, the prognosis of this case was rated as dubious.

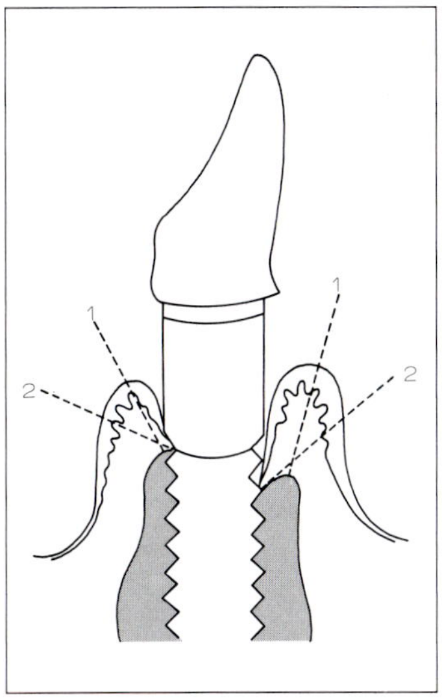

Fig. 281. Schematic flap procedure for resection of gingival hyperplasia.

1 : primary incision 2 : secondary incision

The mucoperiosteal flap is reflected, and the plaque on the fixture and abutment is completely removed with a plastic scaler.

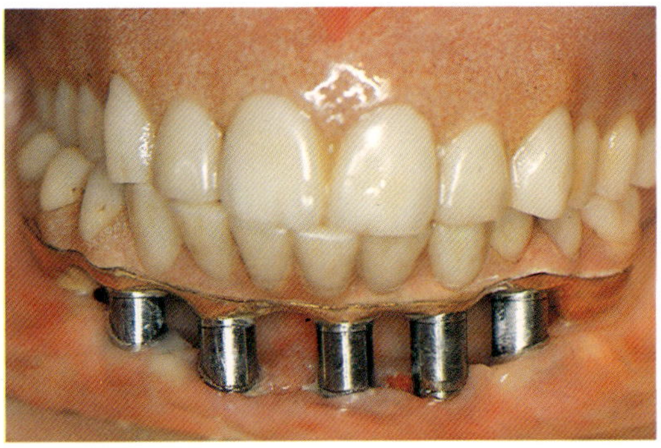

Fig. 282. The clinical situation in Fig. 279, two weeks after the gingival operation.

The height of marginal gingiva has been radically reduced.

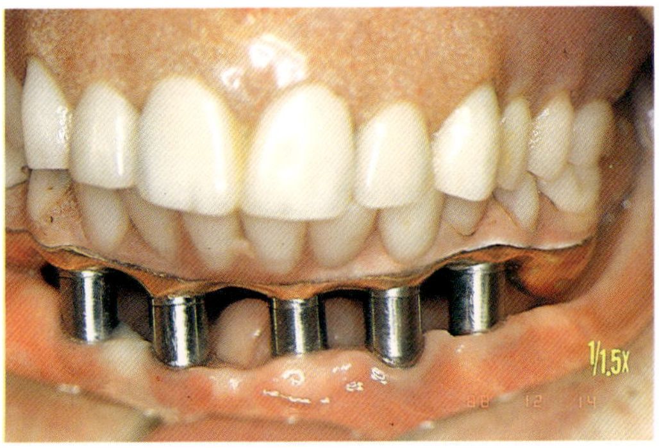

Fig. 283. The situation from Fig. 279, one year after the gingivectomy.

Hyperplasia is no longer evident, mainly due to that mechanical plaque control is combined with irrigation of the peri-implant sulcus with an antimicrobial (CH).

	M	L	D	B
PII	0		0	0
GI	1		1	1
PD	3		3	3
GBI	+		−	−
GCF				17

L / M ⊗ D / B

Table 4. Clinical date after the second operation, showing that the gingival health condition has been improved.

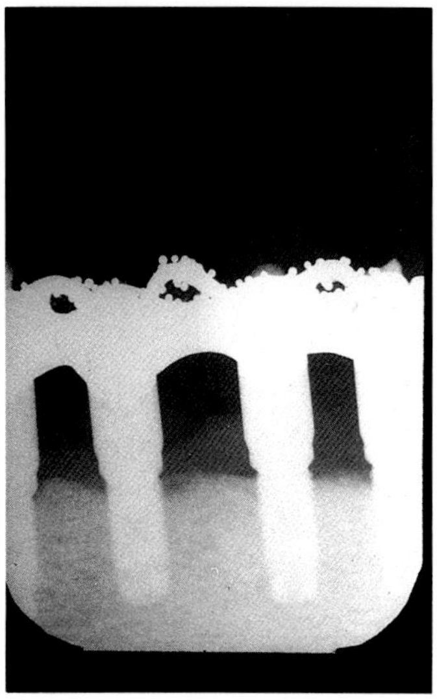

Fig. 284. Radiograph taken after the reoperation, and showing no changes compared with the preoperative film (cf. Fig. 280).

P. gingivalis	−
P. intermedia	−
B. melaninogenicus	−
E. corrodens	−
F. nucleatum	−
Capnocytophaga sp.	−
A. actinomycetemcomitans	++

− : 0/4.5m*l*
\+ : $0 < \times < 10^3$/4.5m*l*
++ : $10^3 \leqq \times < 10^4$/4.5m*l*

Table 5. Results of the bacteriological test performed after the second operation.

Capnocytophaga sp. was not observed ; *A. actinomycetemcomitans* could still be detected though.

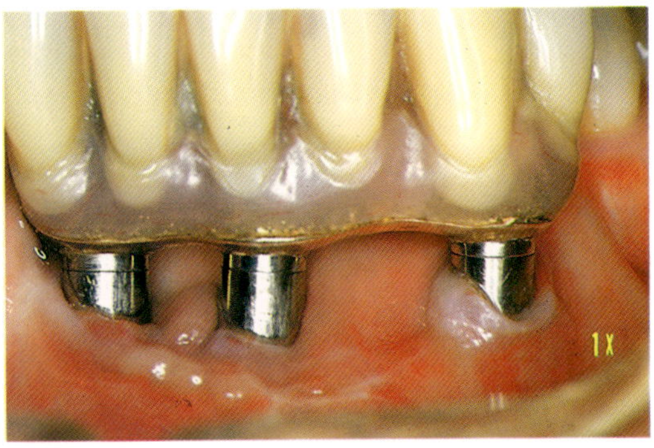

Fig. 285. Clinical situation of a bridge, one year after prosthesis application. Observe the gingival inflammations around the three abutments, which occurred in-spite of the patient maintaining good plaque control.

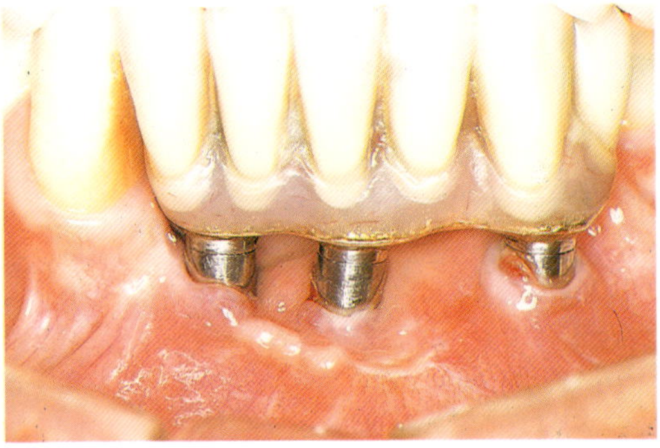

Fig. 286. The gingival condition may be due to the use of long abutments (10 mm or longer), selected because of the thick gingiva, and maybe facilitating the growth of Gram-negative anaerobes. Loosening of the fixture-abutment junction may also be a factor related with the induction of inflammation, because the soft tissue can be infected by microbials living in the component junction.

	M	D	B
P II	0	0	0
G I	1	1	1
PD	10	9	9
GB I	+	+	+
GCF			104

Key: L (top), M (left), D (right), B (bottom) of circle

Table 6. Clinical findings upon detection of gingivitis in the case presented in Fig. 285.

Both the values for PD and GCF are high. The inflammation of the peri-implant sulcus was not decreased by reinforced plaque control.

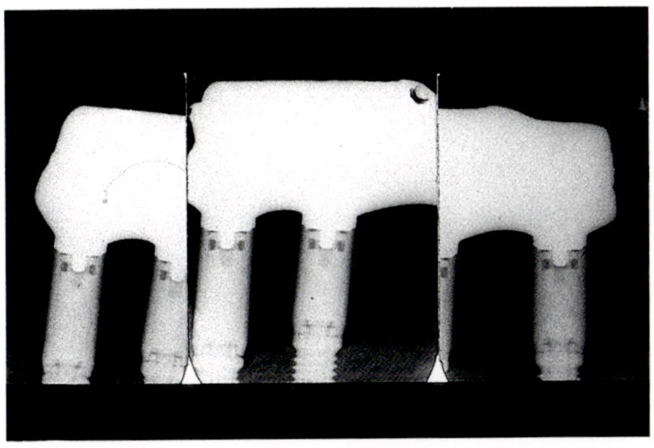

Fig. 287. Radiographs obtained one year after prosthesis application. The density of the bone trabecula around the left fixtures is low and marginal bone loss has occurred.

P. gingivalis	−
P. intermedia	++
B. melaninogenicus	−
E. corrodens	−
F. nucleatum	−
Capnocytophaga sp.	−
A. actinomycetemcomitans	−

− : $0/4.5ml$
+ : $0 < \times < 10^3/4.5ml$
++ : $10^3 \leqq \times < 10^4/4.5ml$

Table 7. Results of the bacteriological test performed at the detection of the gingivitis. *Prevotella intermedia* was found to be strongly positive.

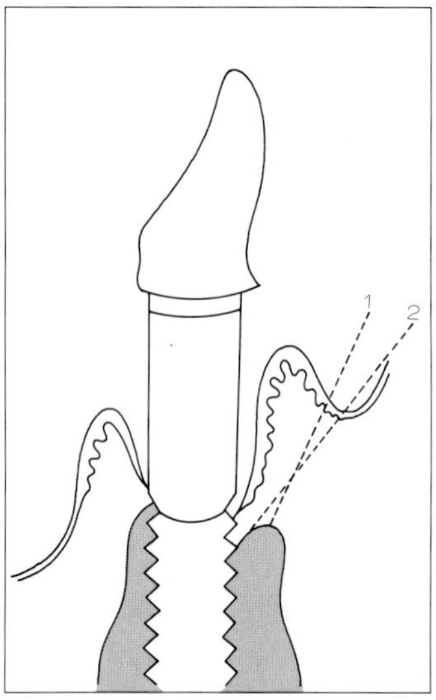

Fig. 288. Schematic representation of the gingival operation.

1 : primary incision 2 : secondary incision

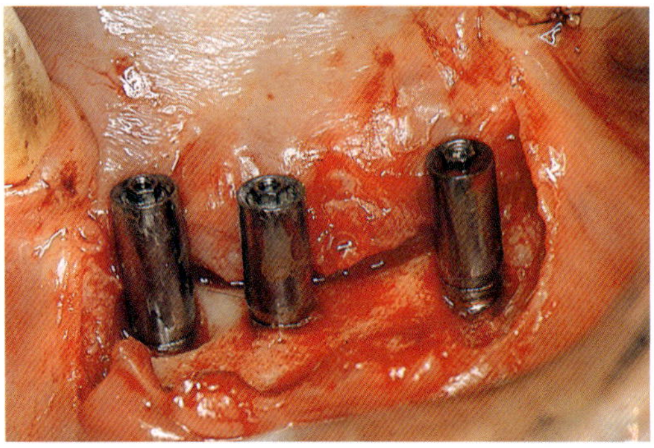

Fig. 289. The mucoperiosteal flaps have been lifted and the crestal bone has been exposed.

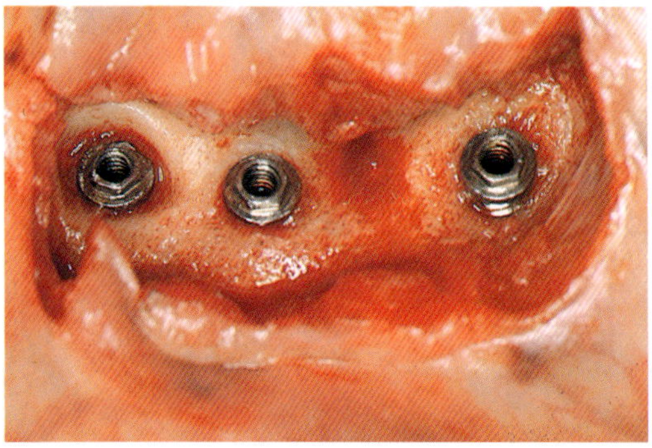

Fig. 290. Because of bone resorption around the implant in the area of the lower left canine, the fixture is slightly exposed on its buccal aspect. Plaque has been completely removed from the exposed fixtures.

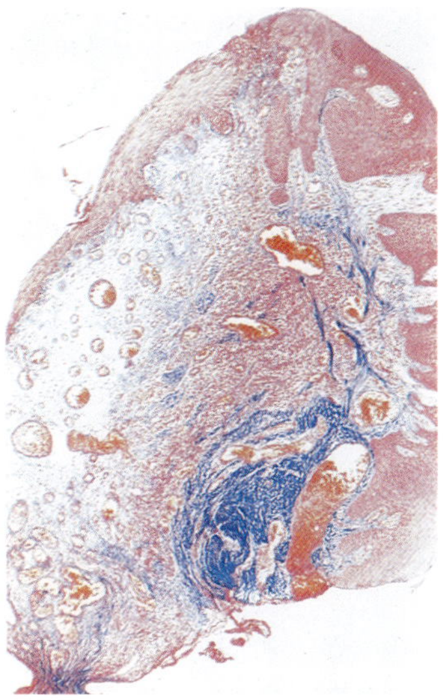

Fig. 291. Histopathological picture of the peri-implant gingiva, removed from the case presented in Fig. 285. The gingival connective tissue immediately below the epithelium is loose, but the infiltration of inflammatory cells is mild. In deeper the connective tissue, part of the infiltration of inflammatory cells (chiefly polymorphonuclear cells) is more pronounced.

	M	B	D	L
PII	0	0	0	
GI	1	1	1	
PD	8	7	6	
GBI	+	−	−	
GCF		85		

(L: top, M: left, D: right, B: bottom of circle)

Table 8. Clinical data two months after operation. The value of PD, gingival bleeding index (GBI), and GCF have improved compared with before treatment.

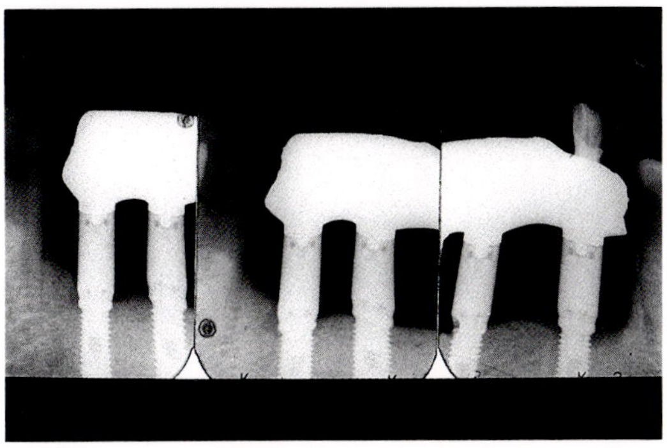

Fig. 292. Radiographs from two months after the gingival operation, showing no change in marginal bone height as compared with the preoperative situation (cf. Fig. 287).

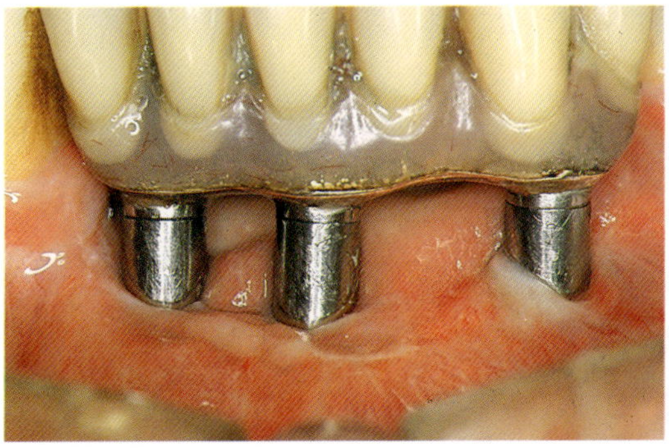

Fig. 293. Clinical condition five months after operation. The gingival health condition has improved. However, plaque control in the region below the gingival margin is essential, because the gingival width is large and the periimplant sulcus depth still remains deep.

P. gingivalis	−
P. intermedia	−
B. melaninogenicus	−
E. corrodens	−
F. nucleatum	−
Capnocytophaga sp.	−
A. actinomycetemcomitans	−

$-$: 0/4.5ml
$+ 0 < \times < 10^3$/4.5ml
$++$: $10^3 \leqq \times < 10^4$/4.5ml

Table 9. Results of the postoperative bacteriological test, showing that *Prevotella intermedia* no longer was detected.

II. TRAINING THE DENTIST

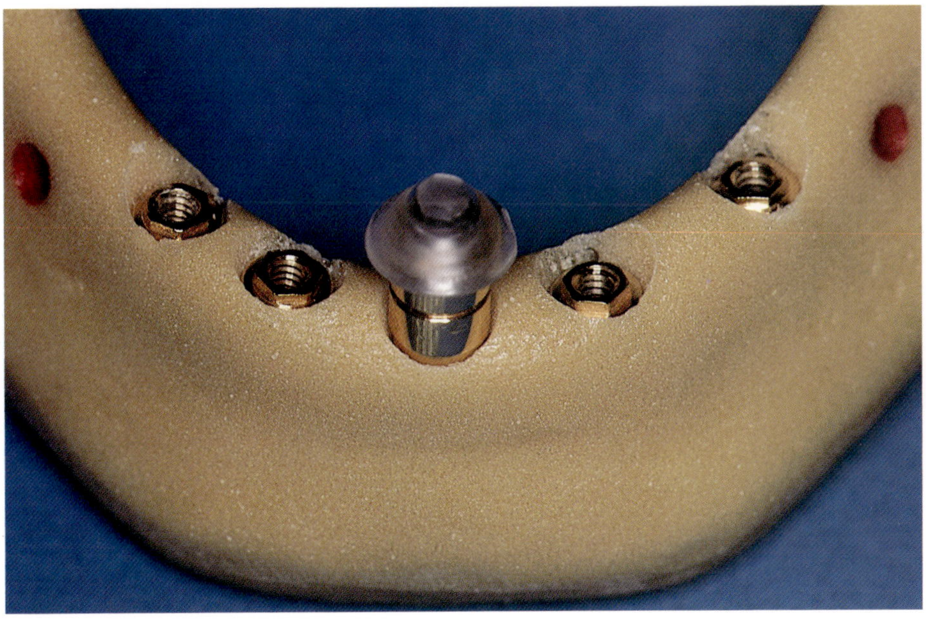

CHAPTER VI

TRAINING IN BASIC SURGICAL PROCEDURES

The Significance of Training and Instrumentation

(1) The significance of training

The Brånemark implant system involves two stages of surgery. Detailed guidelines have been formulated for the materials and instruments to be used at each stage and the order in which they are used. Complete compliance with the guidelines is essential to avoid faulty implant surgery.

To help inexperienced dentists master the procedures for Stage I and Stage II Operations, and to learn how to use the instruments and materials, each step of the operation will be described in detail, while demonstrating the procedure with a polyurethane model of an edentulous mandible. Additional instructions for clinical cases are marked with an asterisk (*) in the text.

(2) General considerations

1. Two trainees, wearing surgical gown and gloves, are to be trained at a time.
2. Five fixtures (3.75 mm in diameter and 10 mm in length) are inserted into 5 different sites between the right and left mental foramens of a polyurethane model of the edentulous mandible. One of the fixtures is provided with an abutment (5.5 mm in length) and a healing cap.
3. While one trainee performs these steps, the other assists in the operation (applying water during drilling, manipulating the control unit, giving necessary advice, etc.).
4. It is very important not to mix or contaminate titanium instruments with stainless steel instruments.

(3) Tools and instruments used for training

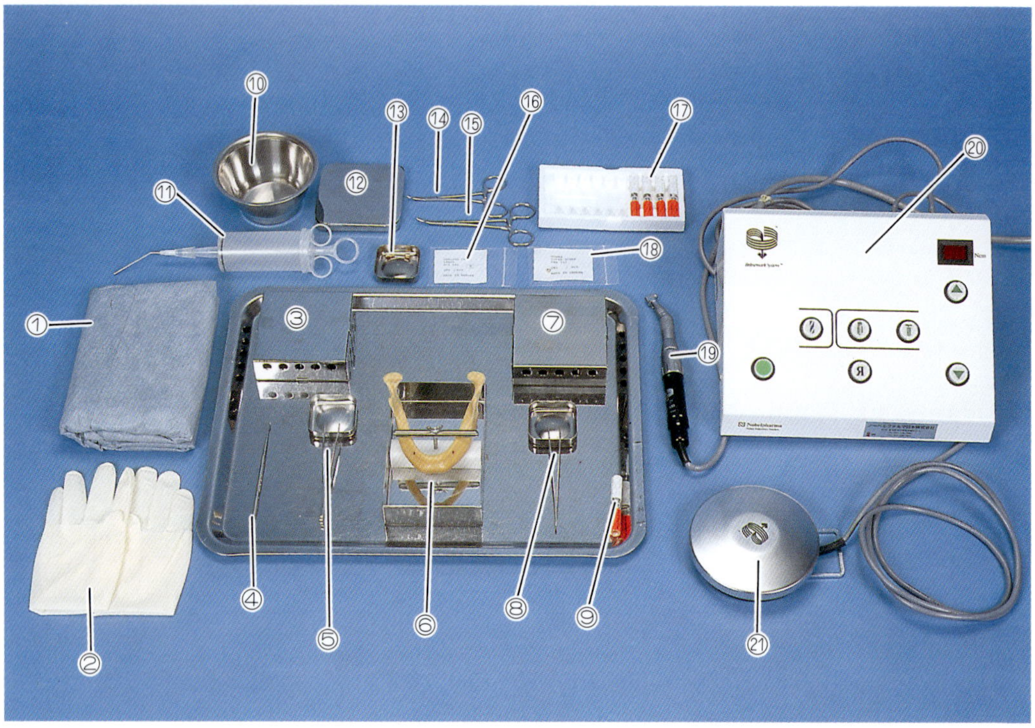

Fig. 294.

① Surgical gown

② Gloves

③ Drill set (stainless steel)

④ Dissector

⑤ Stainless steel bowl and tweezers

⑥ Polyurethane edentulous jaw model + fixed stand

⑦ Fixture insertion set (made of titanium)

⑧ Titanium bowl and tweezers

⑨ A fixture-containing ampoules

⑩ Bowl for receiving applied water

⑪ Syringe for water application

⑫ Abutment set (stainless steel)

⑬ Titanium bowl + abutment (one piece, 5.5 mm long)

⑭ Small abutment clamp

⑮ Large abutment clamp

⑯ Healing cap (1)

⑰ Fixture-containing ampoules (4)

⑱ Cover screw (1)

⑲ Motor + shank + head

⑳ Control unit

㉑ Foot control

(4) **Control unit, foot control, and motor + shank + head**

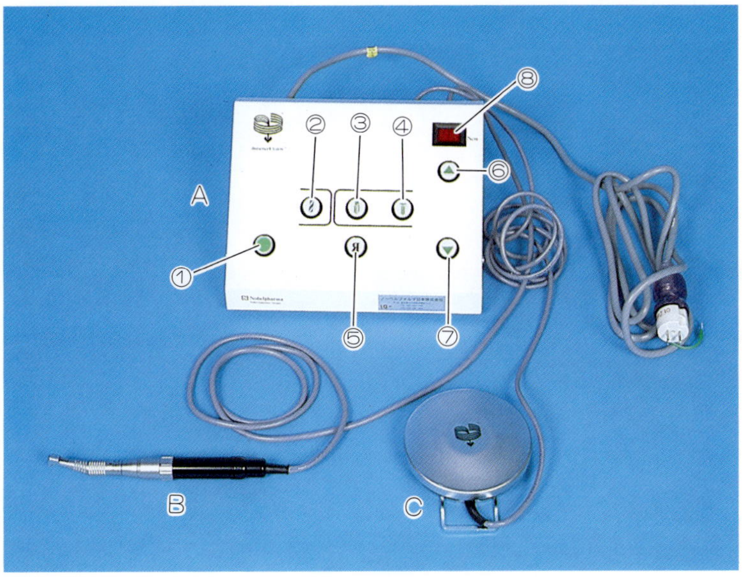

Fig. 295.

A. Control unit

① Control lamp: Goes on when main power button (on back) is switched on.

② Drilling indicator lamp: Goes on when the black point on gear motor is aligned with the blue point on the motor. High speed (0-2000 rpm).

③ Tapping indicator lamp: Goes on when the black point on gear motor is aligned with the green point. Low speed (0-28 rpm). Maximum torque set at 20, 30, 40 or 45 Ncm; when working on the model, use 30 Ncm.

④ Screwdriver insertion button and indicator lamp: This button is pushed keeping the black point on motor gear aligned with the green point. Low speed (0-50 rpm). Maximum torque 15 or 20 Ncm. Function is used for applying and removing cover screws and also for fastening abutment with a machine screwdriver.

⑤ Reverse button and indicator lamp: Reversed function is used in high-speed range (0-200 rpm) and low-speed range (0-50 rpm); Maximum torque, 50 Ncm. Buzzer sounds during use (sound level can be changed with switch on back), its frequency doubles, when the drills are rotating.

⑥ Torque increasing button: Torque can be increased from 20-45 Ncm.

⑦ Torque decreasing button: Torque is decreased the reversed way.

⑧ Display: Maximum torque displayed when motor is set to the low speed range.

B. Foot control

Speed is increased by pressing the pedal. Maximum speed is reached, when the pedal is pressed all the way.

C. Motor + shank + head

Speed is set to the high range (0-2000 rpm), when the black point on the gear is aligned with the blue point on the motor. It is set to the low range (0-50 rpm), when the black point is aligned with the green point.

(5) Drilling, fixture insertion and abutment sets

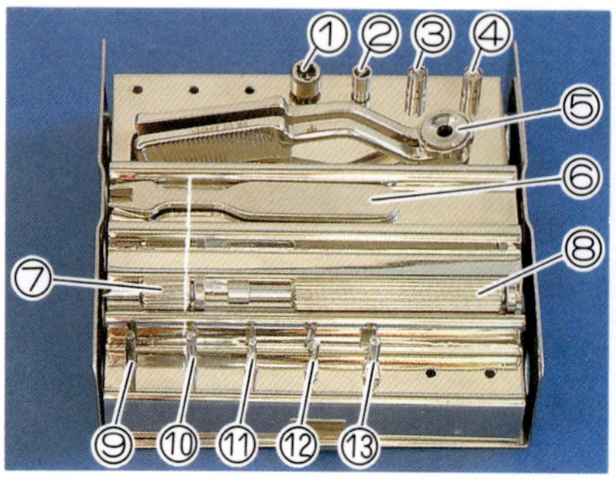

Fig. 296.
Drilling set (stainless steel).

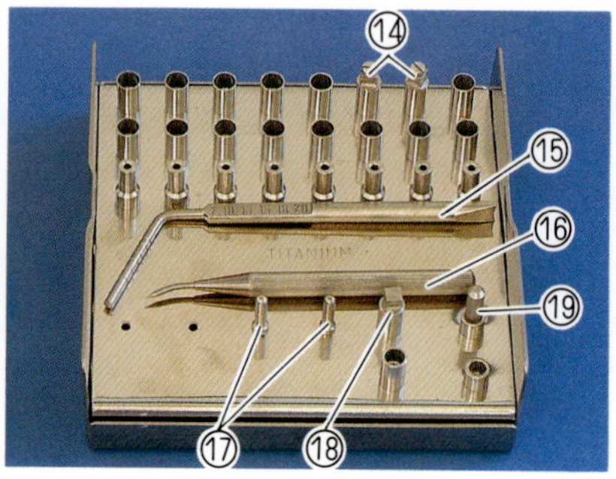

Fig. 297.
Fixture insertion set (titanium).

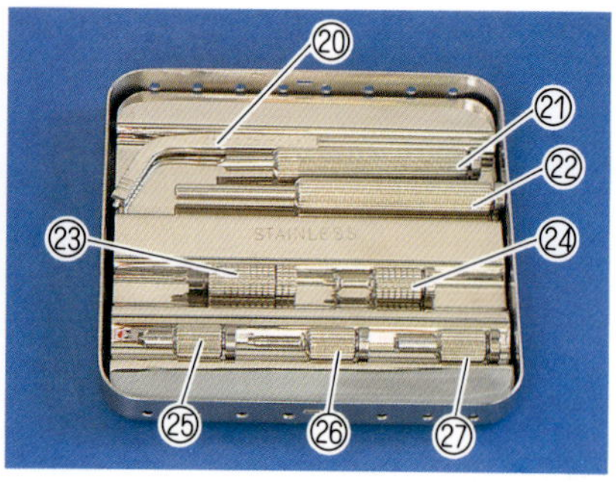

Fig. 298.
Abutment set (stainless steel).

① Connection to contra-angle handpiece
② Machine driver
③ Cover screw inserter (for regular use)
④ Cover screw inserter (for hexagonal cover screw)
⑤ Cylinder wrench
⑥ Open-end wrench
⑦ Short screwdriver
⑧ Long screwdriver
⑨ Guide drill
⑩ Twist drill (2mm in diameter)
⑪ Pilot drill
⑫ Twist drill (3 mm in diameter)
⑬ Countersink
⑭ Fixture mount
⑮ Depth gauge
⑯ Cleaning needle
⑰ Direction indicator
⑱ Tap
⑲ Direction indicator for fixture
⑳ Abutment gauge
㉑ Long screwdriver
㉒ Long hexagonal screwdriver
㉓ Punch
㉔ Cover screw mill
㉕ Short screwdriver
㉖ Short hexagonal screwdriver for cover screws
㉗ Short hexagonal screwdriver

Stage I Operation

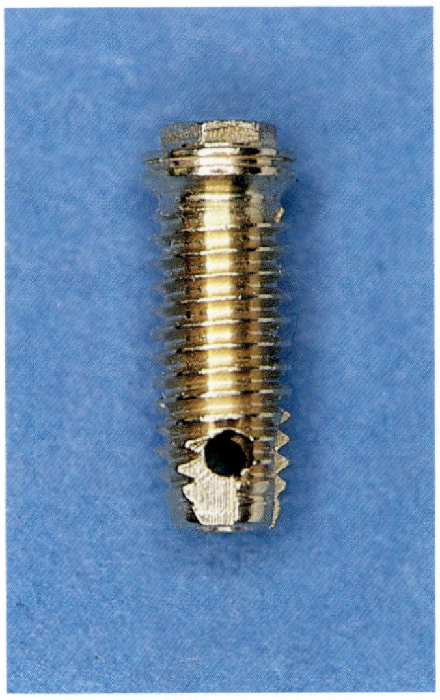

Fig. 299. Fixture: 10 mm long and 3.75 mm in diameter. The diameter of the fixture decreases towards the tip so that a screw thread can be created. The fixture has a hole in the apical portion to make place for bone shavings and to allow bone tissue ingrowth, which reinforces the fixture's stability.

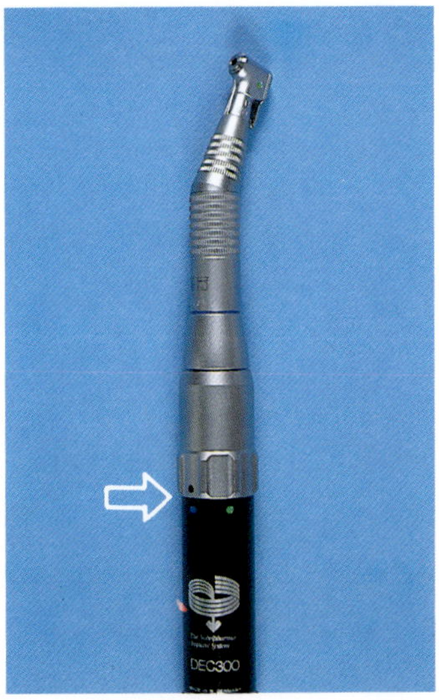

Fig. 300. The main power switch, on the back of the control unit, is turned on and the green light in the left corner of the control panel should light up. The black point on the motor unit is aligned with the blue point (*arrow*), and the light on the control unit should light up. High speed level is used in this and subsequent steps.

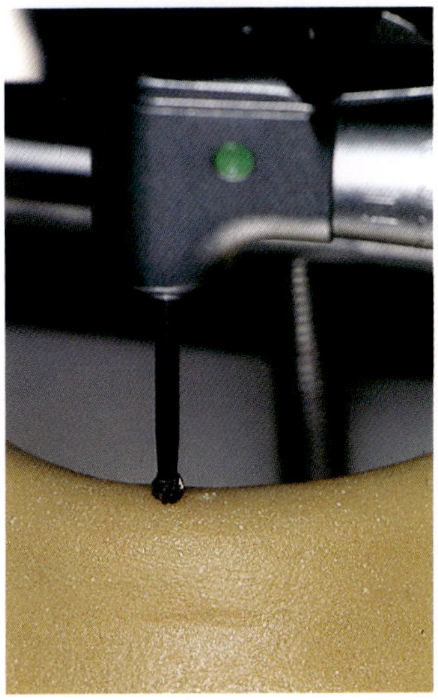

Fig. 301. The starting point for fixture insertion is marked in the midline region of a model of the edentulous mandible with a guide drill.

Remark: If insertion of 5 fixtures is planned, the median insertion point should be marked first and the two most distal sites thereafter.

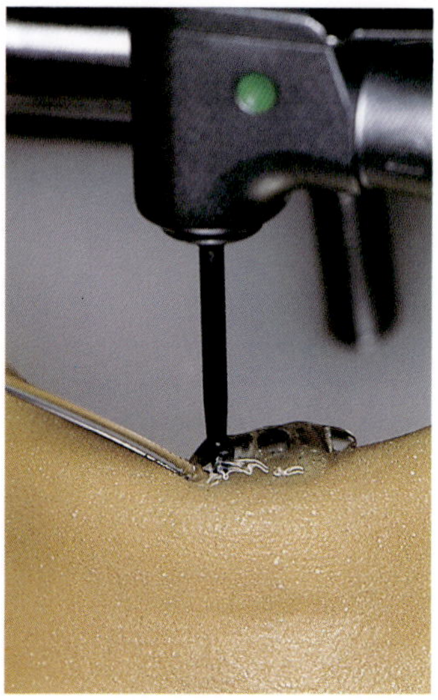

Fig. 302. The drill is moved up and down while profuse irrigation is supplied.

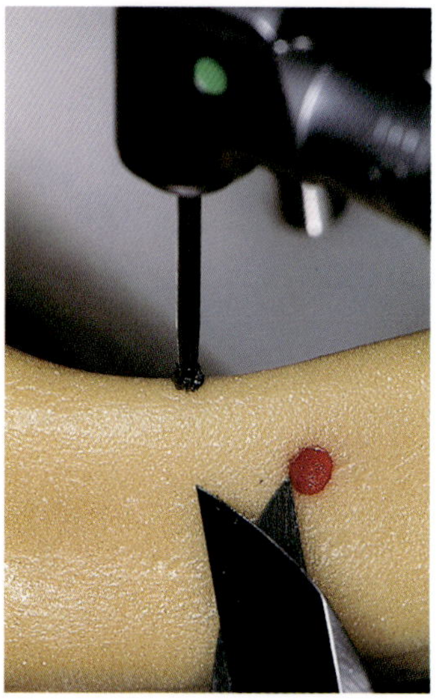

Fig. 303. After marking the midline site, the most distal insertion point is marked approximately 5 mm anterior to the mental foramen (*red*).

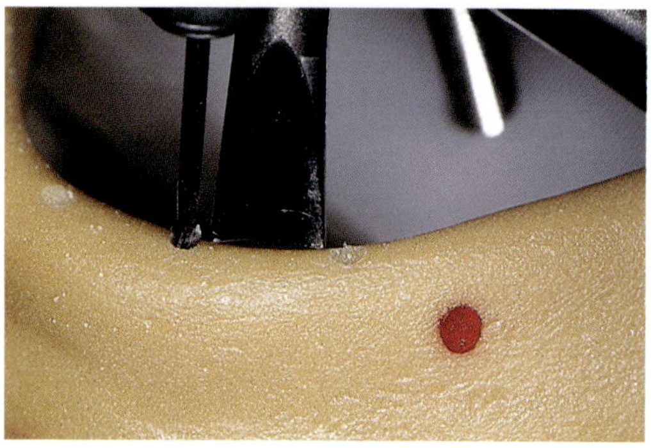

Fig. 304. Mark a third site between the median point and the most distal one, maintaining a distance of at least 7 mm between center to center of the sites. To check the distances the opposite end of the depth gauge is used.

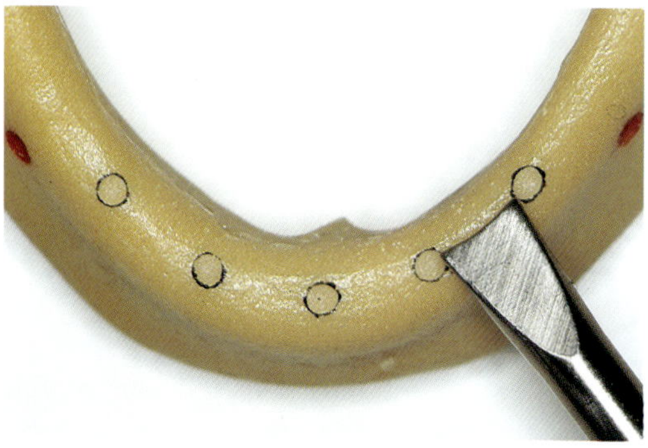

Fig. 305. Also, the most distal site in the right side is marked, thereafter the last site is located between this and the median point. In this way, all 5 fixture insertion points have been marked.

Remark: Take care to place the insertion points along the alveolar crest.

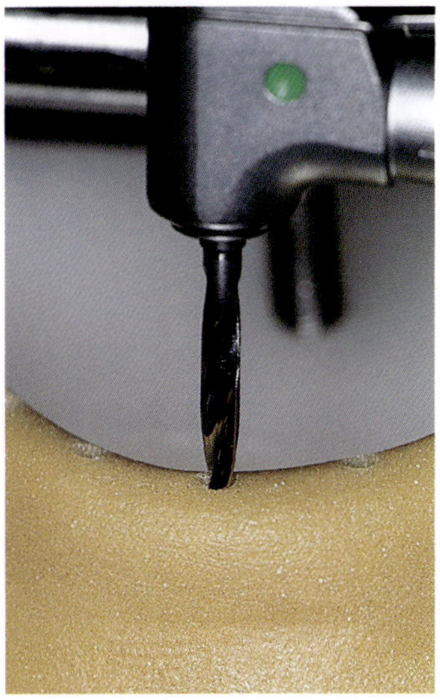

Fig. 306. With a 2 mm diameter twist drill, the midline site is prepared taking care not to break through the cortical plate on the buccolingual surfaces.

Remark: If the drill stops during the preparation, the reverse button (Я) should be pressed to unscrew the drill (a warning sound is heard, when the button is pushed).

* In clinical cases, the direction of natural teeth or artificial teeth in the opposite jaw must be considered when determining the implant directions.

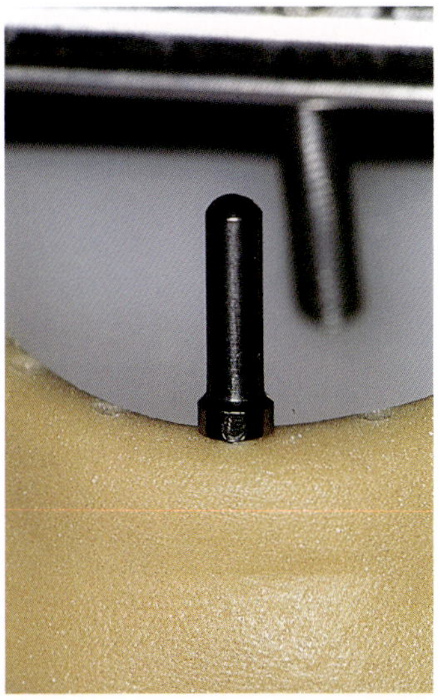

Fig. 307. Upon completion of the preparation in the median region, the direction of the site must be checked, using the narrow end of a direction indicator.

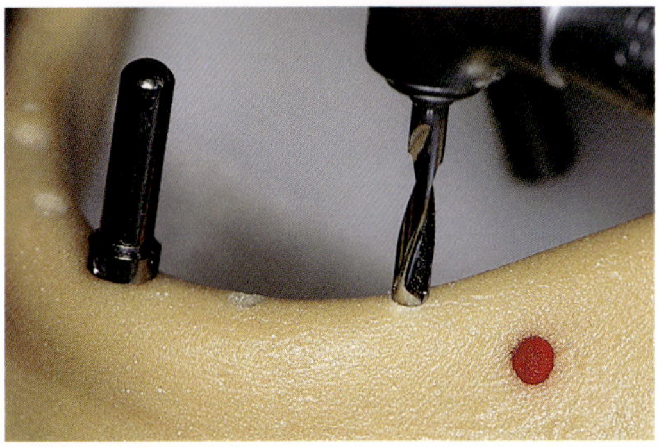

Fig. 308. After the direction indicator has been inserted into the midline region, the most distal site on the left side is prepared with the 2.0 mm diameter twist drill.

Remark: Be careful to follow the direction of the first direction indicator.

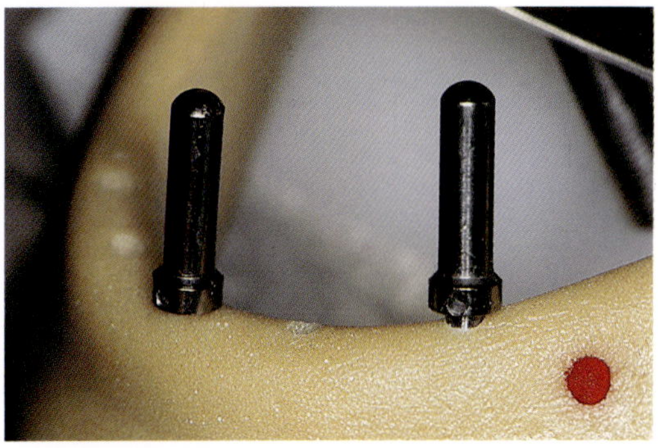

Fig. 309. Parallelism is checked by inserting a second direction indicator into the distal site. The canal must be corrected if not parallel. Finally, the remaining sites are prepared from the midline to the right side.

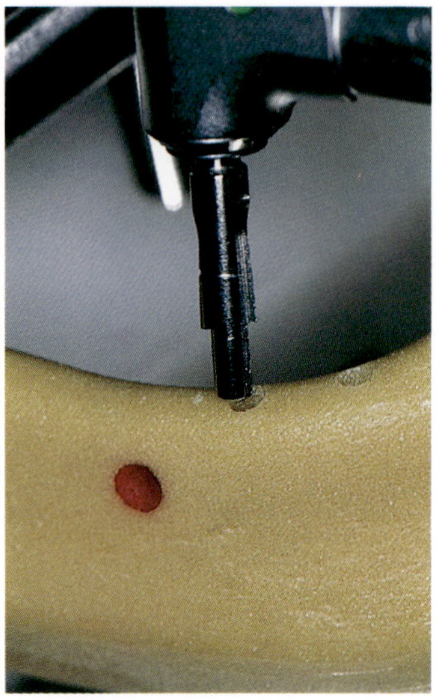

Fig. 310. Using a pilot drill, the entrances of the 2.0 mm canals are enlarged to a diameter of 3.0 mm so that the 3.0 mm diameter twist drill can be used in subsequent steps. The procedure is performed starting with the canals on the right, then moving towards those on the left, taking care to preserve parallelism between the sites.

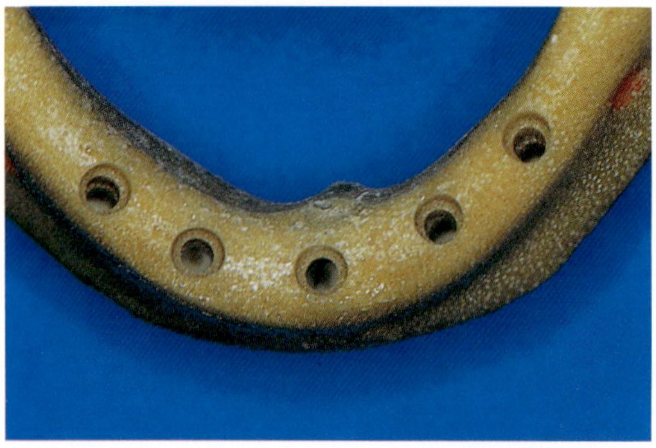

Fig. 311. Completion of the use of the pilot drill.

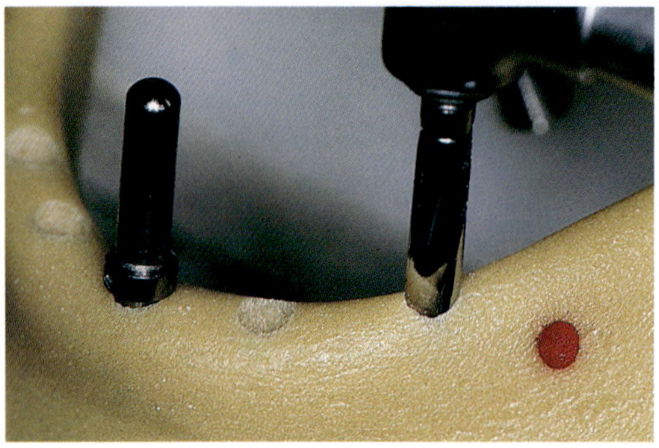

Fig. 312. The thin end of the direction indicator is inserted into the midline site. Referring to this, the canal at the left end side is widened with a 3.0 mm twist drill, keeping the site parallel with the indicator.

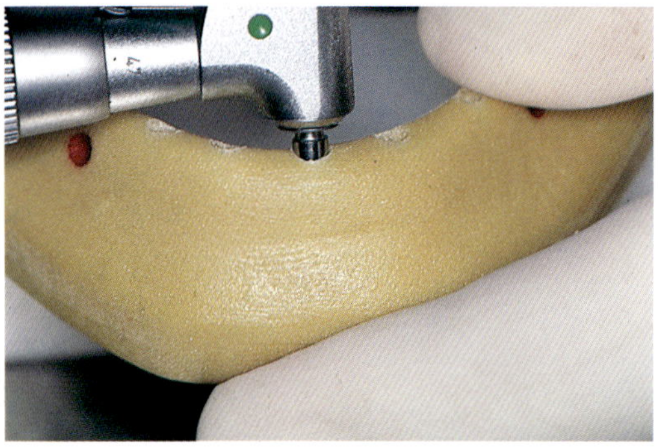

Fig. 313.

* Clinically, the compact bone of the base of the mandible sometimes has to be perforated. In such cases, the index finger of the surgeon is pressed against the skin of the mandibular base during the preparation through the compact bone.

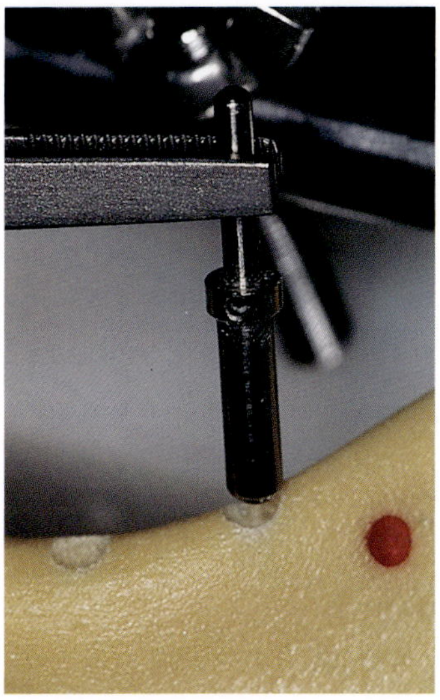

Fig. 314. The wider end of the direction indicator is inserted into the enlarged canal, and the parallelism with the direction indicator inserted into the midline site is checked.

* In cases of massive bleeding from the canal, the direction indicator can be used as a hemostasis.

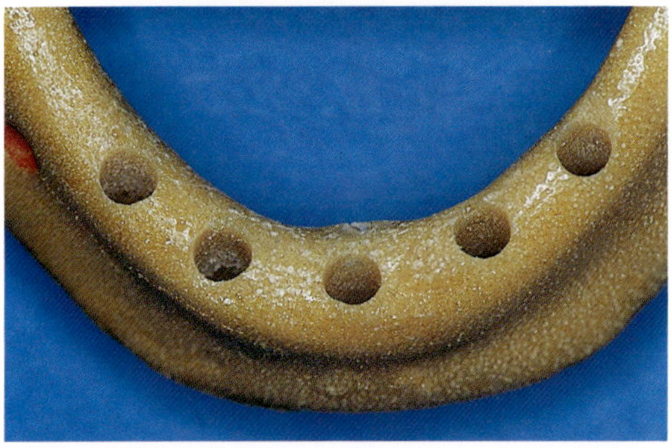

Fig. 315. The remaining canals are prepared with the 3.0 mm twist drill, from left to right. Care is taken to keep good parallelism among the sites.

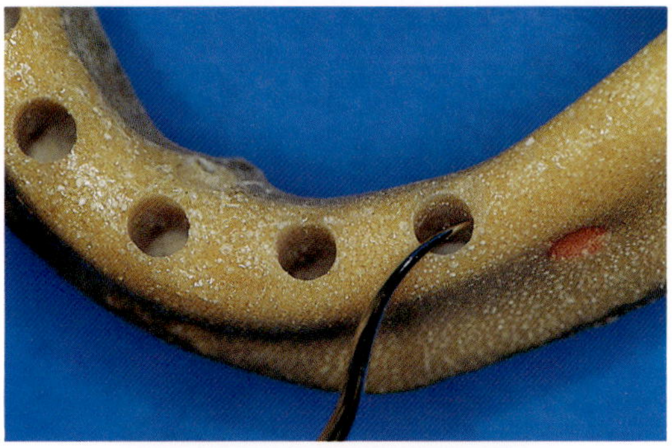

Fig. 316.

* In clinical cases, the thickness of the compact bone in the alveolar crest of all sites is checked with a dissector.

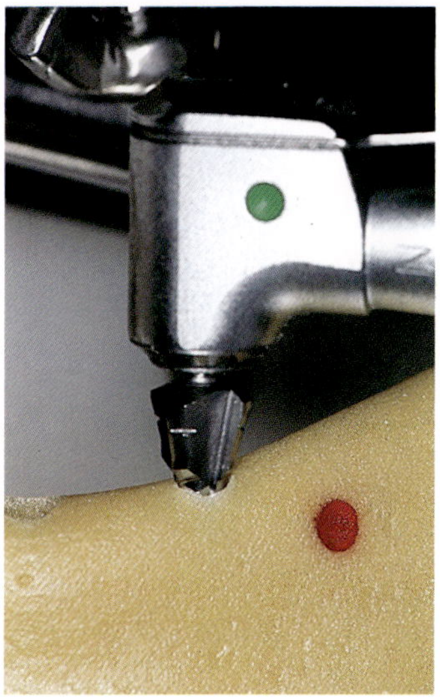

Fig. 317. A conically shaped entrance of the canals is created with a countersink, starting from left to right.

Remark: The mark on the countersink is referred to in creating the shoulder, so that the depth of the drill does not exceed half the thickness of the marginal compact bone layer.

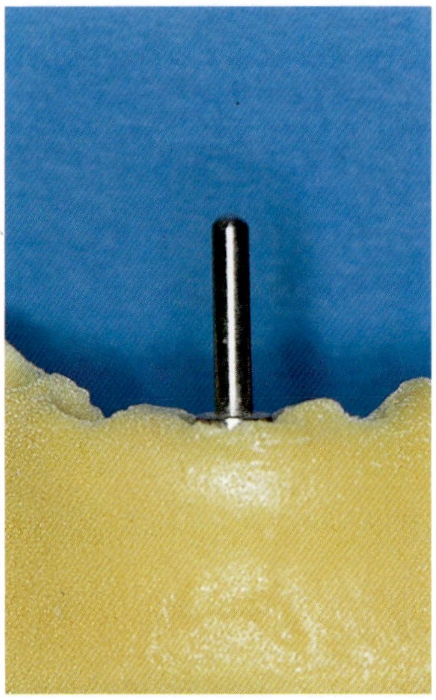

Fig. 318. If possible, the countersinking procedure should be deep enough to accept the cover screw completely. The depth is presumed to be ideal, when the mid ring of the direction indicator becomes leveled with the alveolar crest.

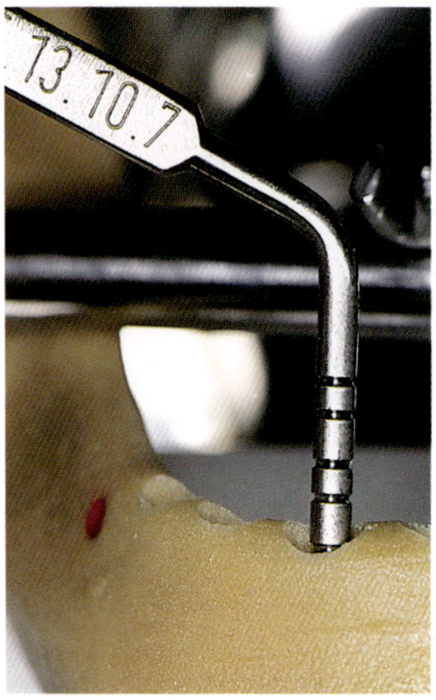

Fig. 319. Using a gauge, the depth of the canal is checked (see Fig. 351 for the comparison).

Remark: The depth gauge is graded for various fixture lengths.

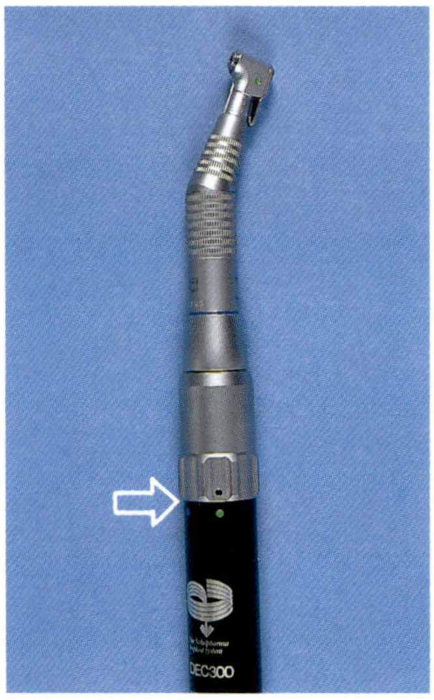

Fig. 320. In subsequent steps, the speed is set at low range (maximum 28 rpm).

Remark: The black point of the motor unit is matched to the green point on the gear (*arrow*) to light the of the control unit.

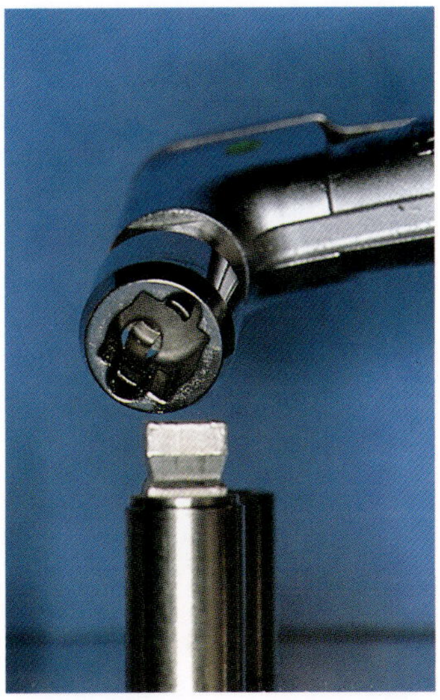

Fig. 321. To create screw threads within the site, a connection to the contra-angle handpiece (hereinafter simply called the "connection") is placed in the head of the handpiece.

Remark: The connection is designed to hold the squared head of the screw tap (hereinafter simply called the "tap") by elastic slip-grip of springs.

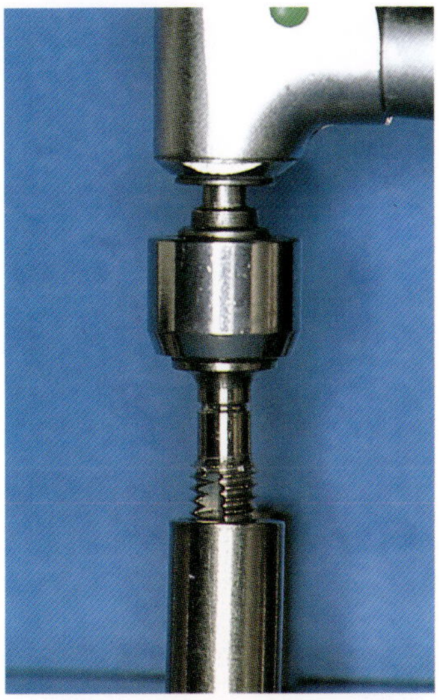

Fig. 322. The tap, carried in the titanium box, is attached to the connection, while rotating the connection slightly and compressing it downward.

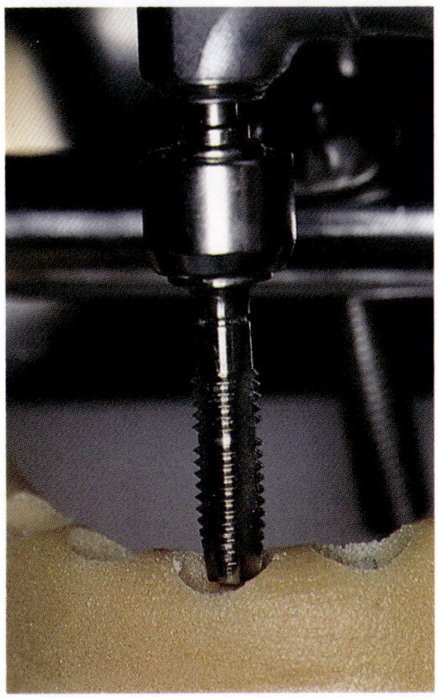

Fig. 323. The tap is inserted into the canal entrances, care being taken to keep good parallelism with the direction of some other site. During this procedure, the tap is rotated and pressed towards the bottom of the site in order to start the cutting.

Remark: The torque level is put on 30 Ncm when cutting in the plastic model.

* In clinical cases, profuse irrigation with saline solution is indispensable during this procedure. Depending on the bone density, the torque is set from 20-45 Ncm by pushing the buttons marked with ▲ and ▼.

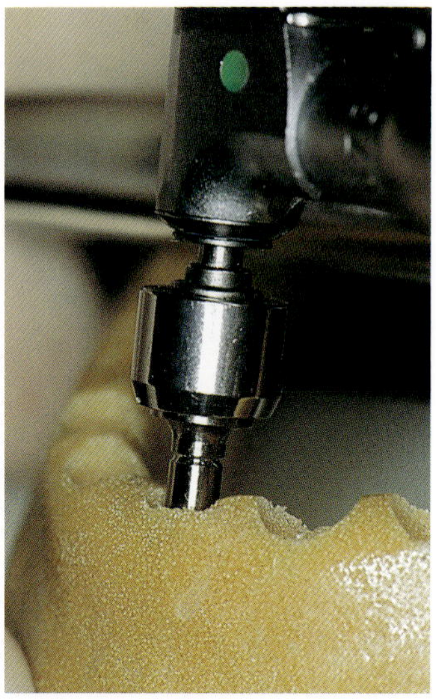

Fig. 324. When the tap has cut to a sufficient depth, strong resistance can be felt and the rotation of the tap should be stopped. Push the reverse rotation button Я (a sound is heard, when this is pushed) and unwind the tap slowly.

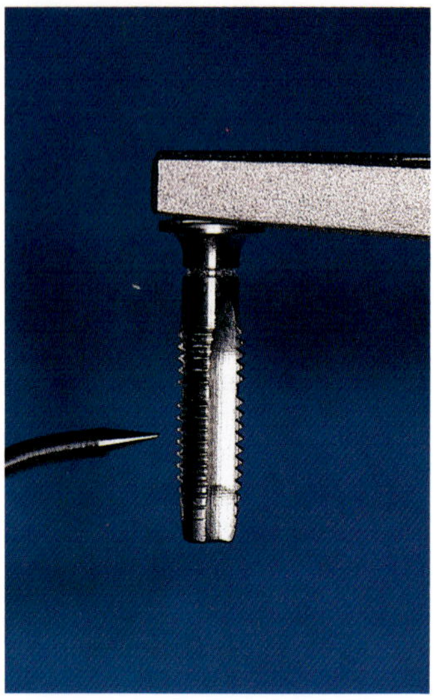

Fig. 325. Shavings in the tap grooves are removed with a cleaning needle.

Remark: The tap is cleaned after each site threading.

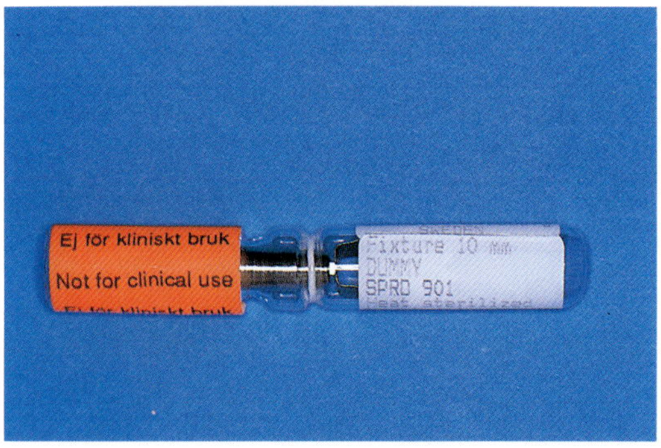

Fig. 326. A fixture-containing ampoule.

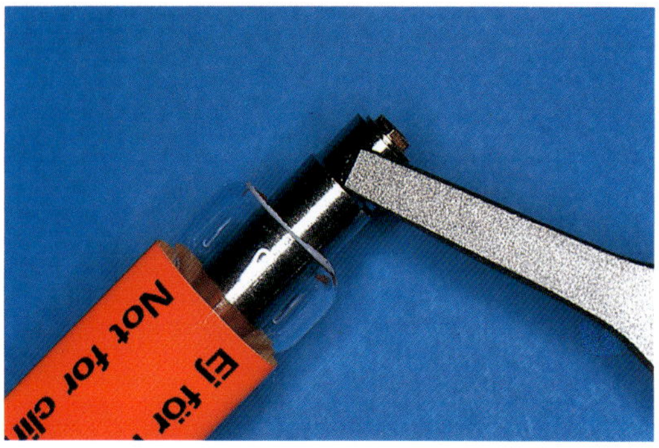

Fig. 327. The ampoule is broken, and the cylinder, containing the fixture is lifted out and placed into the titanium organizer.

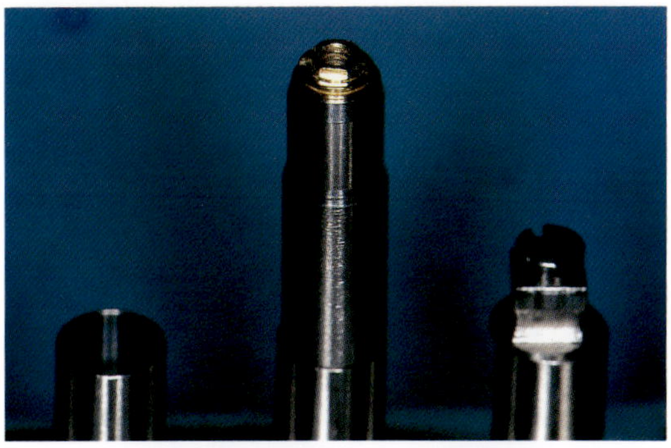

Fig. 328. Using titanium tweezers, the cylinder carrying the fixture is placed into the supporting cylinder of the titanium organizer.

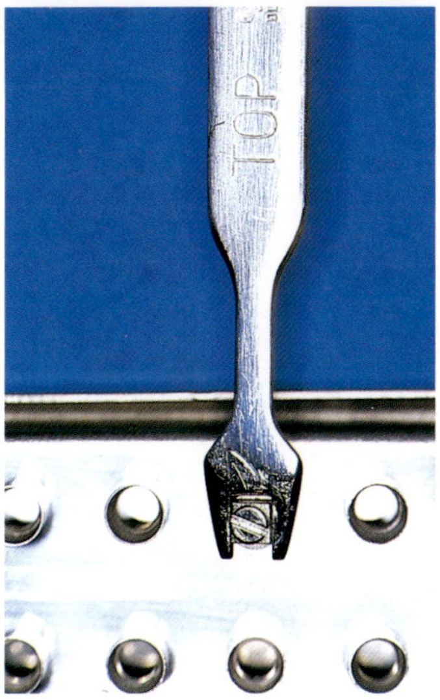

Fig. 329. The fixture mount is taken out of the box, using an open-end wrench.

Remark: In using the open-end wrench, the side marked "TOP" should be turned upwards.

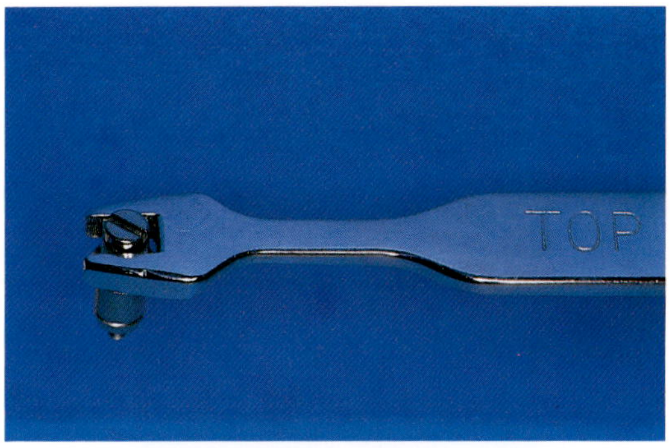

Fig. 330. The wrench is slightly tapered in its branches so that the fixture mount cannot fall off, while being carried.

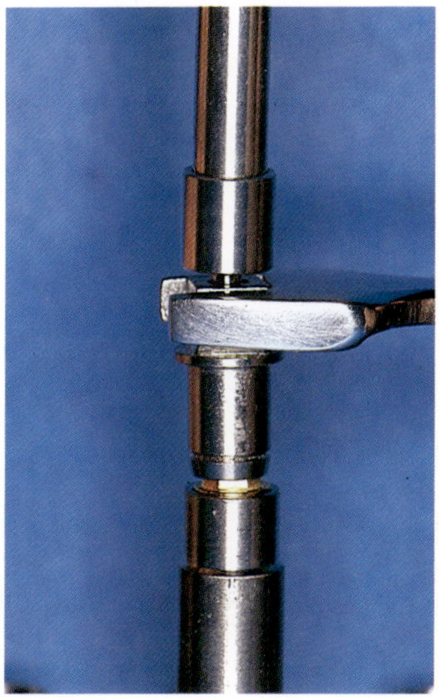

Fig. 331. While being held by the wrench, the fixture mount is attached to the fixture head using a long screw-driver.

Remark: After tightening the mount screw, the screw mount is rotated back about 1/4 a turn and then tightened again.

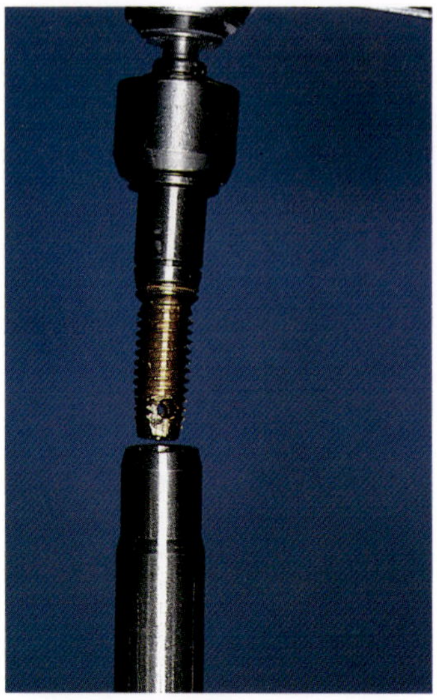

Fig. 332. The mount + fixture is connected to the connection in the handpiece, and lifted out of the cylinder.

Remark: The connection is rotated slightly and compressed downward when seated on the fixture mount.

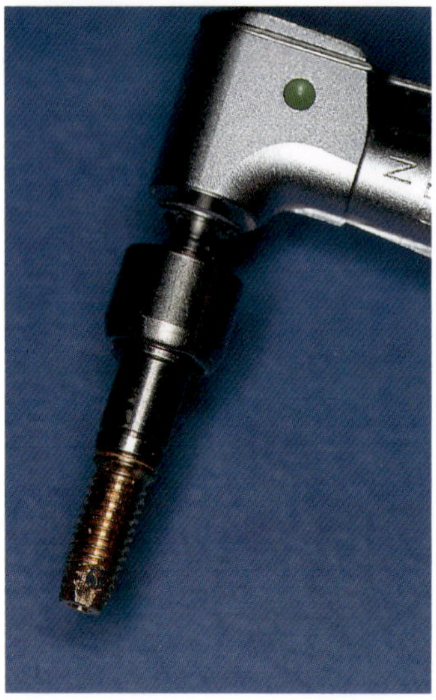

Fig. 333. The fixture mount + fixture is carried to the fixture site, inclining the components slightly to prevent them from falling off.

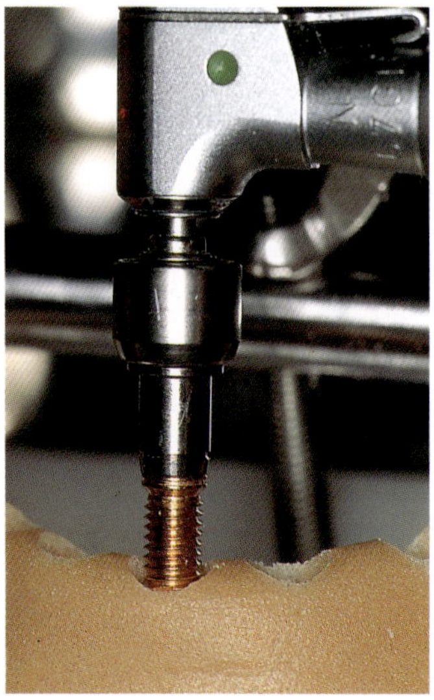

Fig. 334. In training, the fixture is first inserted into the mid fixture site. Irrigation is not applied until the region of the fixture's horizontal hole in the tip has entered the bone site.

Remark : The torque is set at the level used for the tap i.e. 30 Ncm.

* In clinical situations, the fixture is first inserted in the most distal site in the left side.

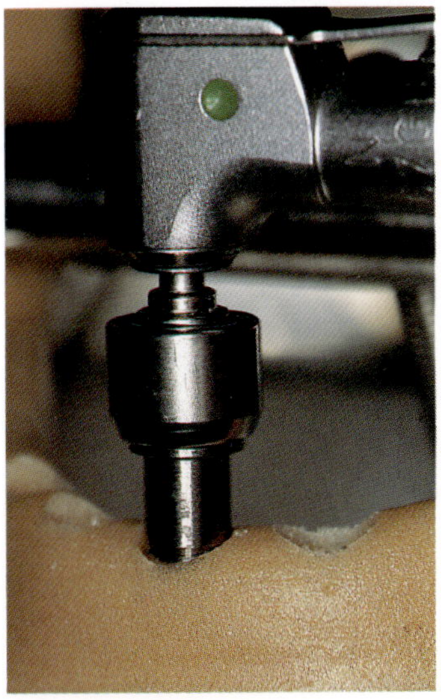

Fig. 335. When the fixture has entered to almost the proper depth, a strong resistance can be felt, and the motor stops rotating.

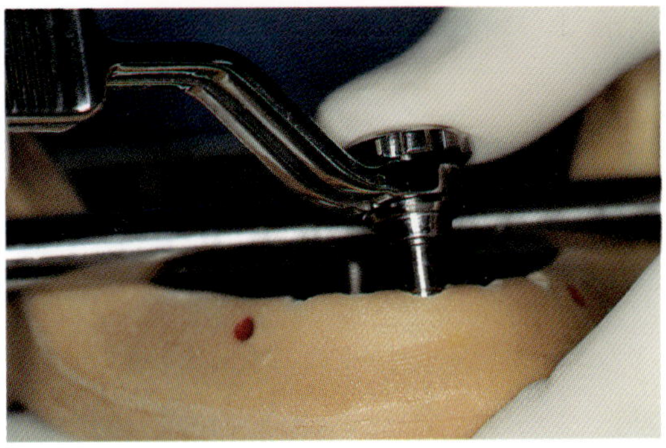

Fig. 336. After removing the connection, the fixture is completely inserted manually, using a cylinder wrench. The thumb is placed on the head of the wrench and the index finger on the lower margin of the mandible. Tightening is performed, while compressing the wrench grip. The fixture tip is designed to allow self tapping of a few mm.

Remark: Irrigation is applied during this procedure. Tightening is performed until a good resistance is felt.

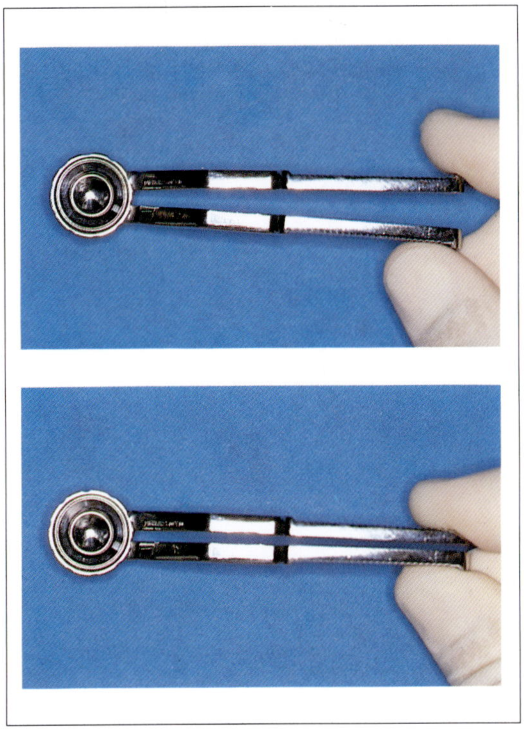

Fig. 337. The way to use the cylinder wrench : Close the branches with your fingers, and the cylinder will be locked in working position.

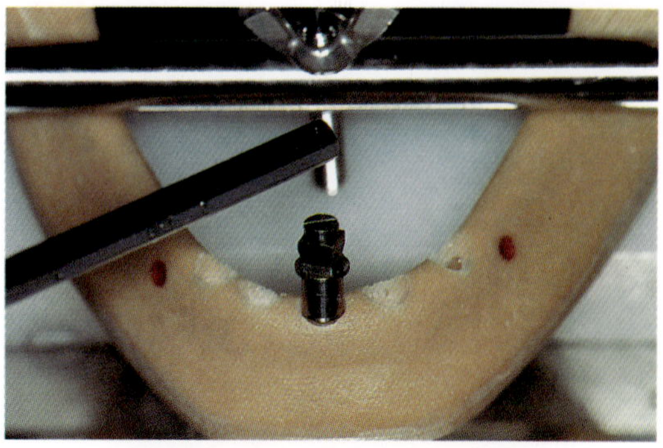

Fig. 338. With a fixture mount applied to the fixture, the percussion sound from a dissector is checked (from a distance of about 3 cm).

* In clinical cases, a high metallic sound is heard when the fixture is surrounded with dense bone tissue.

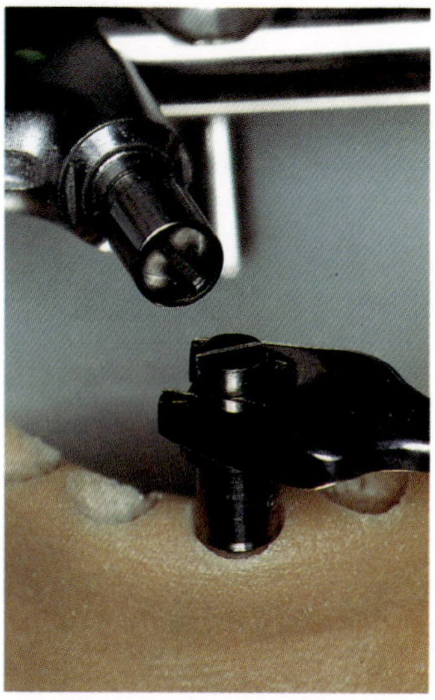

Fig. 339. A machine screwdriver is connected to the contra-angle head and is used together with an open-end wrench in order to remove the mount from the fixture.

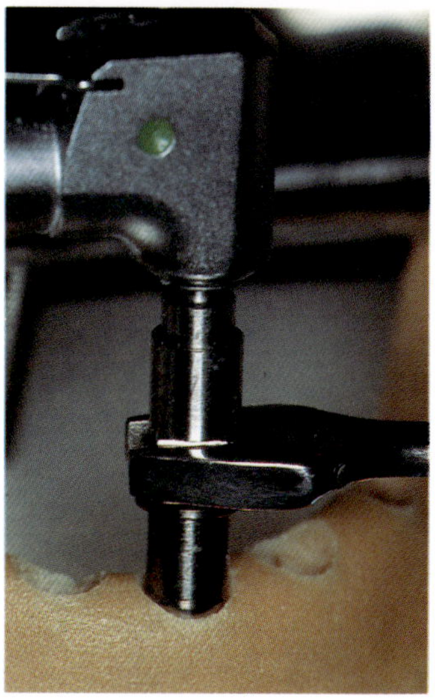

Fig. 340. Push the (Я) marked button of the control unit (a sound is heard) and loosen the fixture mount screw by reversed rotation of the motor. During this procedure, the open end wrench is attached to the squared head of the fixture mount to prevent the fixture from rotating.

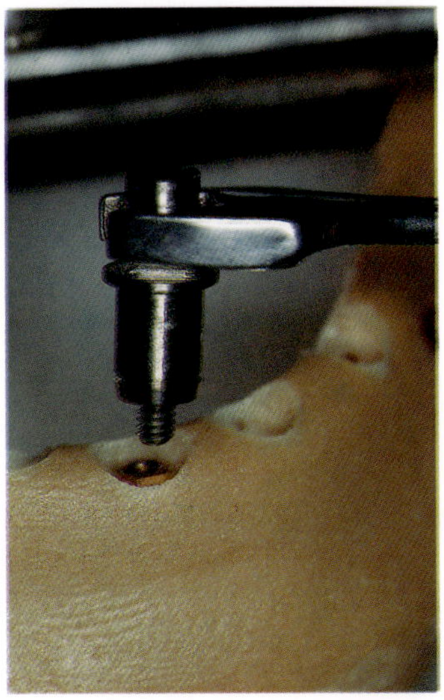

Fig. 341. When the fixture mount has been unscrewed, it is removed by lifting it away with the open-end wrench.

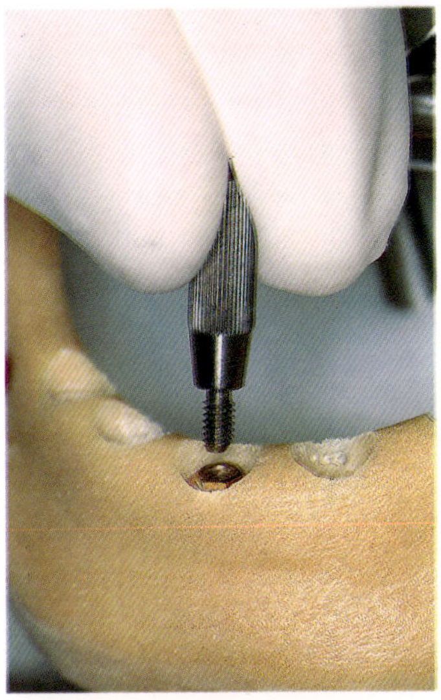

Fig. 342. The direction indicator for fixture is attached manually into the internally threaded canal of the fixture.

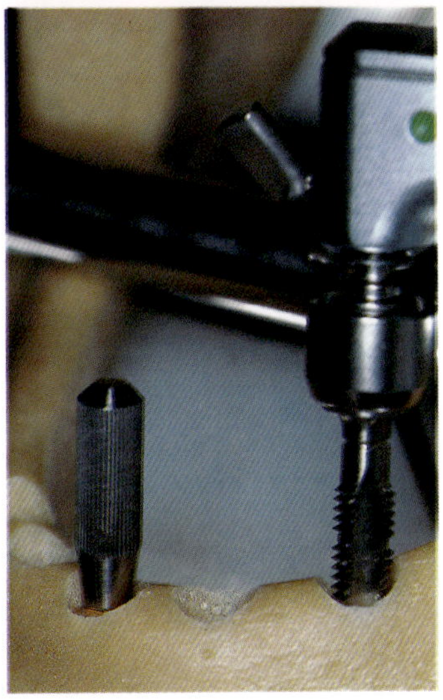

Fig. 343. Referring to the direction indicator set in the first site, the remaining canals are tapped and consecutively, fixtures are inserted from the left to the right side.

* In clinical cases, tapping and fixture insertion start in the most distal site on the left side. In training, the first site to be treated in the one in the midline, whereafter the distal site on the left hand side is treated.

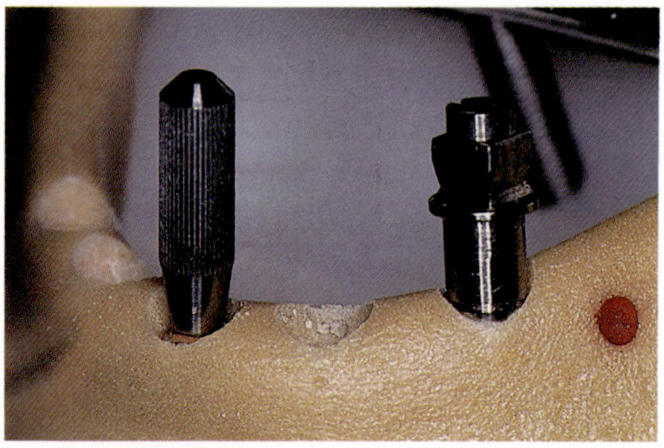

Fig. 344. If possible, the fixtures should be parallel with each other. However, deviation of less than 30 degrees can be accepted.

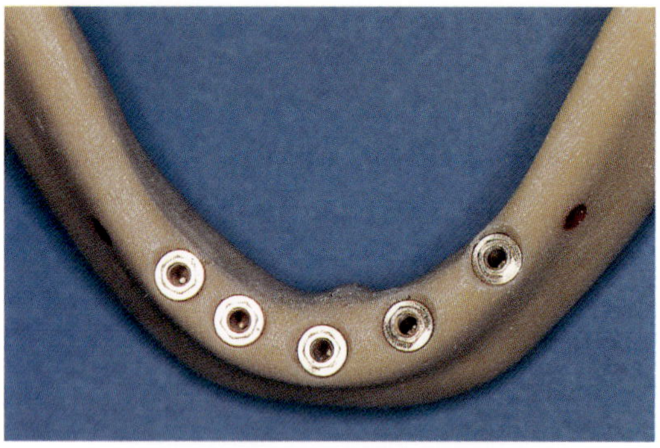

Fig. 345. Completed insertion of 5 fixtures.

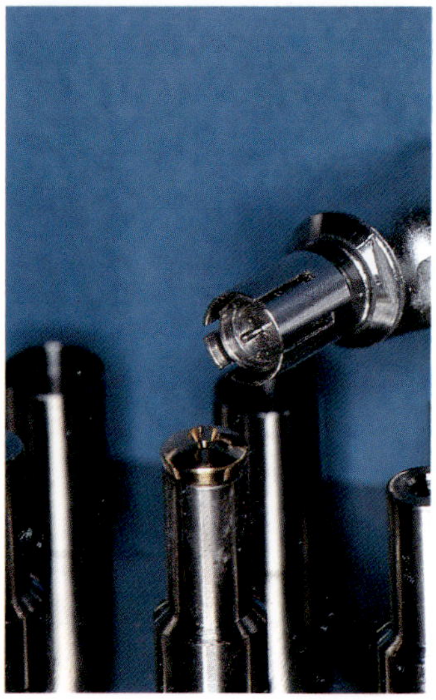

Fig. 346. Cover screws, contained in a glass ampoule are placed into a titanium bowl. Using titanium tweezers, the cover screw is lifted and placed in the titanium box. The button marked (T) of the control unit is pressed. The cover screw is lifted with a screw inserter, connected to the head of the contra-angle handpiece.

Remark: The screw inserter is designed to have a slip-grip onto the cover screw, when it is strongly pushed onto the head of the screw.

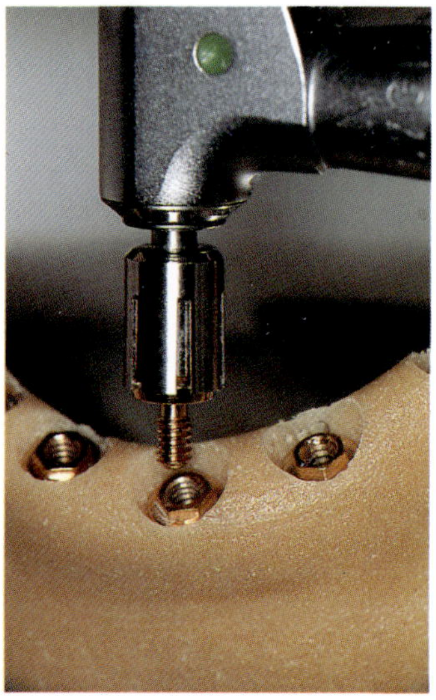

Fig. 347. The cover screw is placed into the central canal of the fixture, and is inserted with the machine at the lowspeed setting.

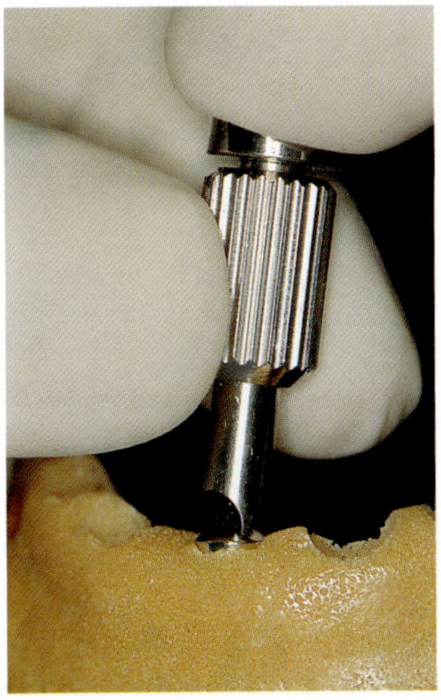

Fig. 348. When the cover screw is almost in position, it is finally tightened with a short manual screwdriver.

Remark: The screwdriver is kept in position by keeping a thumb on top of its head, while rotating the grip of the screwdriver with the other thumb and the index finger.

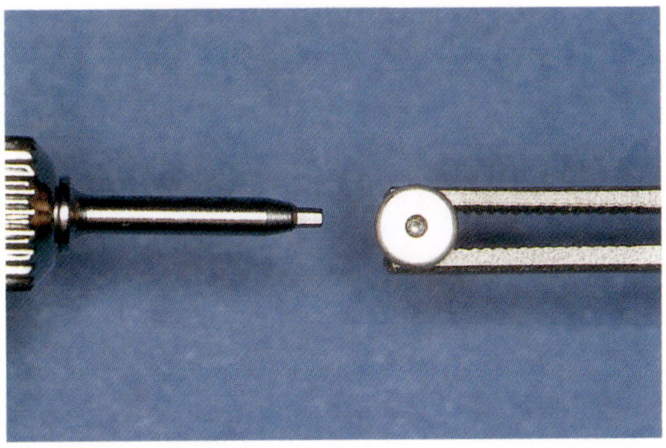

Fig. 349.

* In clinical cases, where the width of the upper jaw or alveolar crest is not sufficient, a cover screw with a flat head is used. This screw has an inhex in the center. It is tightened with a hexagonal screw driver, specially designed for this purpose.

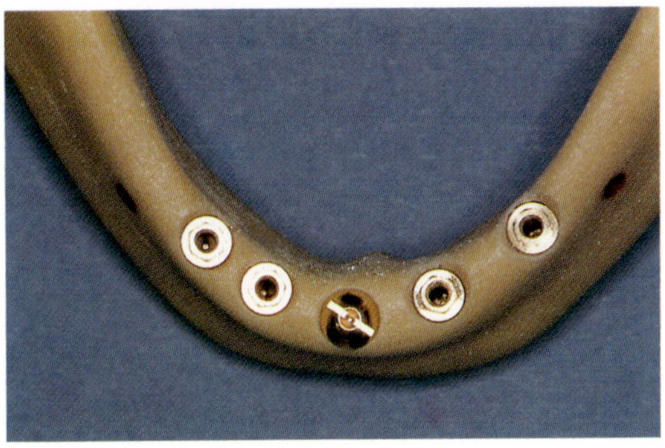

Fig. 350. The stage I operation has been completed in the model.

Lengths of drills, depth gauge, countersink, tap, fixture mount, cover screws and fixture.

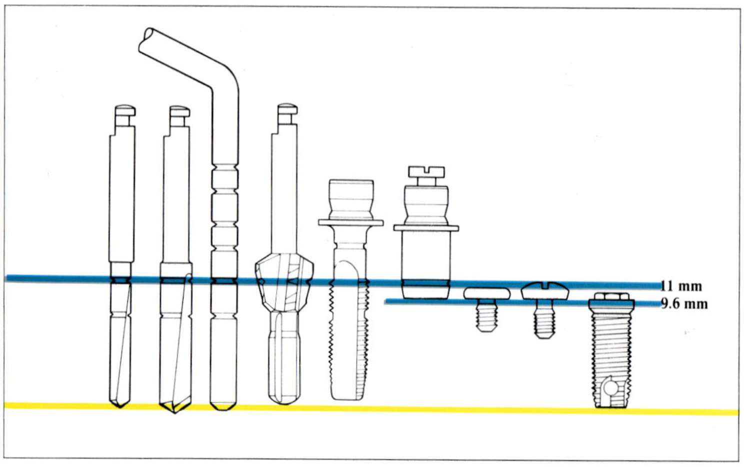

Fig. 351.

The lengths of the tools and instruments used for insertion of 10 mm long fixtures (3.75 mm in diameter) are shown in Fig. 351. The following conditions can be noted:

1. The depth determined with a depth gauge indicates the fixture length + the height of the cover screw head, and does not represent the length of the fixture itself.
2. The mark on the fixture mount represents the level of the upper surface of the cover screw head.
3. The mark of the tap does not indicate that the bottom of the canal has been reached. A safety margin is placed in the bottom region to minimize the risk of destruction of the bone threads, in cases of fragile bone marrow. Even when no screw thread has been created in this region, the fixture can be inserted to the predesignated depth, utilizing the self tapping function of the fixture tip.

Stage II Operation

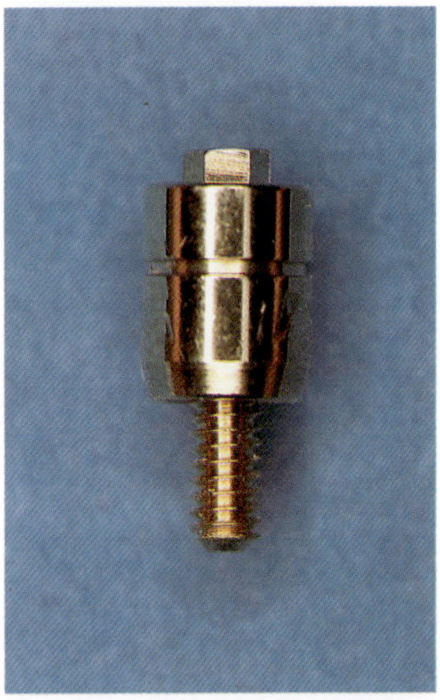

Fig. 352. A 5.5 mm long abutment, marked with a ring indicating that it is a dummy.

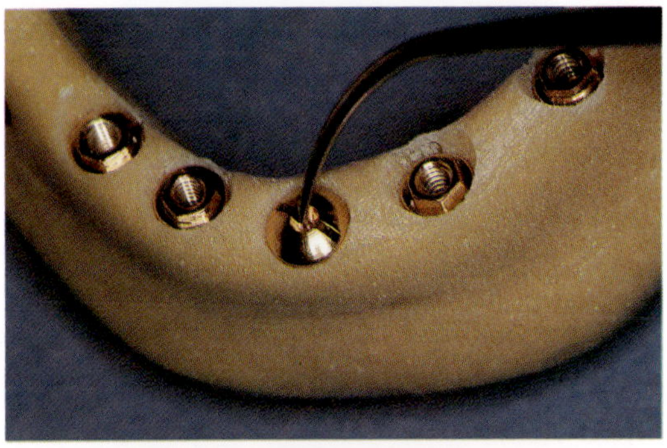

Fig. 353.

* In clinical situations, the position of the cover screw is checked by palpation and via probing through the mucosa.

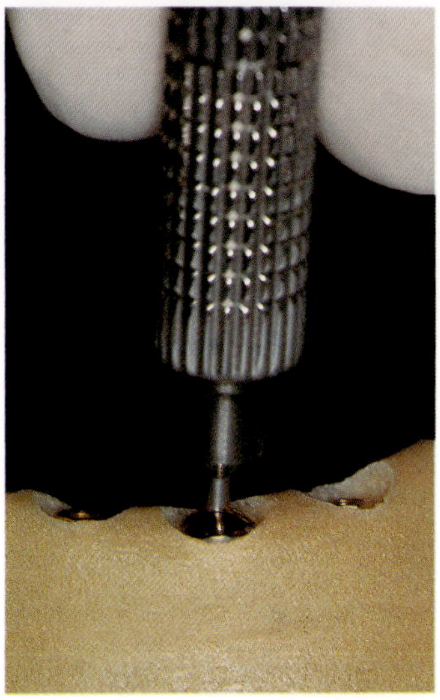

Fig. 354.

* After incising the alveolar crest mucosa, the central hole of the cover screws is located, and the central guide peg of the punch is inserted into the cover screw hole.

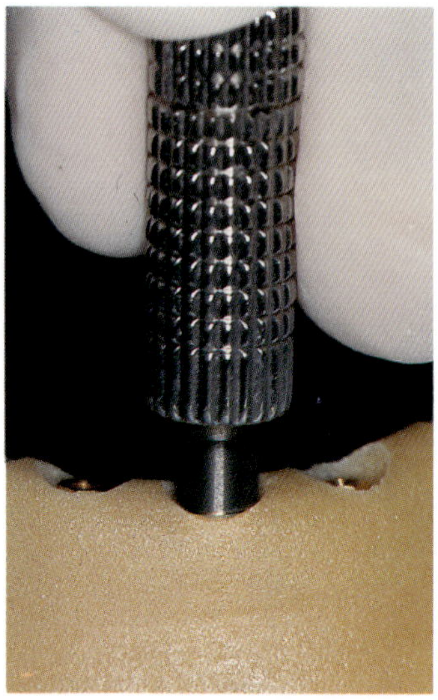

Fig. 355.

* The punch is used in the following way. With the right thumb and index finger, the punch grip is pushed down while turning the instrument strongly in the direction of the cover screw, cutting the mucoperiosteum in a cylindrical form. During this process, the thumb is fixed on the punch head.

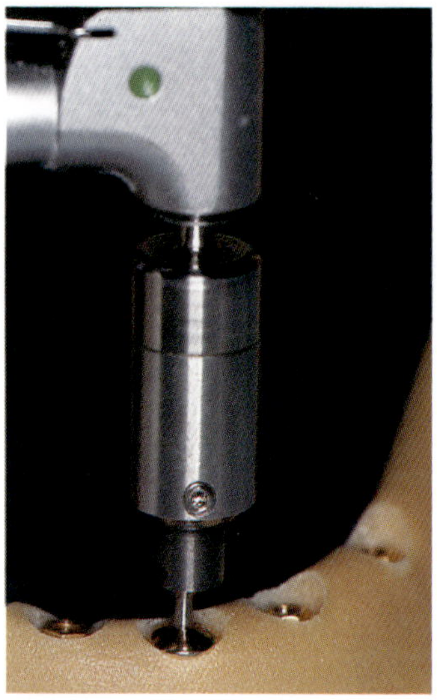

Fig. 356.

* Instead of a manual punch, a machine punch (from the special instrument catalog) can be used to make this procedure easier.

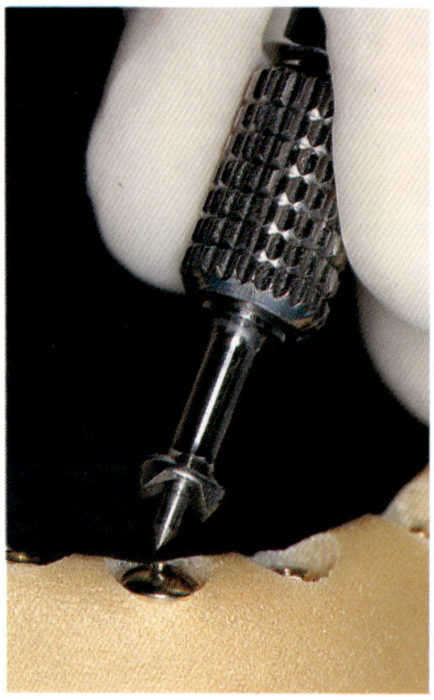

Fig. 357.

* In cases, showing bone overgrowth of the cover screw, the bone needs to be removed with a cover screw mill. This instrument should only be used in the presence of a cover screw.

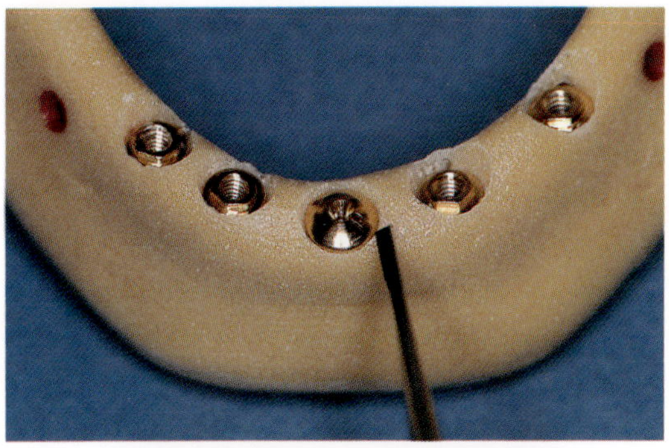

Fig. 358.

* If the bone, covering the screw head, cannot be completely removed with a cover screw mill, a fine chisel or small round bur is recommended.

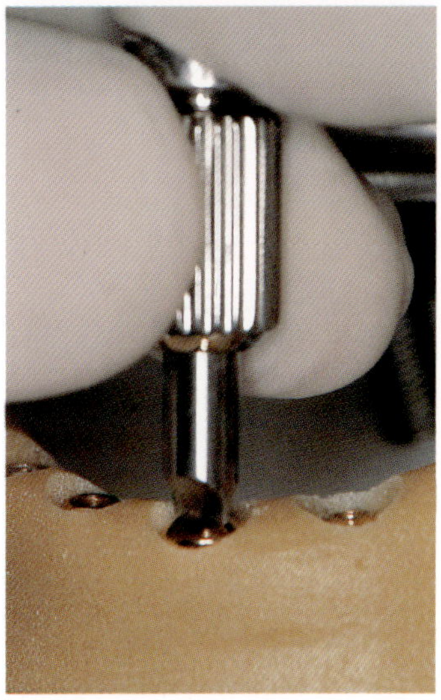

Fig. 359.

* After removing the cover screw, using a short manual screwdriver, the fixture head is checked for fibrous connective tissue or bone tissue surrounding the hex part. If so, they have to be completely removed with a second cut of the punch. This is one of the most important steps in the stage II operation.

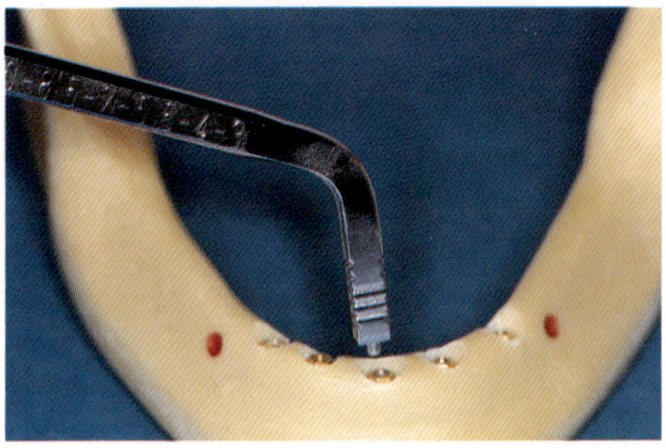

Fig. 360.

* The tip of an abutment gauge is inserted into the central hole of the fixture head, and an abutment with an appropriate height is selected depending on the thickness of the mucosa. The upper margin of the abutment should protrude through the gingiva by about 2 mm (lower jaw) or 1 mm (upper jaw), respectively.

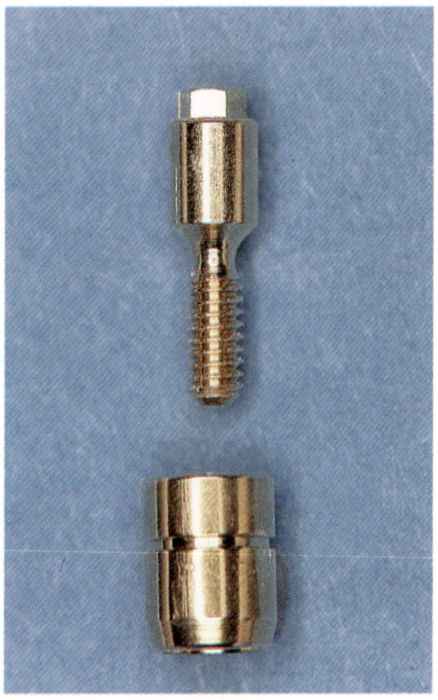

Fig. 361. The abutment screw is inserted into the abutment cylinder.

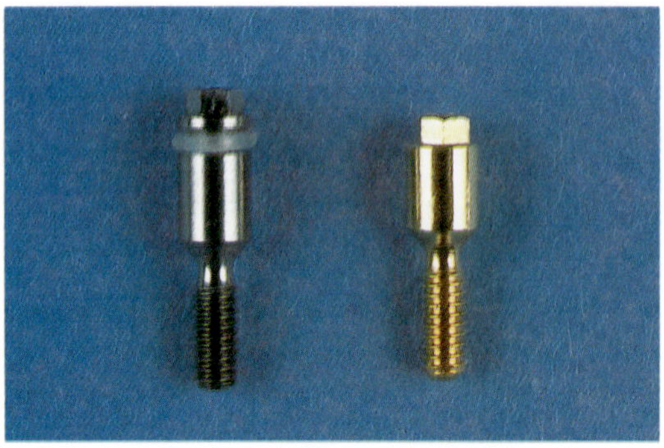

Fig. 362.

∗ In the clinical situation, the head of the abutment screw has an O-ring around the neck to prevent invasion of saliva and other materials into the central canal of the fixture.

Left: for clinical use

Right: for training

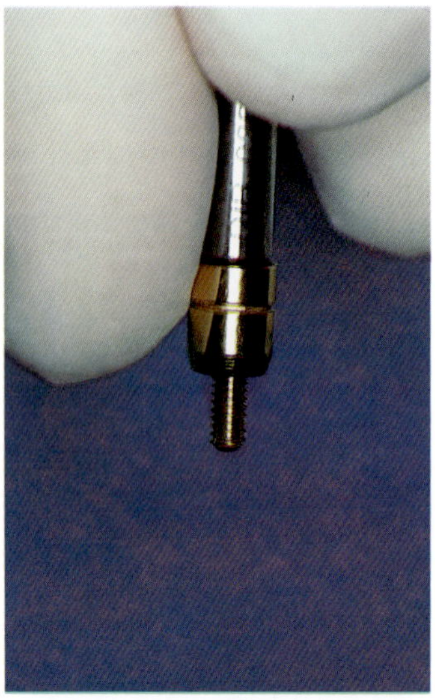

Fig. 363. An abutment is connected to a short hexagonal screwdriver.

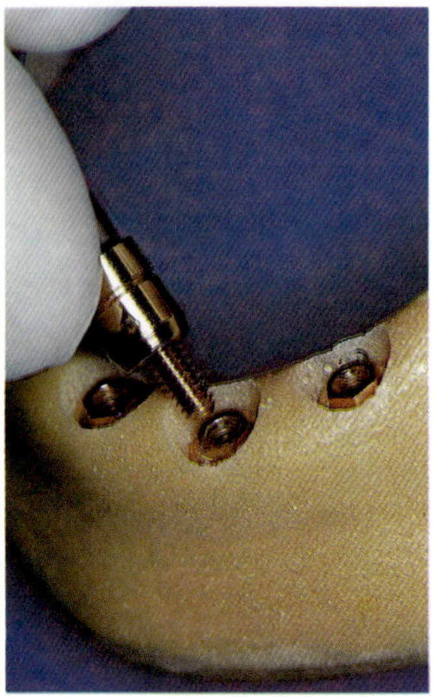

Fig. 364. The abutment screw is inserted into the canal of the fixture head and tightened lightly.

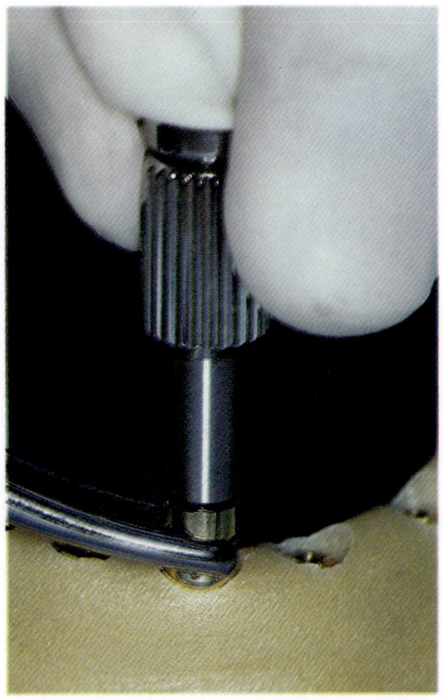

Fig. 365. Check with a small abutment clamp that the abutment can be rotated freely above the head of the hex. The clamp is rotated and pushed towards the fixture so that the hexagonal head of the fixture fits into the inhex of the abutment (Fig. 75). The screw of the abutment is tightened, keeping a firm grip of the cylinder with a large abutment clamp.

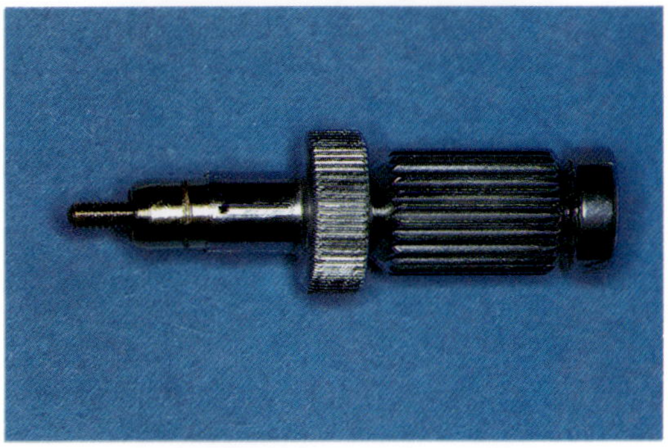

Fig. 366.

Remark: An abutment holder is useful, when applying the abutment, into which a short hexagonal screwdriver is inserted. With the holder, it is not possible to counteract apical torque, when tightening the not screw.

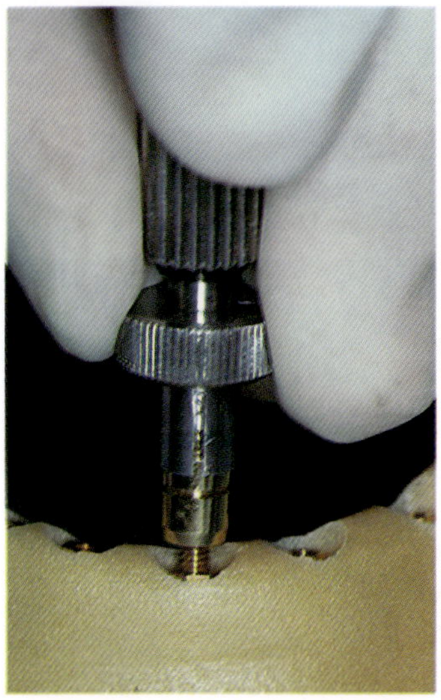

Fig. 367.

Remark: An abutment screw is inserted into the canal of the fixture and lightly tightened. The holder is rotated and pushed towards the fixture so that the abutment fits onto the fixture. After tightening the abutment screw, the holder is removed and the screw is finally tightened while the abutment is held with the large abutment clamp.

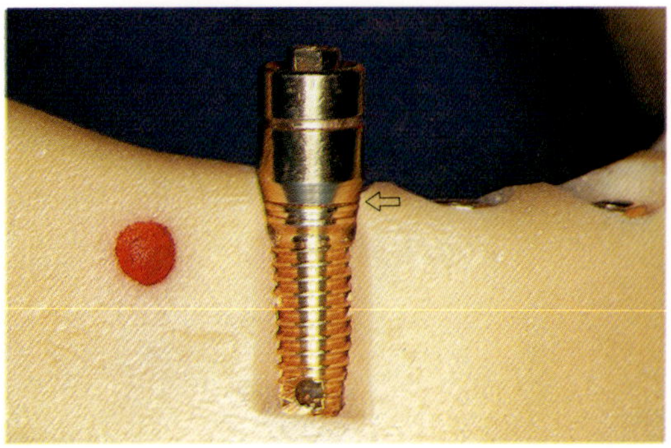

Fig. 368.

Remark: The seating of the abutment cylinder onto the fixture head is one of the most important steps in the stage II operation, and is shown in this picture by the *arrow*.

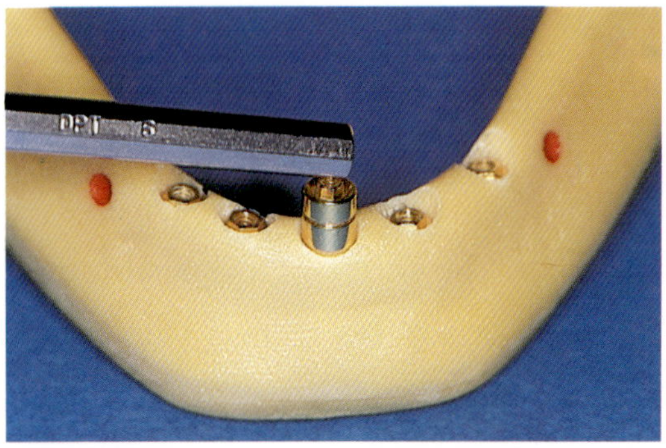

Fig. 369. The percussion test is performed, when the abutment is seated on the fixture.

* In clinical cases, a high metallic sound is heard if osseointegration has occurred between the fixture and the surrounding bone.

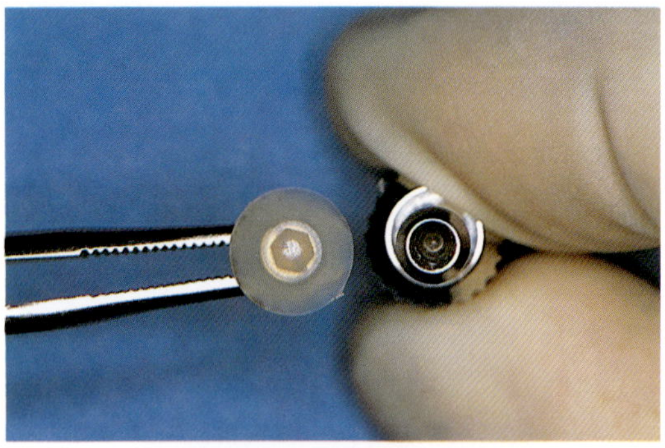

Fig. 370. The healing cap is carried via the hexagonal process of its head, joined to a short hexagonal screw-driver.

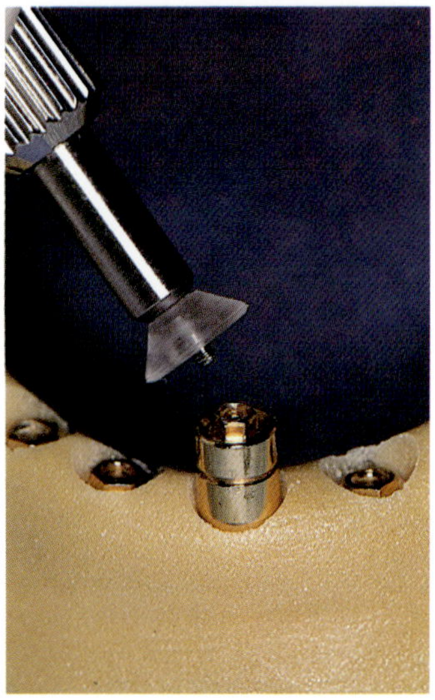

Fig. 371. The healing cap is attached to the abutment screw.

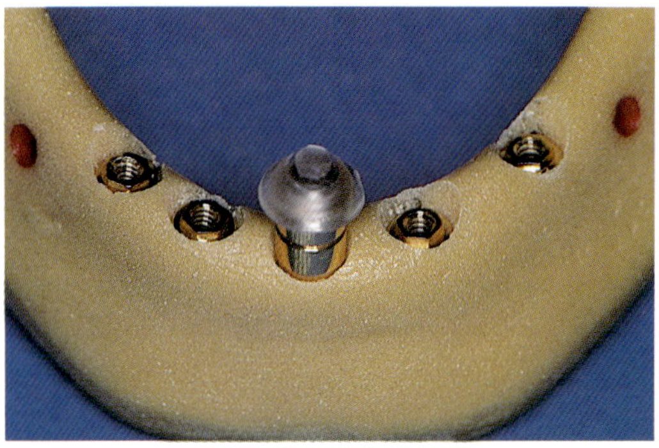

Fig. 372. The simulated surgical training, using a model, is completed, when five fixtures, one abutment and the healing cap have been applied.

CHAPTER VII

TRAINING IN BASIC PROSTHETIC PROCEDURES

The aim of this training is to understand the composition and handling of each component, and to practice impression technique, bite registration and application of a try-in denture and framework, using a training model.

Pretreatment

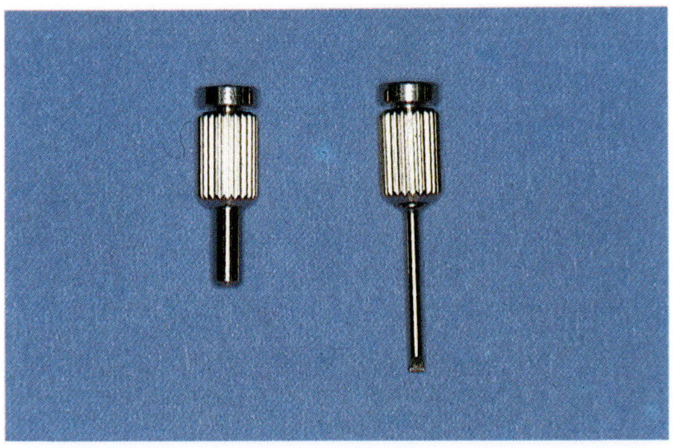

Fig. 373. Screwdrivers:
Left: hexagon screwdriver (inhex)
Right: screwdriver

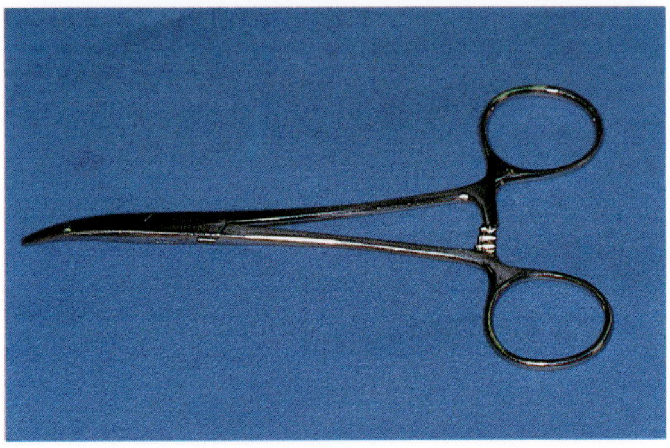

Fig. 374. Large abutment clamp.

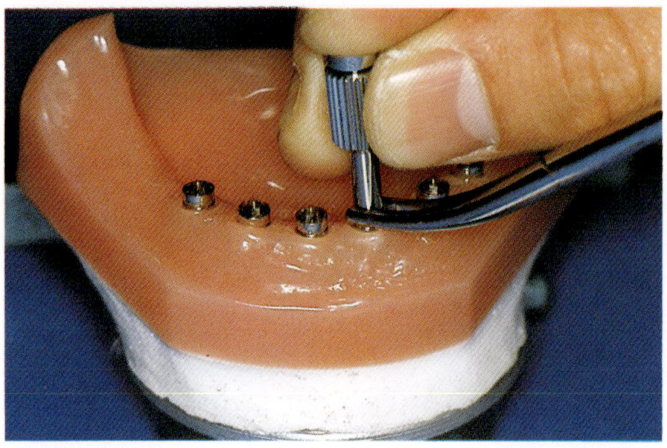

Fig. 375. Before starting any prosthetic treatment, the tightness of all abutment screws is checked. An abutment clamp is secured around the abutment while checking. If the abutment screw is loose, the accurate fit of each abutment to fixture is checked radiographically, after the abutment screw has been sufficiently tightened.

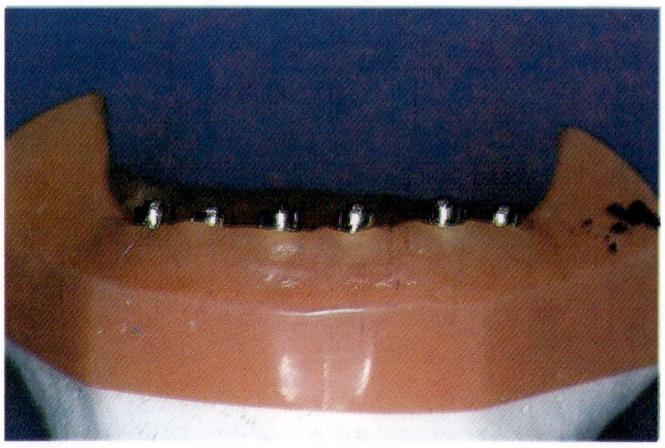

Fig. 376. When the mucosa has healed completely after the stage II operation, the height of the abutments above the resin mucosa is equal. If the height of the abutments is not uniform, the abutment cylinders can be replaced. If needed, after replacement, the fit of the components is checked radiographically.

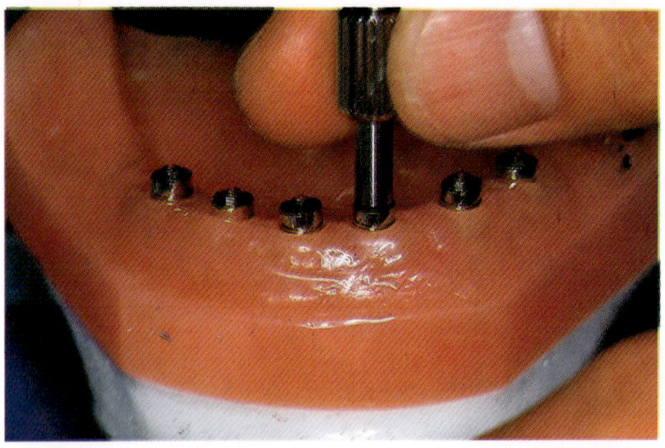

Fig. 377. An abutment screw is loosened, and the abutment cylinder is removed.

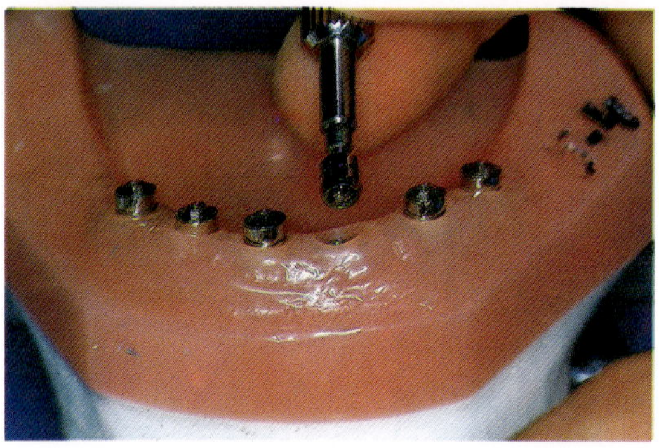

Fig. 378. Abutments of various lengths are available, from 3.0mm to 10mm.

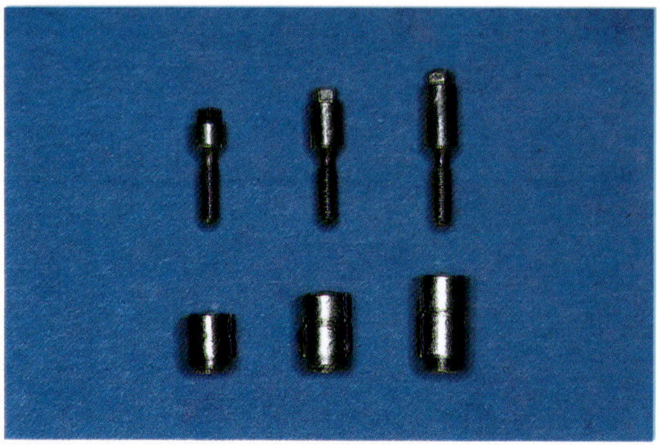

Fig. 379. Paired abutment cylinder and abutment screw are used.

Impression Taking

(1) Pick-up technique

This impression technique employs squared impression copings.

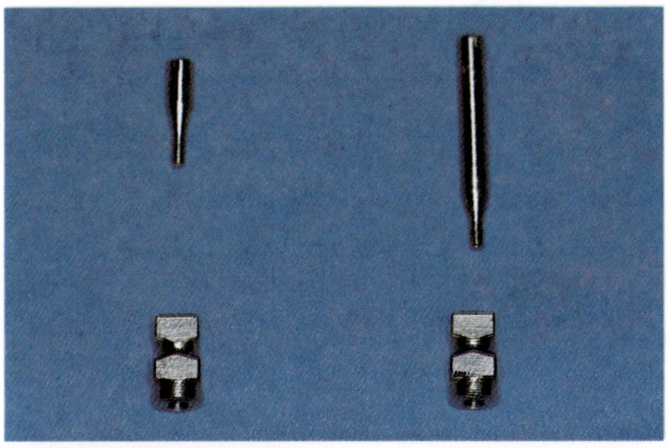

Fig. 380. Long and short guide pins and squared impression copings.

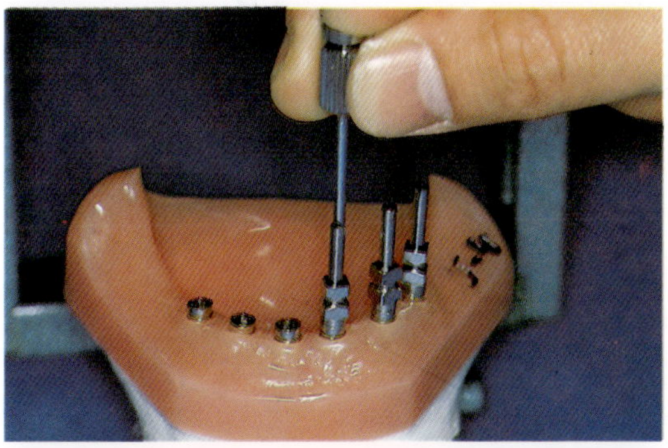

Fig. 381. The squared impression coping is screwed into position, using a guide pin. The fit between the coping and the abutment cylinder is checked.

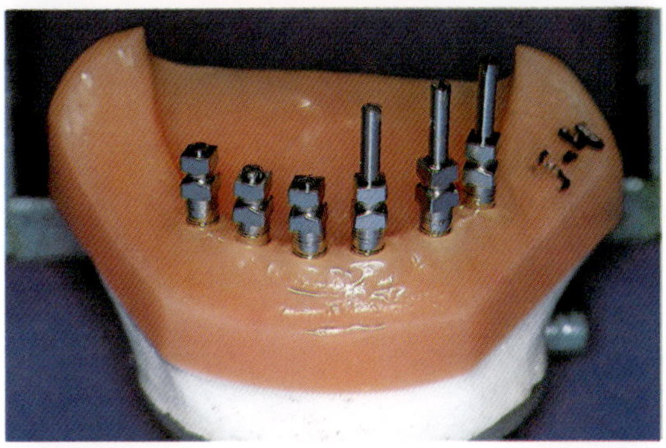

Fig. 382. If possible long guide pins are used, however, if the space to the antagonistic teeth is limited, short quide pins are used instead. For the training, three long guide pins and three short ones are available.

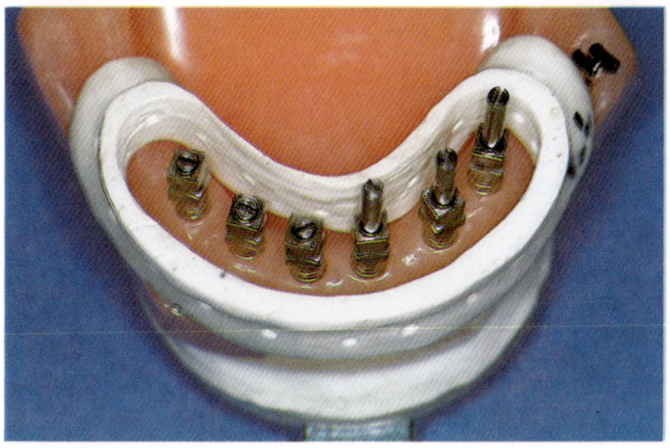

Fig. 383. An impression tray with the upper side open is fabricated and adjusted so that the space between the tray and the copings is appropriate.

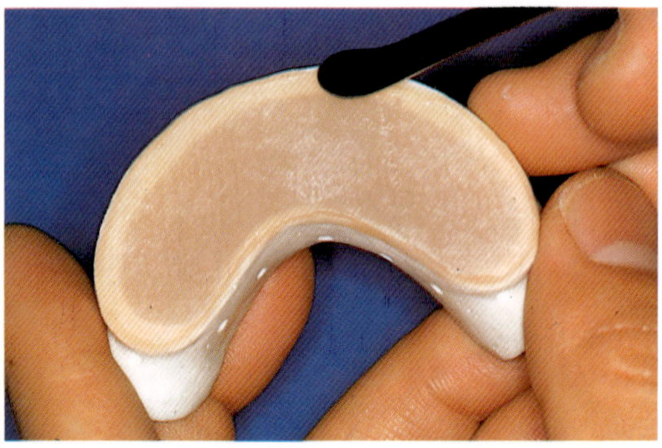

Fig. 384. A layer of paraffin wax is applied to close the open side of the tray.

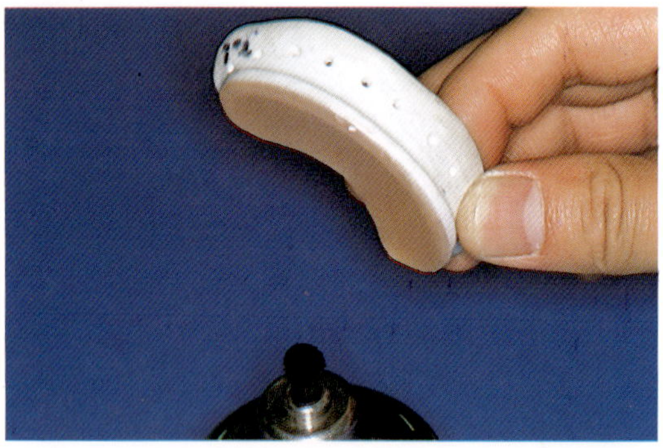

Fig. 385. The wax is softened over a flame.

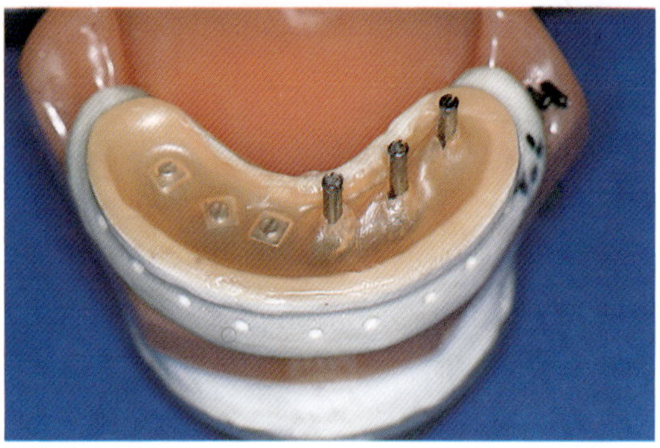

Fig. 386. The tray is placed back on the model, with the long guide pins protruding through the wax, and the tip of the short guide pins touching the wax.

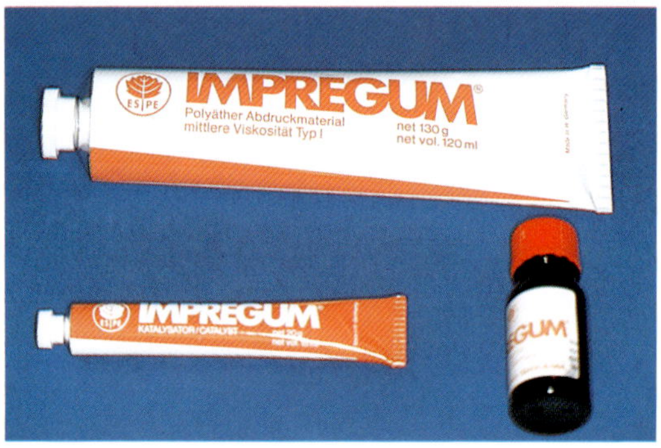

Fig. 387. Impression plaster is used in totally edentulous jaws, to provide the most accurate impressions. In partially edentulous jaws polyether rubber is used instead. In the present training session, *Impregum* ®(a polyether rubber impression material) is available.

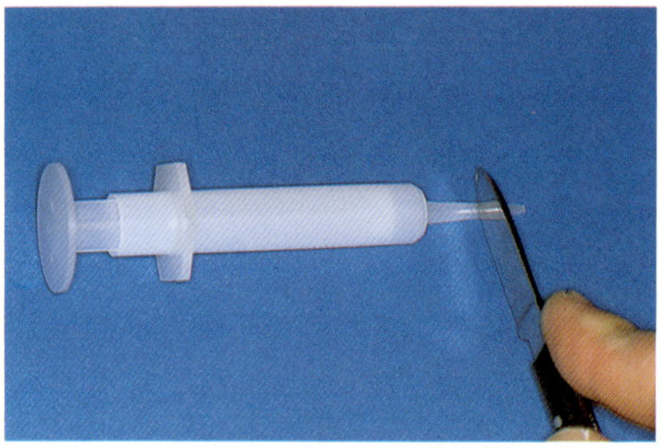

Fig. 388. A syringe with a cut tip is used when taking the impression.

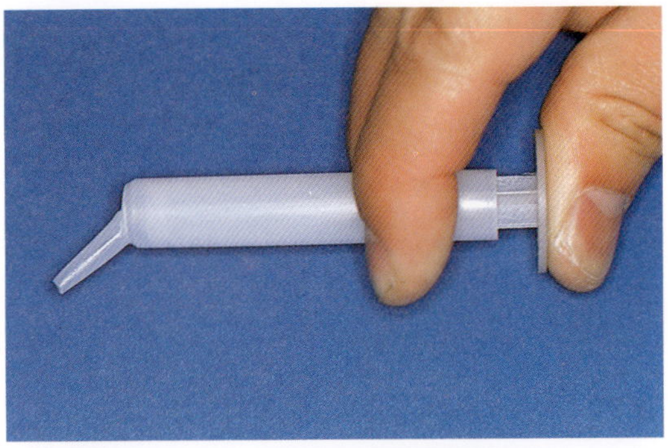

Fig. 389. The syringe tip can be angulated to allow smooth injection of the impression material.

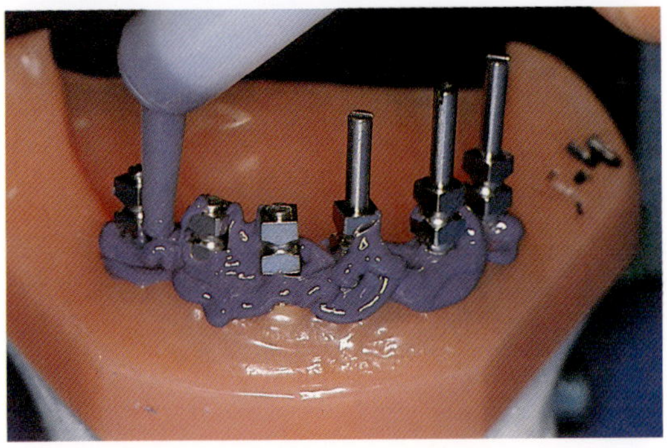

Fig. 390. Impression material is applied with the syringe, starting at the posterior squared impression coping. In clinical situations, care is taken to avoid any compressing of the peri-abutment mucosa that has not healed completely.

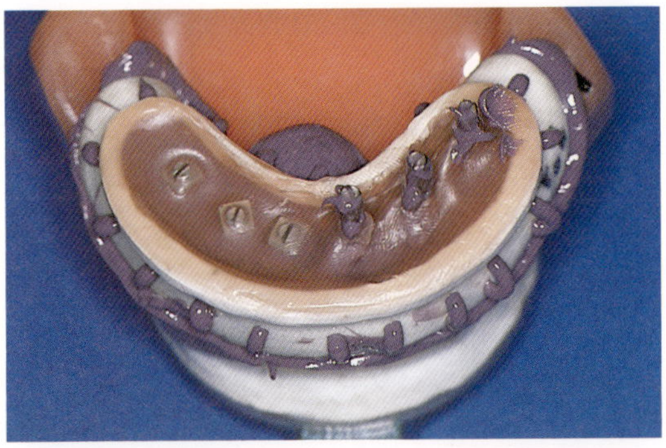

Fig. 391. The tray, carrying impression material, is fitted onto the model.

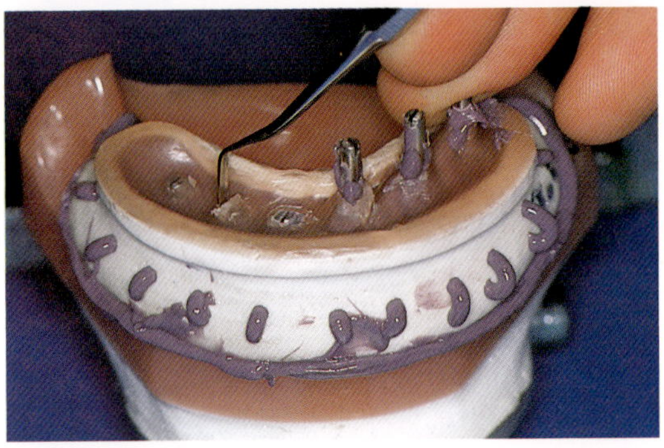

Fig. 392. Wait until the impression material has hardened completely, before starting to manipulate the tray.

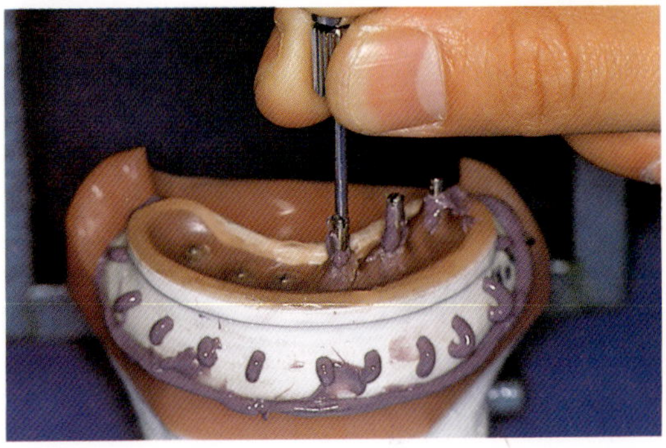

Fig. 393. Loosen the guide pins with a screwdriver.

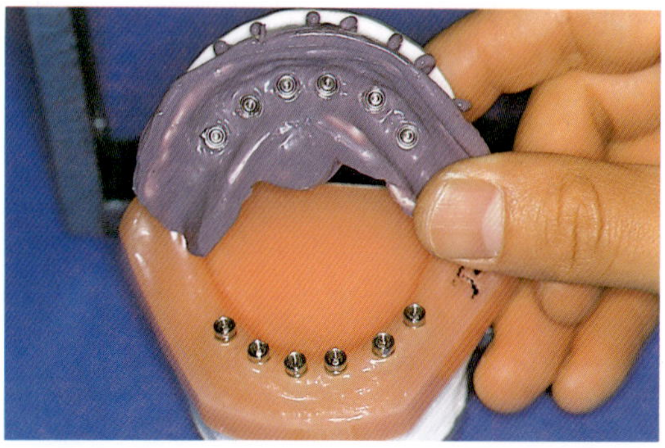

Fig. 394. The tray is removed together with the squared impression copings and the impression material.

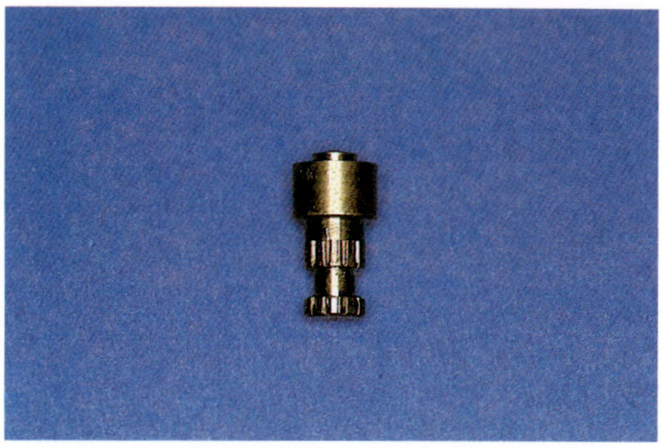

Fig. 395. A brass replica of an abutment is shown.

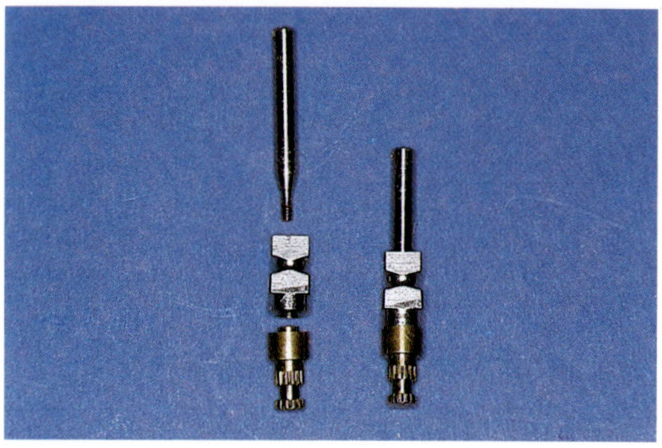

Fig. 396. The combination of an abutment replica and a squared impression coping and a guide pin.

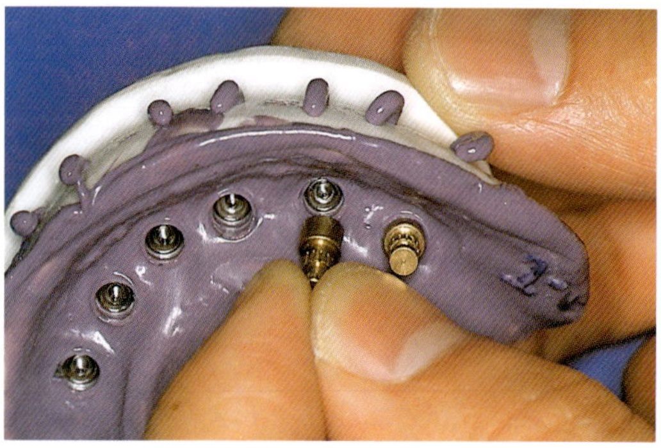

Fig. 397. The abutment replicas are attached to the squared impression copings within the impression, using guide pins.

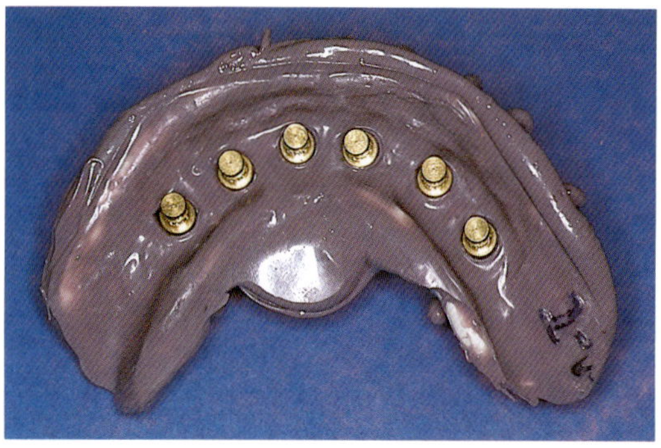

Fig. 398. All abutment replicas are in place within the impression.

(2) Reseating technique

This technique for taking impressions employs tapered impression copings. The procedure was originally developed for taking impression with hydrocolloid materials. At present, the use of rubber impression materials is recommended, due to its higher precision level.

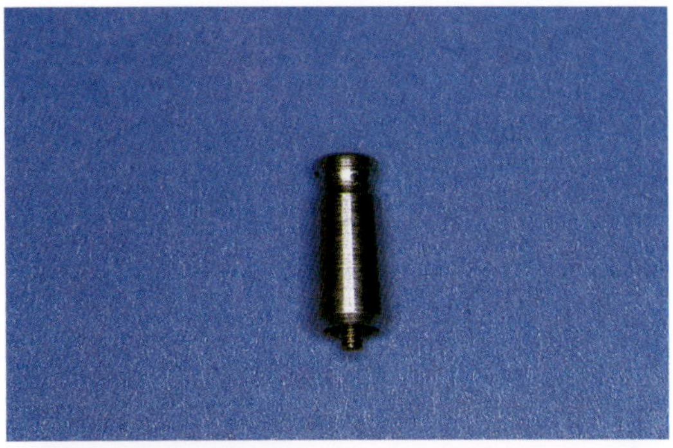

Fig. 399. A tapered impression coping with attached screw is shown.

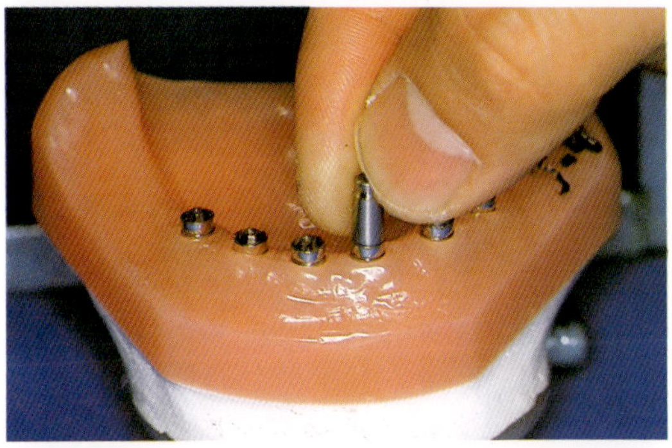

Fig. 400. The tapered impression coping is attached onto the abutments, manually.

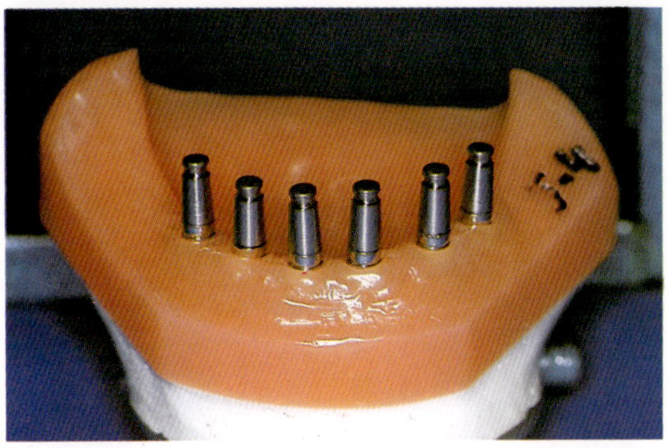

Fig. 401. When all copings are placed on the abutments, their fit to the abutments is checked carefully.

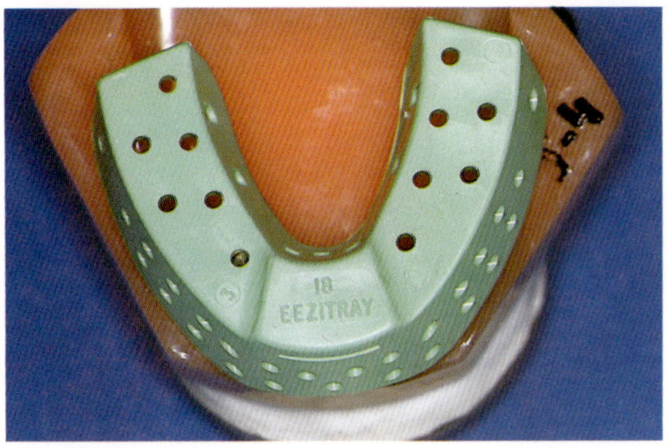

Fig. 402. An impression tray is tested on the model.

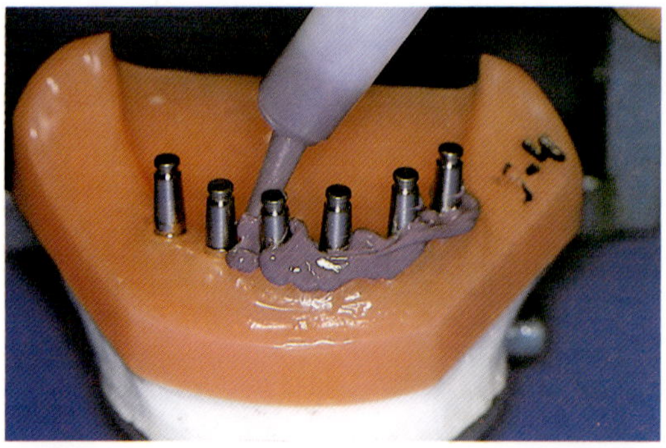

Fig. 403. Using a syringe, impression material is applied around the impression copings.

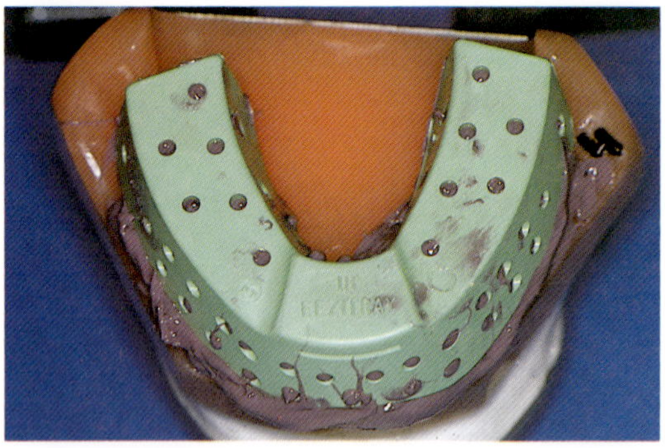

Fig. 404. The tray, carrying impression material, is pressed onto the model.

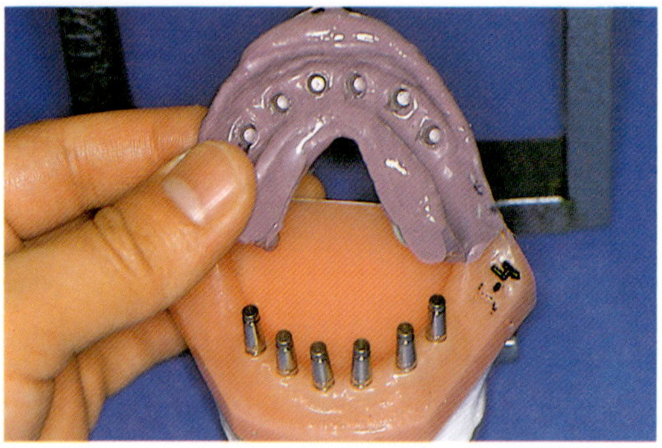

Fig. 405. After the impression material has hardened properly, the tray with the impression material is removed from the model. The copings remain connected to the abutments, when removing the tray, but are thereafter removed from the abutments.

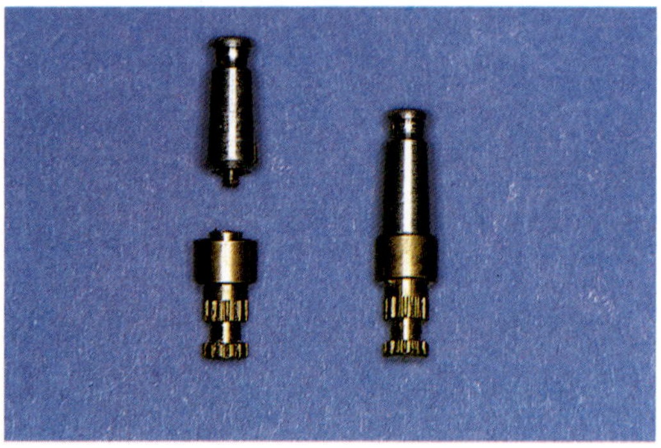

Fig. 406. The combination of the tapered impression coping and the abutment replica. The coping is manually joined to the abutment replica.

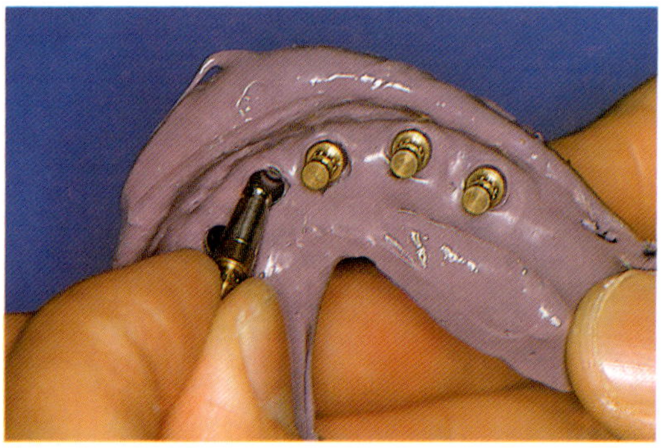

Fig. 407. The joined coping and abutment replica is replaced in the impression material, taking care that a good fit is obtained in the undercut region of the coping tip.

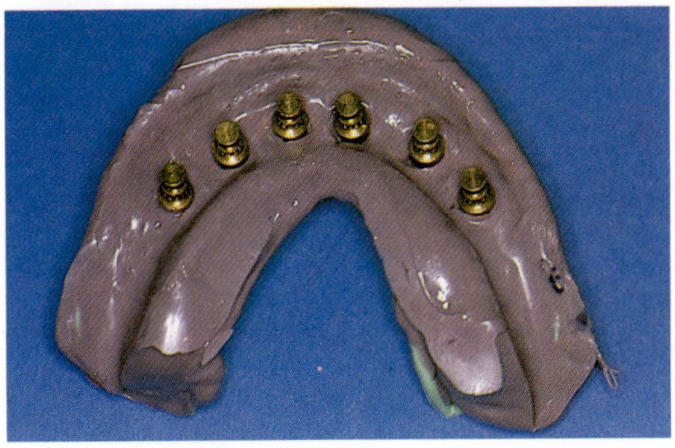

Fig. 408. All abutment replicas, are in place in the impression. The reseating technique is advantageous in that it provides a good fit between the abutment replica and the tapered impression coping. The technique is also applicable to cases in which the use of guide pins is difficult. However, the previously presented pick-up technique is the procedure of first choice.

Bite Registration

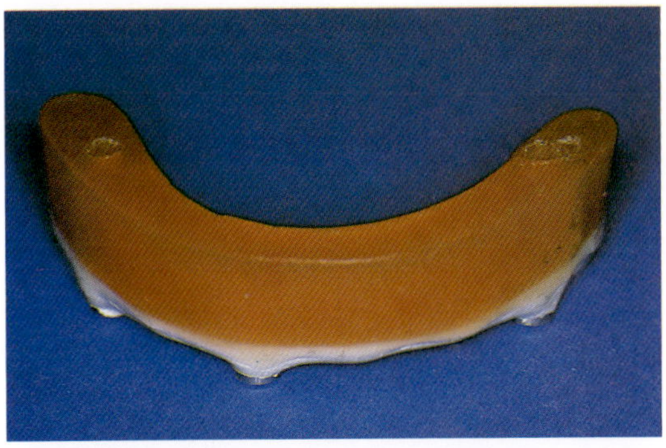

Fig. 409. A complete occlusion rim is created.

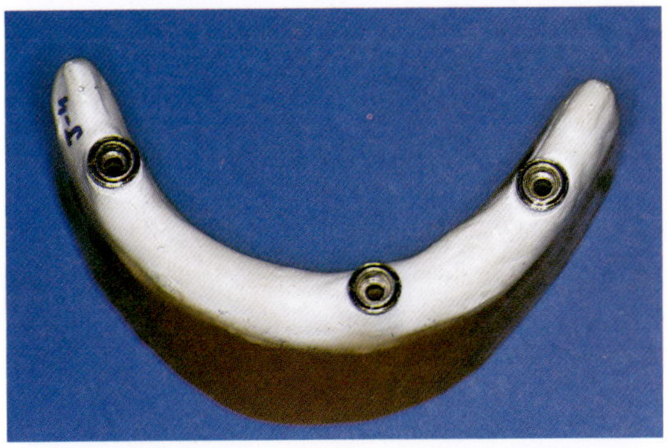

Fig. 410. The base of the occlusion rim is designed to include the gold cylinders and to allow a check of the fit of the cylinders towards the abutments.

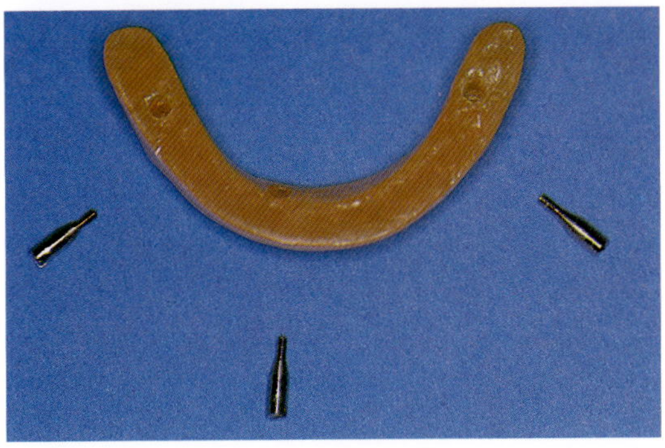

Fig. 411. To retain the occlusion rim onto the abutments, guide pins of lengths that does not hamper occlusion are chosen.

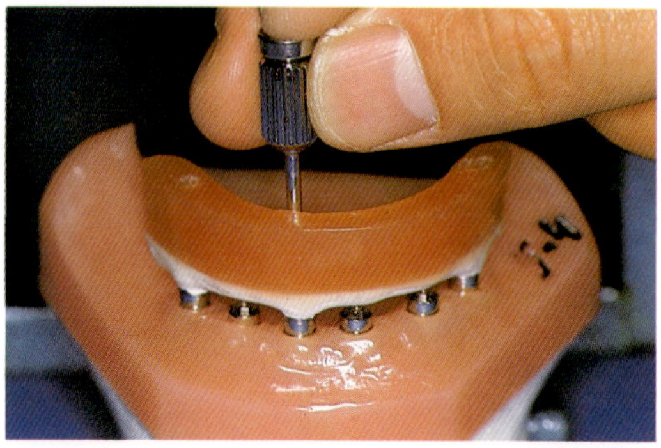

Fig. 412. The occlusion rim is joined to the abutments, using guide pins. In clinical cases, at least 3 pins are used for the attachment.

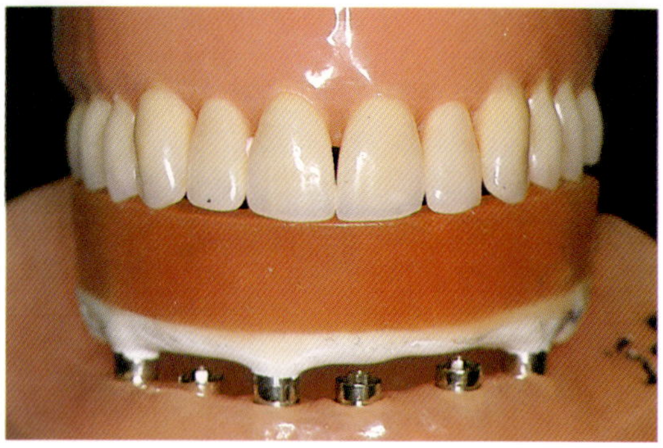

Fig. 413. The bite registration is carried out by routine methods.

Application of a Wax-Up Denture

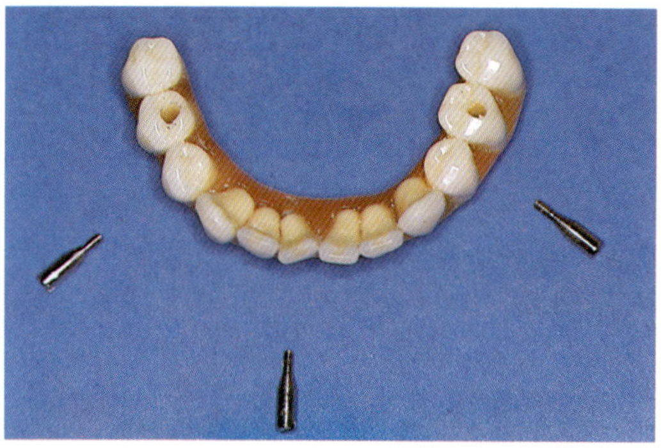

Fig. 414. A wax-up denture has been manufactured. It is applied to the abutments via guide pins.

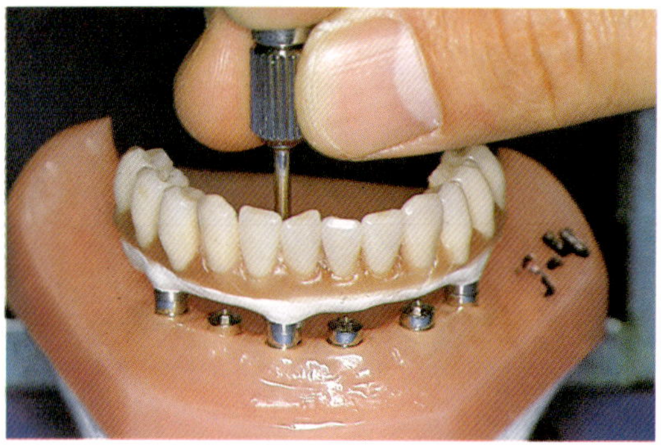

Fig. 415. The wax-up denture in place on the abutments, and being fixed via short guide pins.

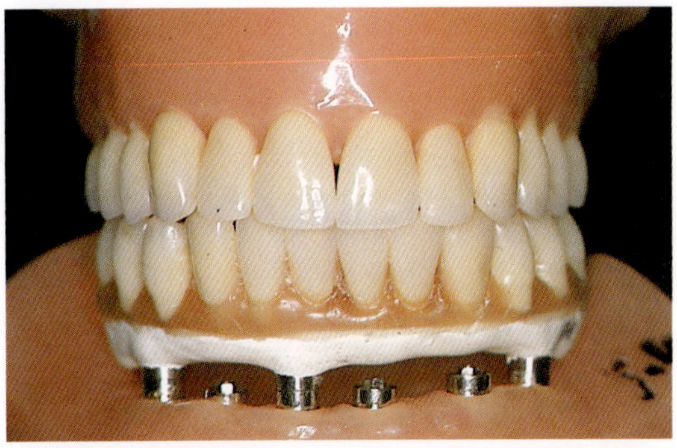

Fig. 416. The position of implants and artificial teeth together with the occlusal relationship are checked. The use of composite resin or acrylic resin teeth is recommended for the occlusal surface, because these materials absorb shock well during occlusion.

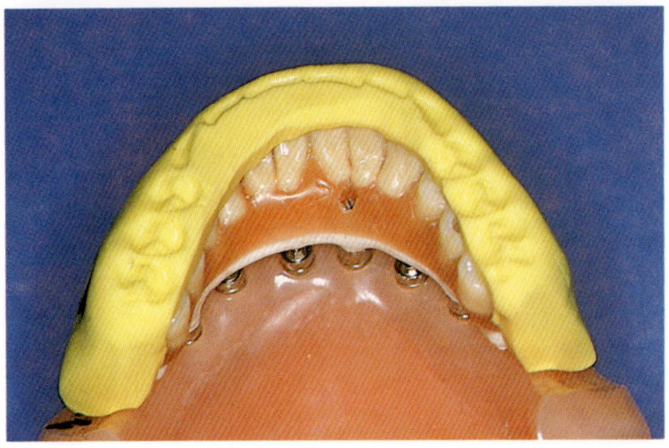

Fig. 417. Using a Labial Index, the position of the artificial teeth is recorded.

Try-In of the Cast Framework

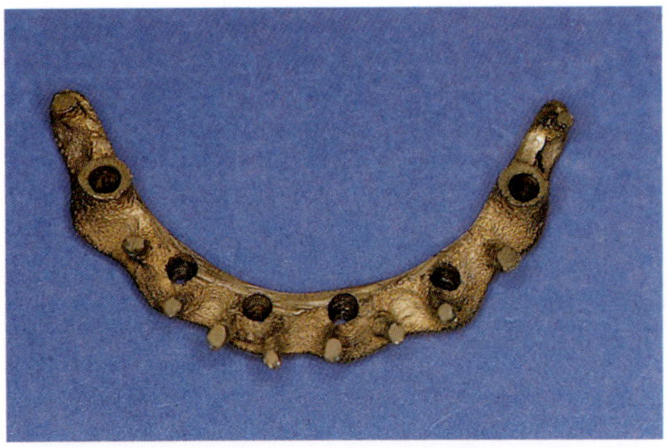

Fig. 418. The superior surface of a complete cast framework. As a rule, one retention is required for each artificial tooth.

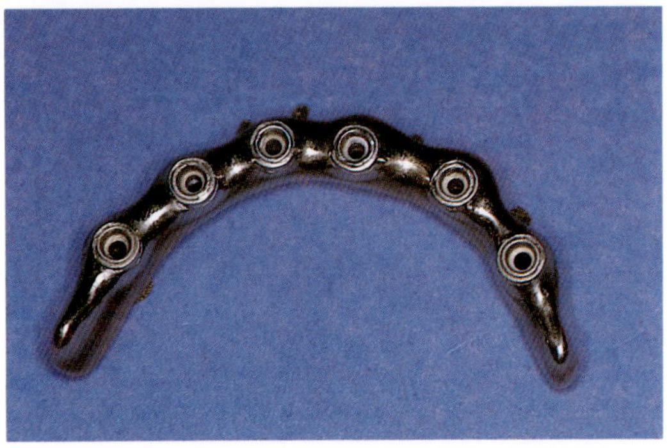

Fig. 419. The mucosal side of a complete cast framework. The extension of a bridge from the distal abutment can be approximately 10 mm in the upper jaw, and about 20 mm in the lower. This difference between the two jaws is due to the difference in bone quality.

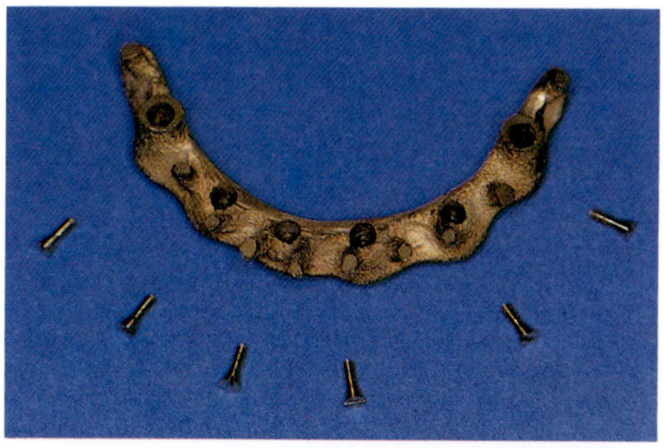

Fig. 420. The framework is attached to the abutments, using gold screws.

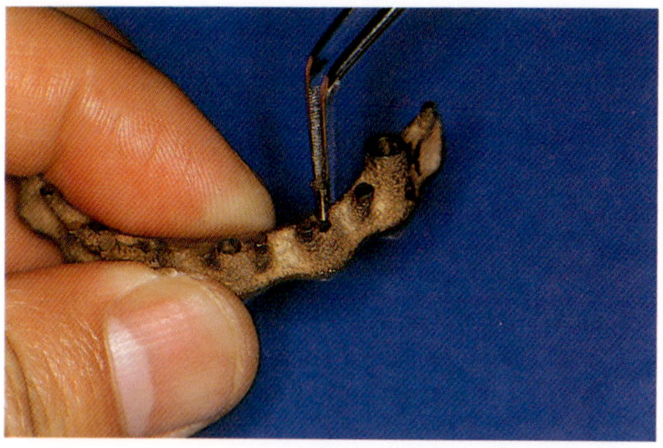

Fig. 421. All gold screws are seated in the screw holes before the framework is fitted onto the abutments of the model.

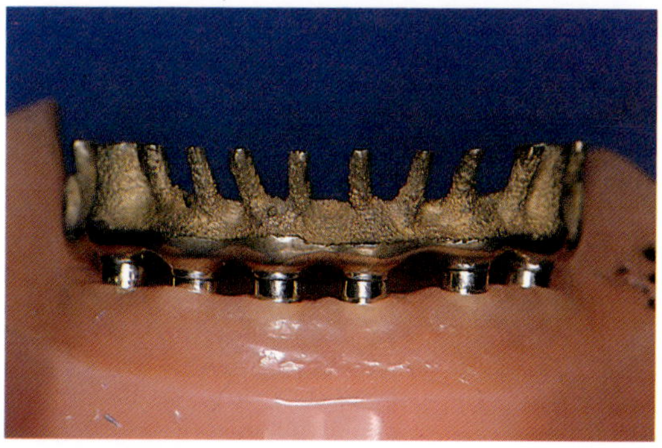

Fig. 422. After placeing the framework onto the abutments it should be checked that there is a passive fit between the abutments and the gold cylinders.

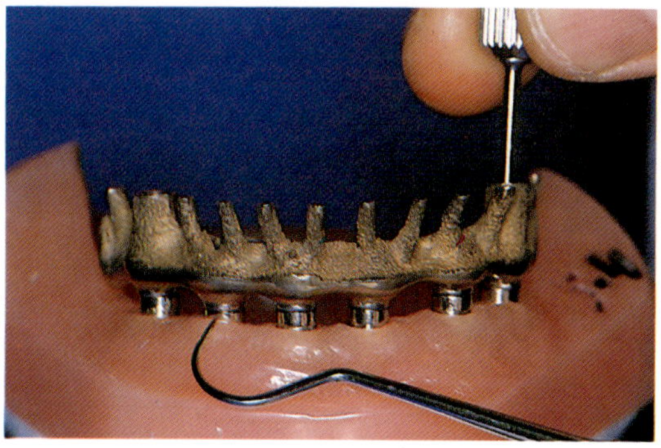

Fig. 423. Thereafter, the most posterior gold screw on one side is tightened to make sure that there is no elevation of the framework on the opposite side. The same procedure is repeated on the other side.

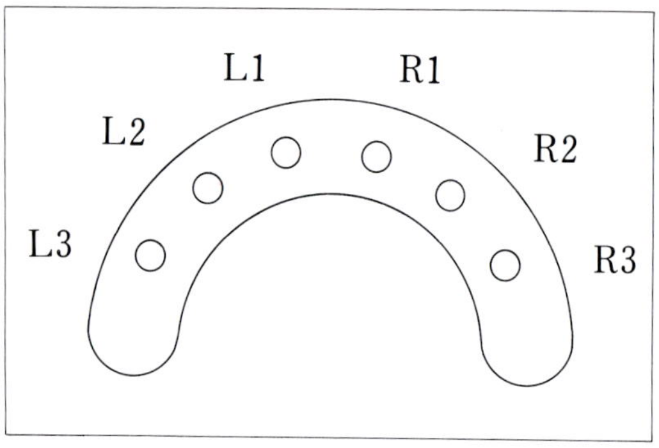

Fig. 424. Usually, the gold screws are tightened in the order of right No. 2, left No. 2, left No. 3, right No. 1, left No. 1 and then right No. 3. Each screw is securely fastened. If the fit of the framework is not good, the order of screw tightening is changed. If a good fit still cannot be obtained, the framework is sectioned, and the parts are placed back on the abutments and joined with Duralay®(Reliance Dental Mfg. Co., Worth, Ill., U. S. A.). The framework is thereafter removed for re-soldering.

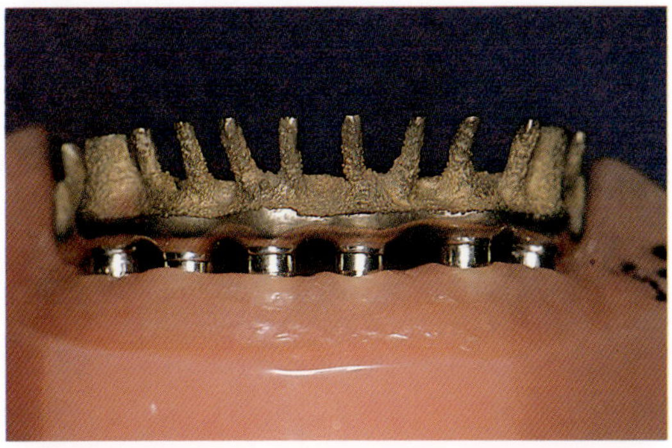

Fig. 425. When the framework has been tightened via all the gold screws, the fit between the gold cylinders and abutments is checked.

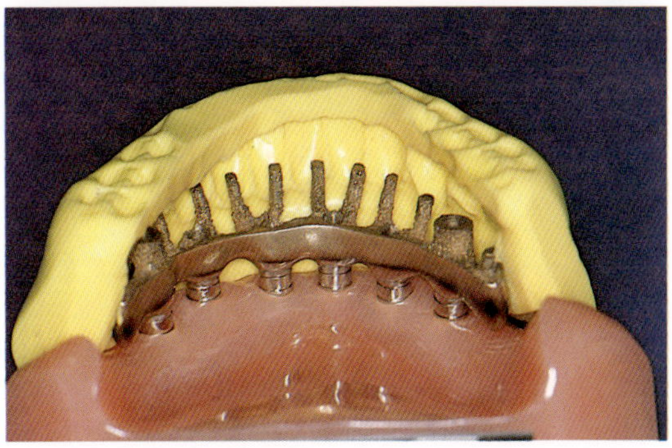

Fig. 426. The relationship between the Labial Index and the framework is thereafter assessed.

> For training in basic procedures, the model shown below is used. Prosthetic procedures have already been described.

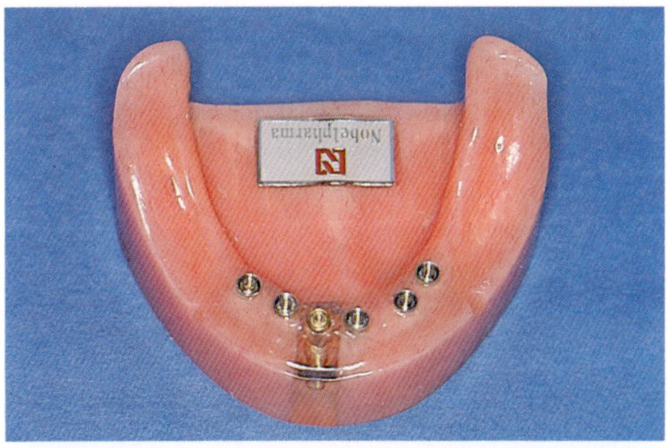

Fig. 427. Lower jaw model. Although this model differs slightly from that used in this text, the prosthetic procedures are the same as those described in the text.

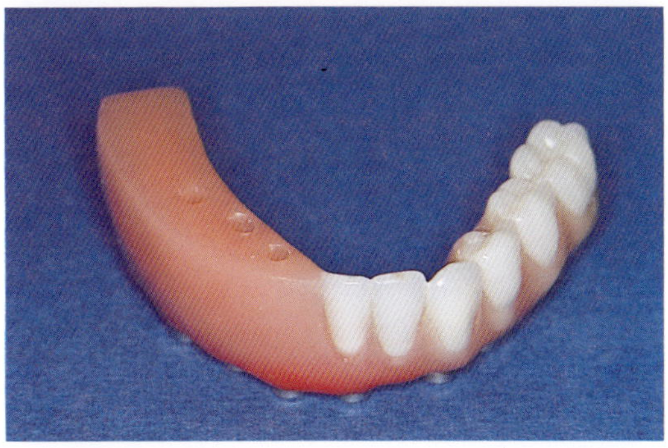

Fig. 428. A occlusion rim with a complete arch of artificial teeth on the left side is shown.

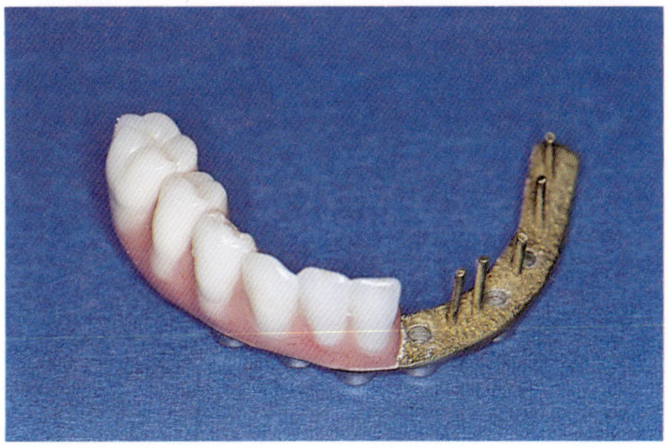

Fig. 429. A metal frame with a complete arch of artificial teeth on the right side is shown.

III. TRAINING THE TECHNICIAN

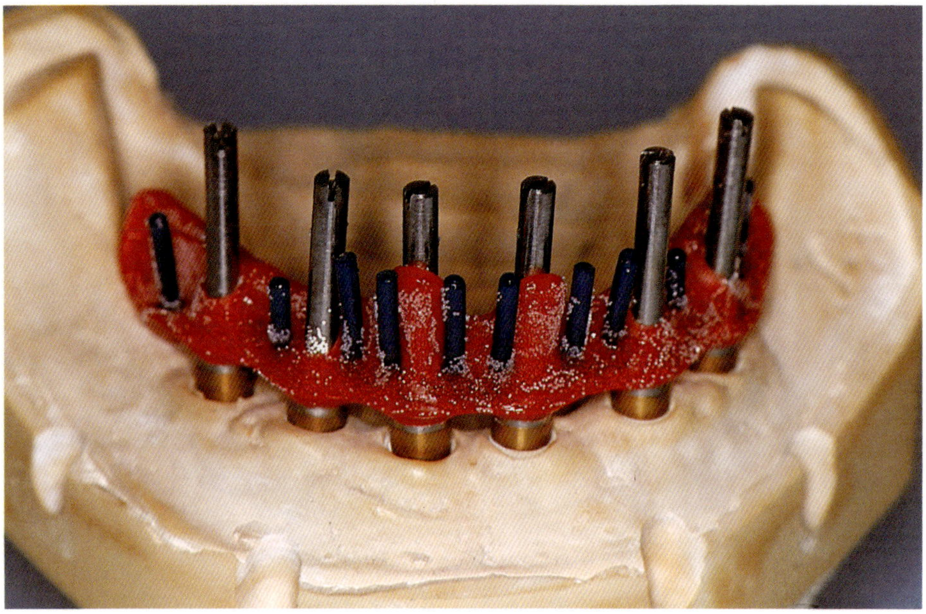

CHAPTER Ⅷ

BASIC TRAINING IN LABORATORY PROCEDURES PART 1

Part 1 includes the following: (1) understanding the composition and handling of the components, needed for the production of implant dentures; and (2) preparation of custom trays, working models, trial bases, arrangement of artificial teeth and the labial index, as well as formation of the wax framework, investing, casting, resin polymerization and polishing, with the use of training models.

Preparation of Custom Trays

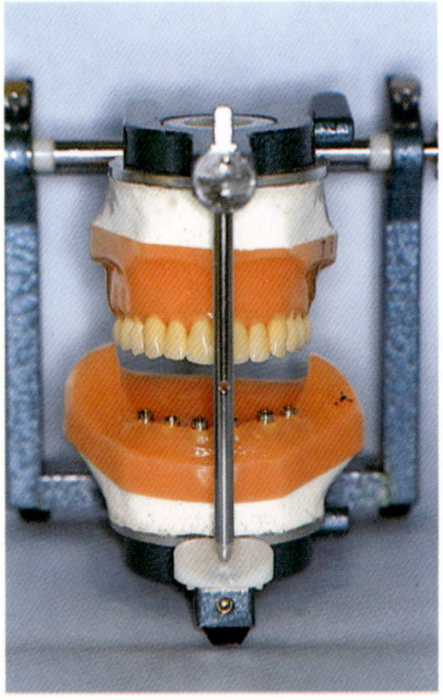

Fig. 430. A model used for training.
The lower jaw model has six inserted fixtures connected with abutments.

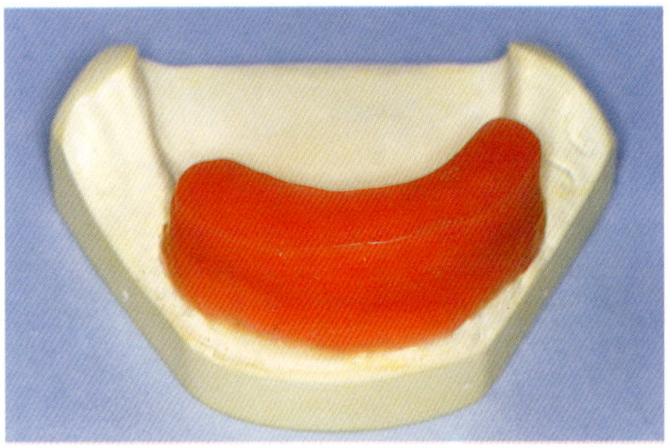

Fig. 431. An impression of the lower jaw model is taken with an alginate impression material. A study cast model is made, on which a wax rim is prepared and fixed to the area of the abutments. The height of the wax rim is made about 1 mm shorter than the length of the guide pins. The labio-lingual width of the wax rim is made 1.5 mm wider than the squared impression copings.

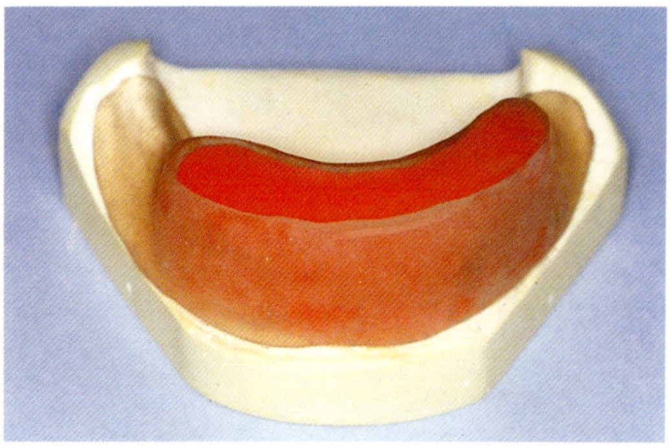

Fig. 432. According to the routine method for creating distal extensions of partial dentures, a tray resin material is compressed to the wax rim and alveolar ridge, maintaining a window on the upper side of the wax rim.

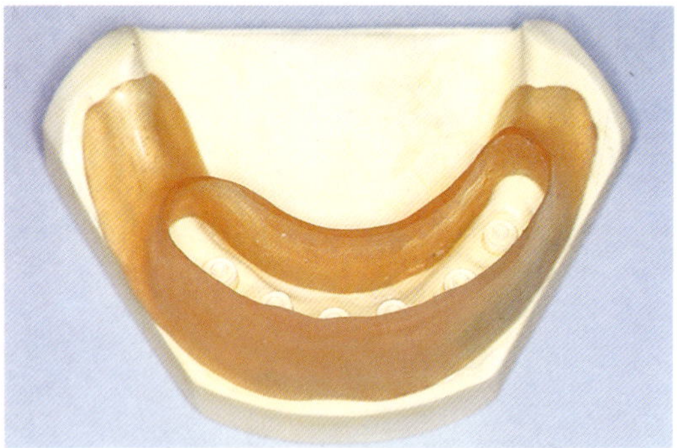

Fig. 433. After removing the waxrim, a complete custom tray has been fabricated.

Fabrication of a Working Model

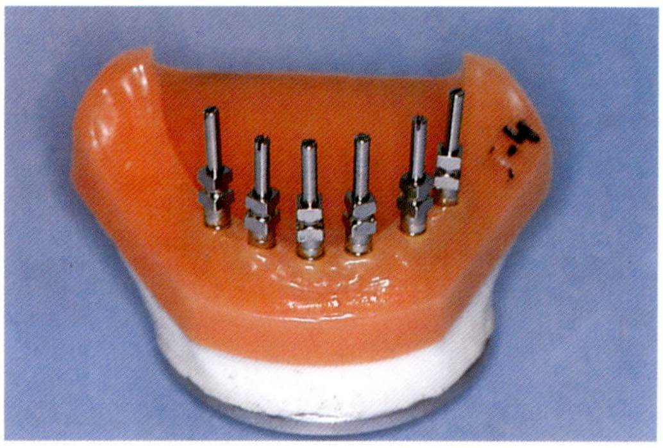

Fig. 434. Using long guide pins, the squared impression copings are connected to the abutments on the resin working model.

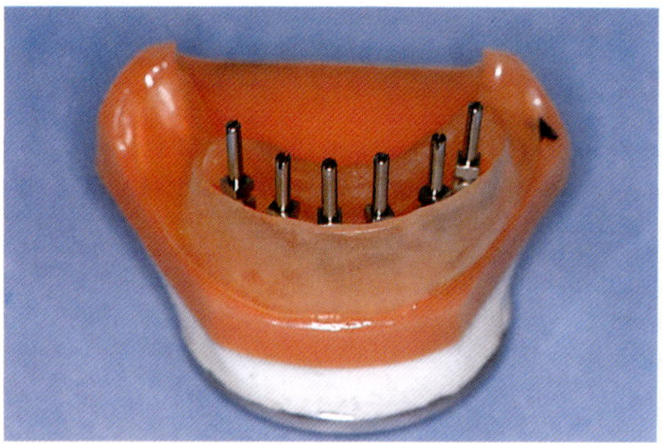

Fig. 435. The fabricated custom tray is placed on the working model. Confirm that an appropriate space is present between the custom tray and the squared impression copings and guide pins.

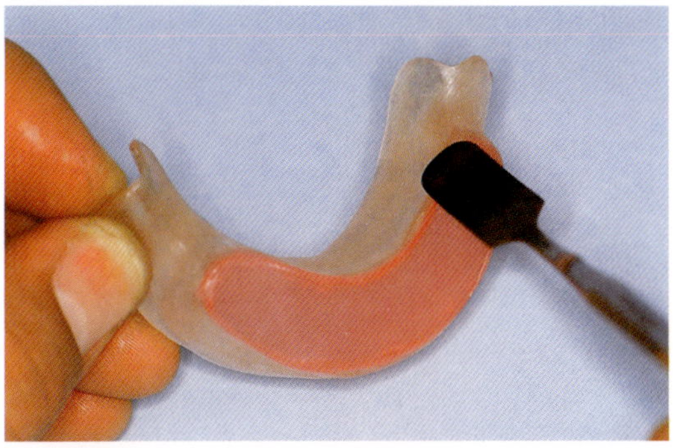

Fig. 436. The window of the tray is closed with paraffin wax.

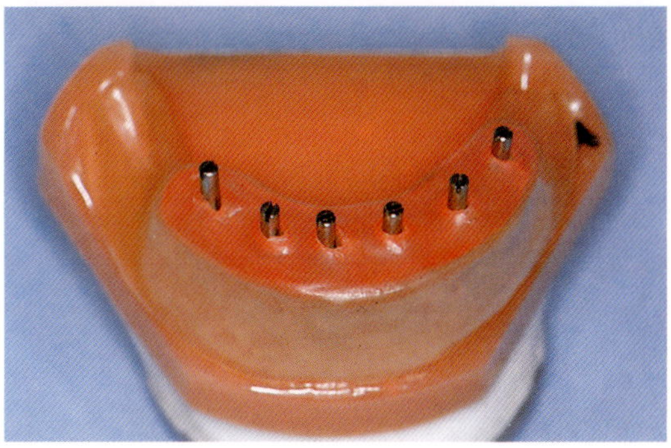

Fig. 437. After softening the paraffin wax over a flame, the tray is applied to the model. The tips of the guide pins are allowed to perforate through the wax so their positions are marked.

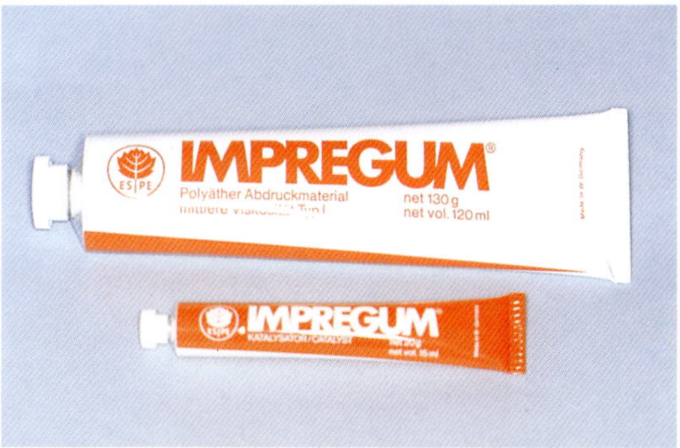

Fig. 438. Preparation of impression material.

A polyether rubber impression material (*Impregum*®) is used. In clinical cases, the impression is taken by dentists. In this training, the dental technicians take the impression of the model to prepare a working model.

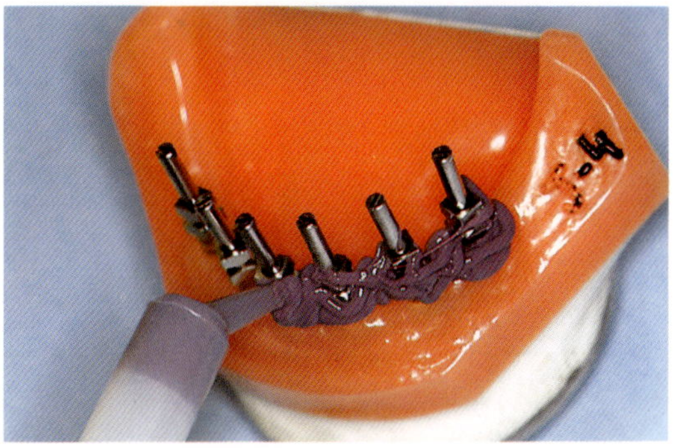

Fig. 439. First, the impression material is applied around the abutments, using a syringe.

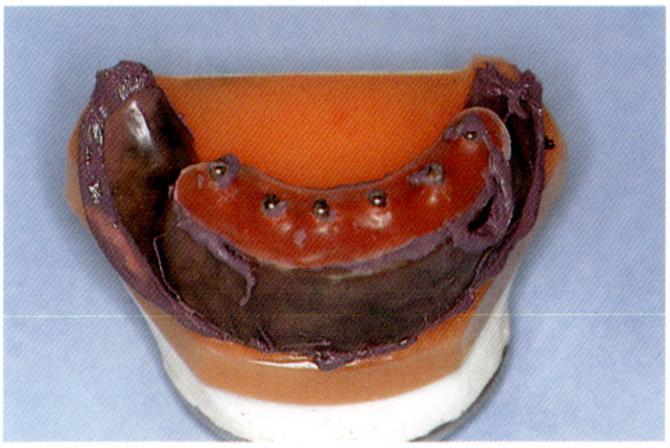

Fig. 440. The impression material is then applied to the tray, which is pressed onto the model in such a way that the guide pins fit the perforations in the wax lid.

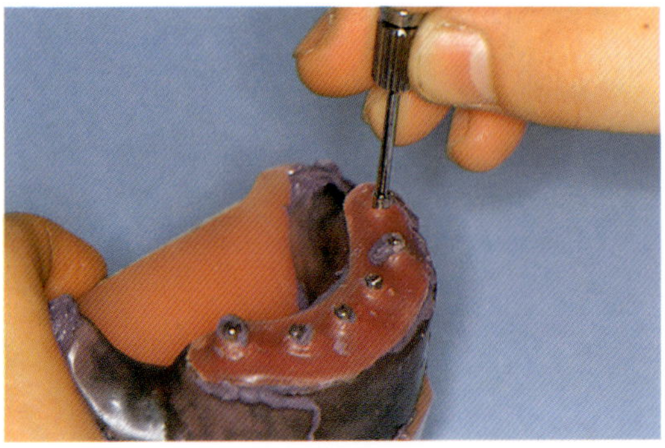

Fig. 441. After the impression material has set the guide pins are loosened with a screwdriver to remove the tray and the impression material from the model.

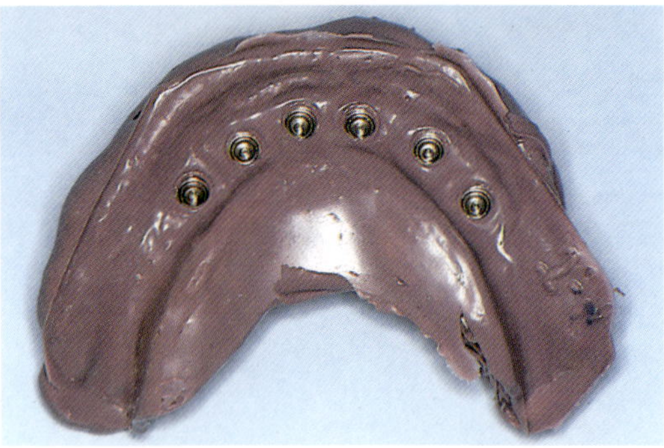

Fig. 442. Detailed inspection of the impression is carried out.

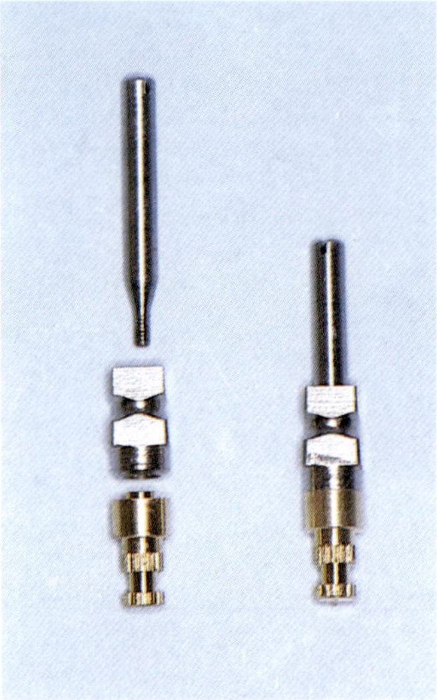

Fig. 443. Preparation of abutment replicas.

This figure shows the relationship between the squared impression copings and the abutment replicas.

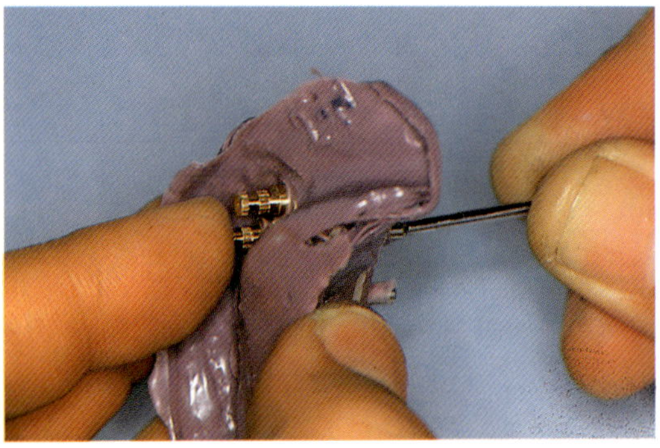

Fig. 444. Using guide pins, the abutment replicas are screwed onto the squared impression copings of the impression.

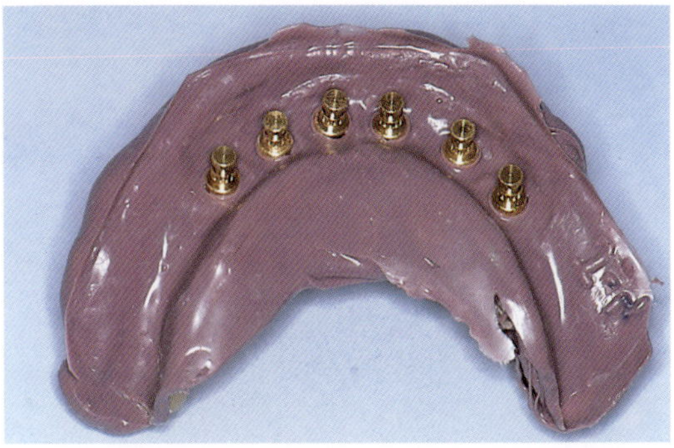

Fig. 445. Completed application of the abutment replicas.

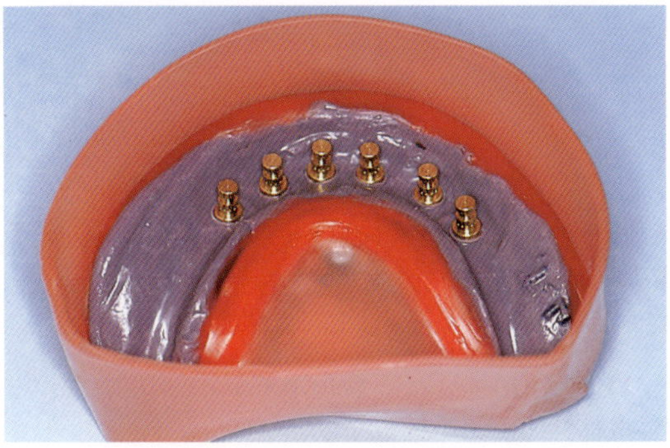

Fig. 446. Routine boxing of the impression is performed.

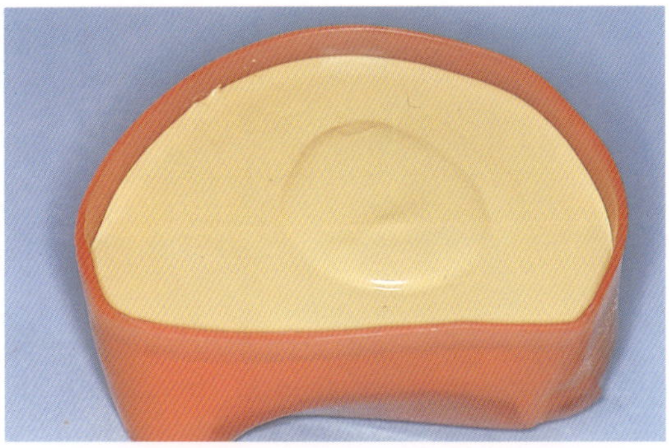

Fig. 447. Plaster (ultrahard plaster) is poured into the box to a thickness of at least 15 mm from the base of the impression.

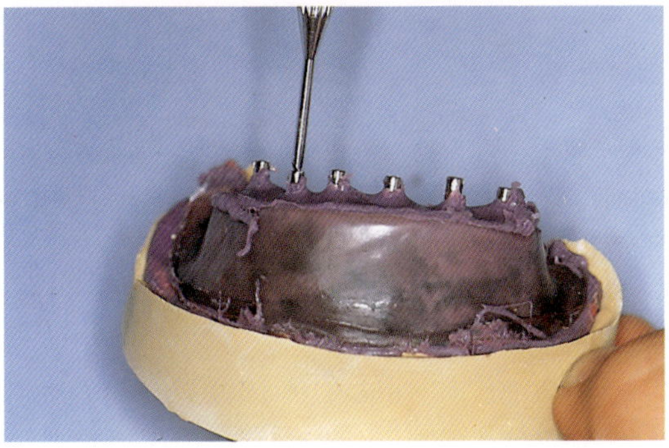

Fig. 448. When the plaster has set, the guide pins are loosened with a screwdriver to remove the tray and the impression material from the model.

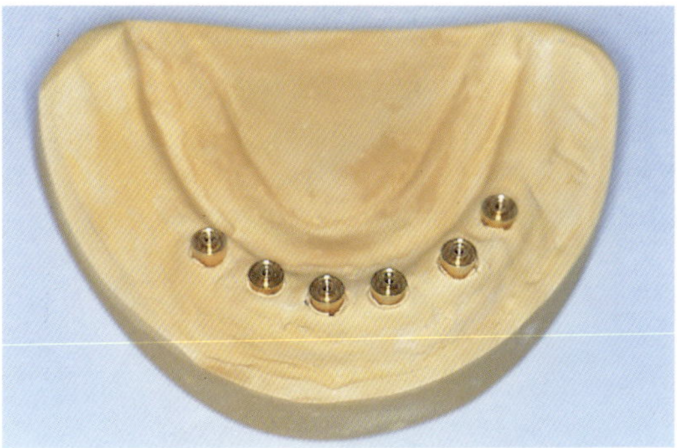

Fig. 449. Excessive plaster is trimmed to complete a working model, in which the positions of the abutments are accurately reproduced.

Preparation of the Occlusion Rim

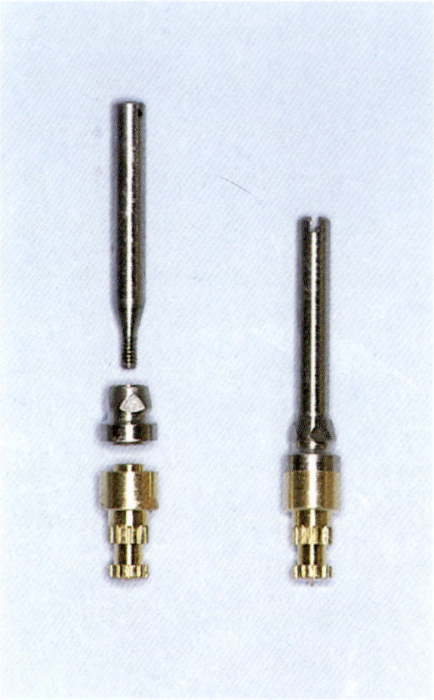

Fig. 450. Preparation of gold cylinders.

The figure shows the relationship between gold cylinders, guide pins and abutment replicas.

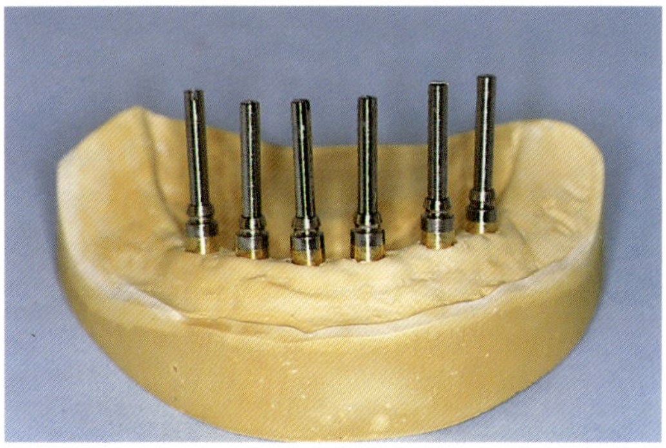

Fig. 451. Using the guide pins, the gold cylinders are connected to the abutment replicas of the working model.

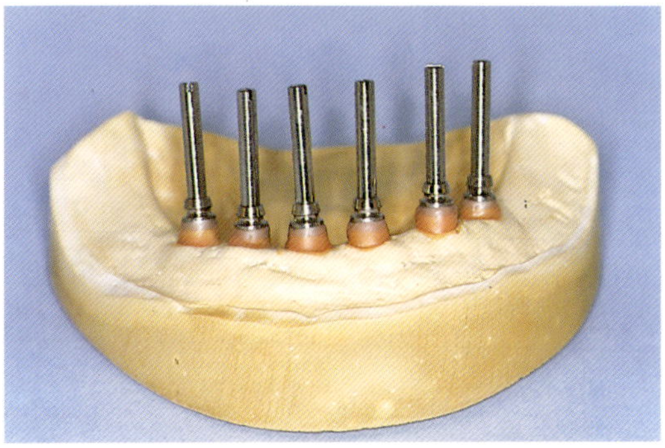

Fig. 452. Paraffin wax is applied around the abutment replicas to serve as a relief of under cuts.

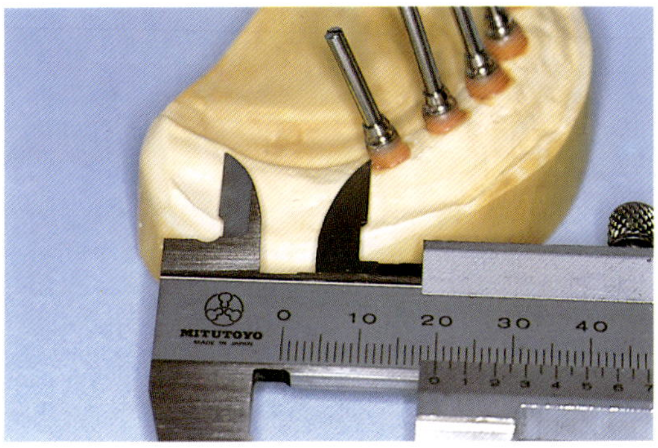

Fig. 453. Determination of the position of the posterior margin of the occlusion rim.

As a rule, the length of the free end of an implant denture from the most distal abutment must be within 20 mm for the lower jaw and within 10 mm for the upper jaw. In this training session, the required length is 20 mm.

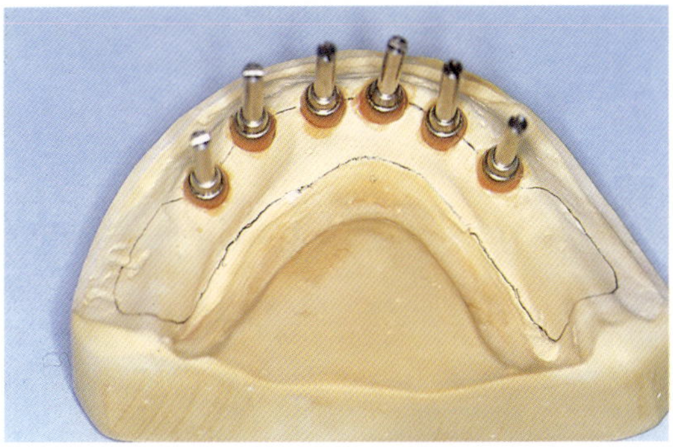

Fig. 454. Contour of the base plate.

To enable checking of the fit between the gold cylinders and the abutments, the labial side of the gold cylinders should not be covered by the base plate. In other regions, the base plate is designed similarly to what is used for routine free-end partial dentures.

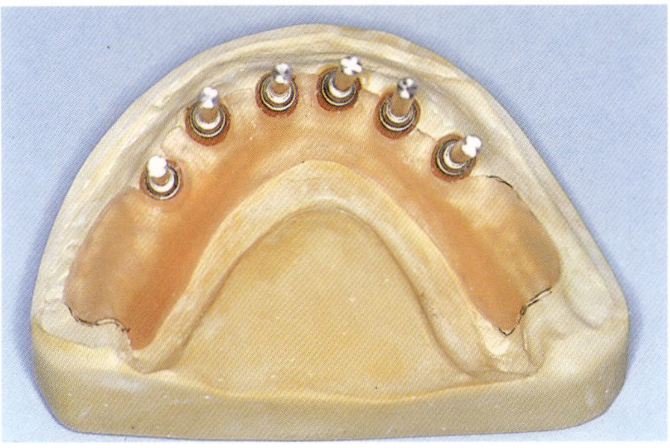

Fig. 455. A self-curing resin is applied to the model, within the marks for the base plate and to a thickness of about 1 mm. The resin is compressed along the contour line, and excess material is trimmed away.

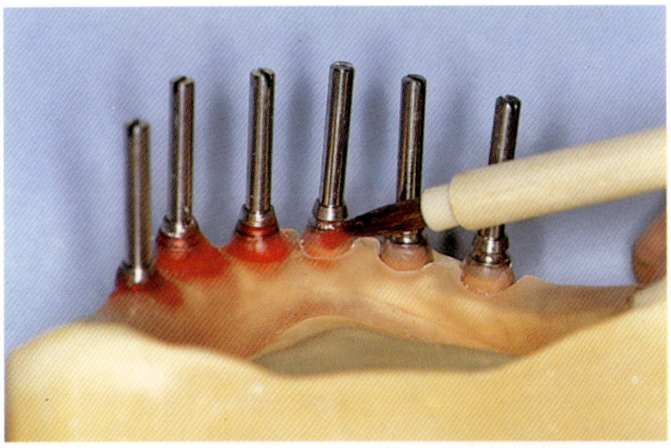

Fig. 456. After preparing the base plate, *Duralay*® is applied to the contact surfaces with the gold cylinders, linking them to the base plate.

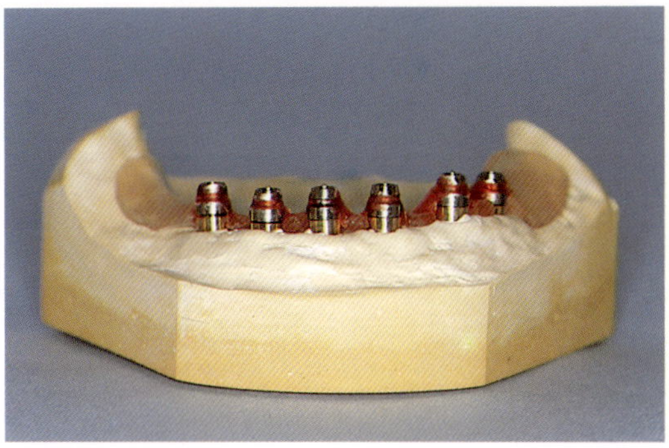

Fig. 457. After linking the base plate to the gold cylinders, the fit between the gold cylinders and the abutment replicas is checked.

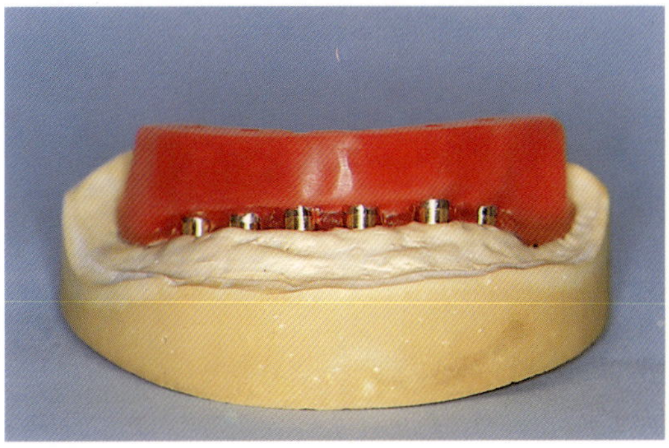

Fig. 458. Using paraffin wax, an occlusion rim is prepared onto the base plate. The labial side of the base is kept open so that the fit of the gold cylinders to the abutment replicas can be checked at any time.

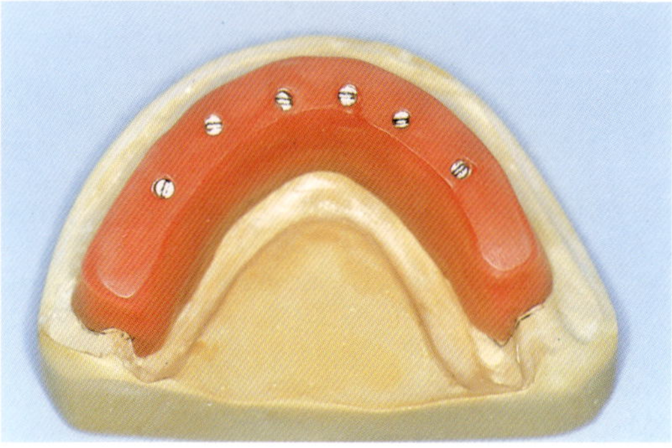

Fig. 459. A complete wax occlusion rim, together with its guide pins.

Mounting of the Working Cast in the Articulator

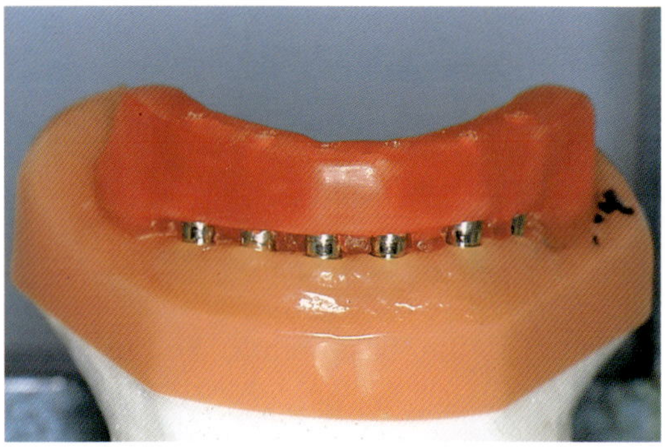

Fig. 460. Using guide pins, the occlusion rim is connected to the abutments of the model.

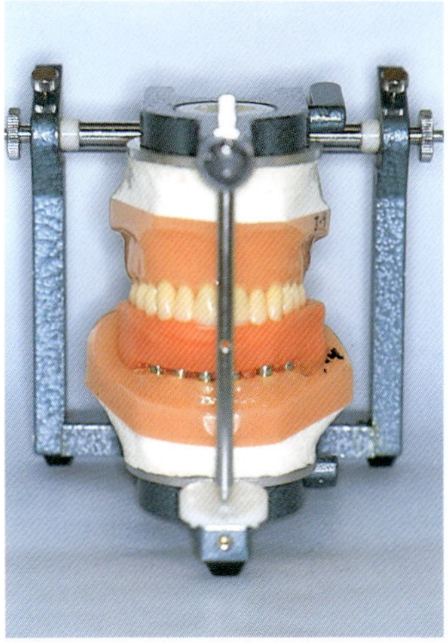

Fig. 461. The occlusion rim is adjusted, and the jaw relationship is checked.

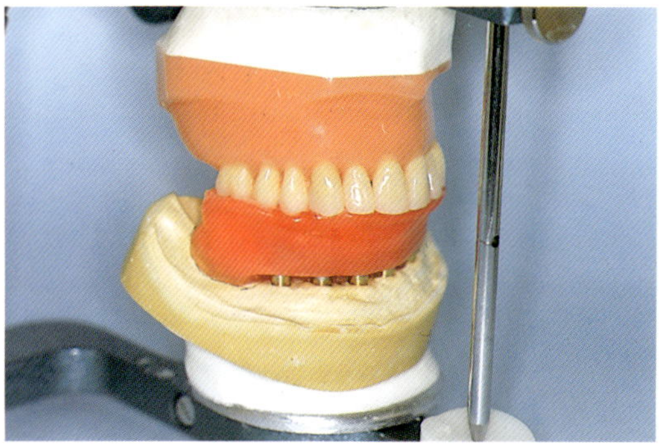

Fig. 462. The occlusion rim is transferred to a working cast, and the model is mounted in the articulator.

Arrangement of Artificial Teeth

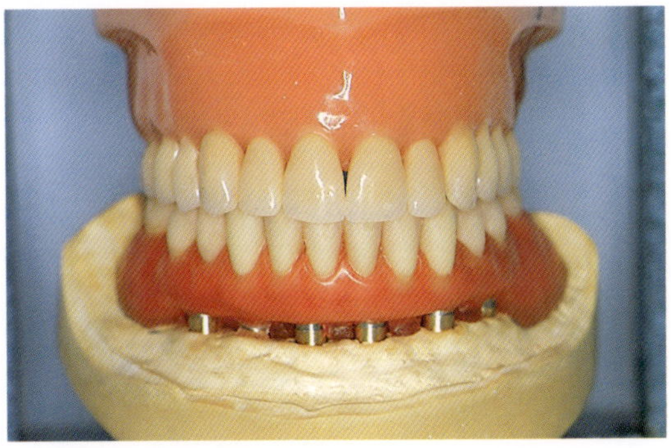

Fig. 463. The artificial teeth are arranged in accordance with instructions from the dentist. Occlusion during lateral movement must be cuspid-protected, if the antagonistic teeth are natural teeth, and full-balanced if a removable denture is used in the opposite jaw. Acrylic resin teeth are utilized in order to absorb occlusal shock forces.

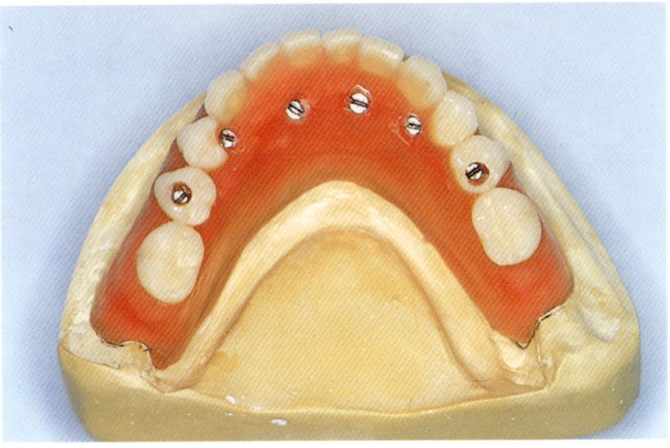

Fig. 464. The relationship between the guide pins and the artificial teeth.

If the guide pins interfere the positions of the artificial teeth, these are adjusted accordingly, to create the bridge locking screw canals.

Preparation of a Labial Index

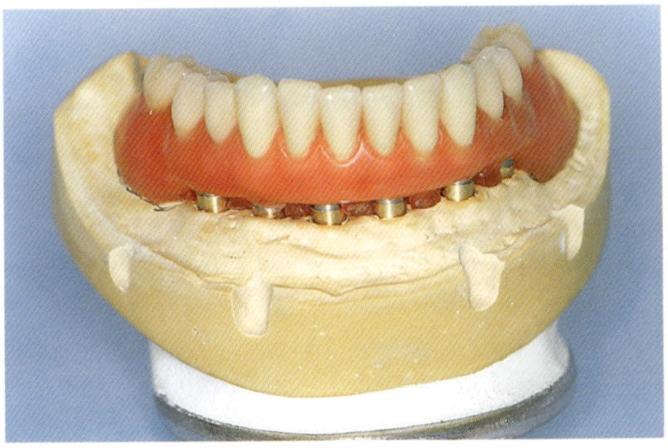

Fig. 465. When the trial denture has been completed, grooves to determine the position of the labial index are created on the bucco-labial side of the working model.

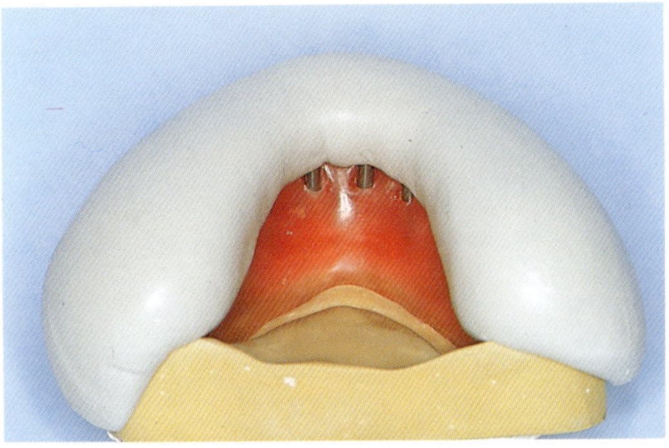

Fig. 466. Using a silicon impression putty material, a labial index for the artificial teeth and bucco-labial gum is prepared.

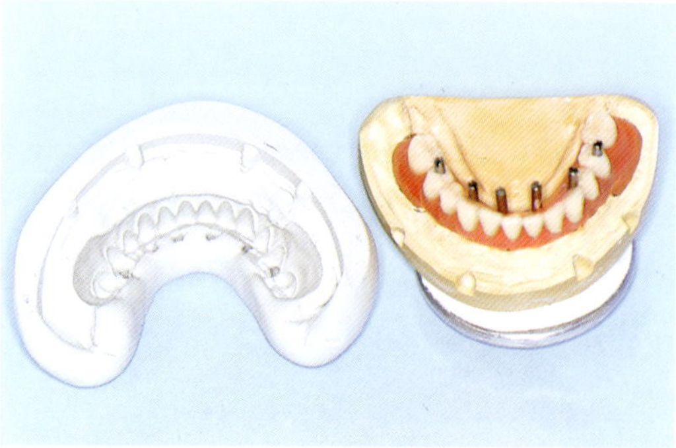

Fig. 467. A complete labial index.

Wax-Up of the Framework

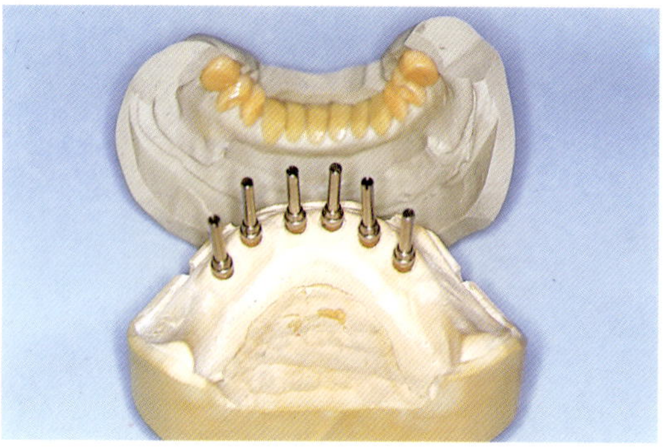

Fig. 468. The wax is removed from the artificial teeth and base plate, and the artificial teeth are replaced in the labial index.

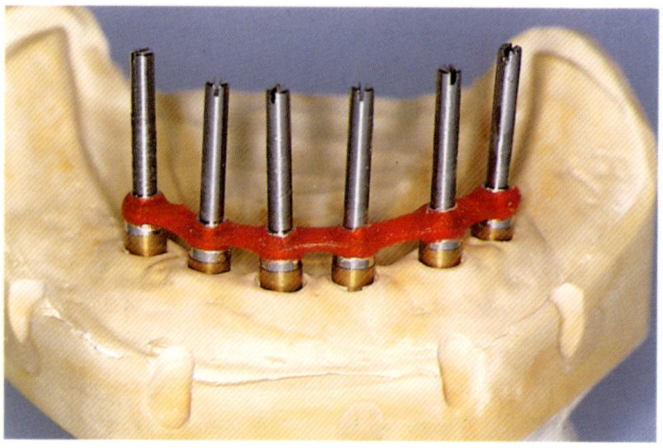

Fig. 469. *Duralay* ® is applied around the gold cylinders in a circular form to connect and fix the cylinders.

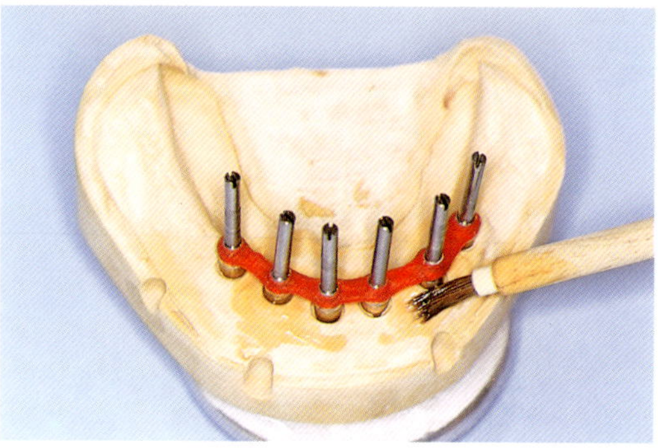

Fig. 470. A wax-separating agent is applied to the surface of the plaster model.

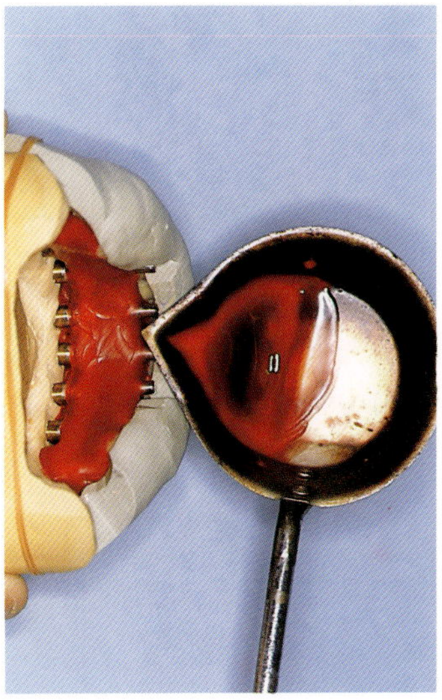

Fig. 471. The labial index together with the artificial teeth are replaced on the model. In preparation for the framework of the prosthesis, inlay wax is poured into the area corresponding to the denture from the lingual side.

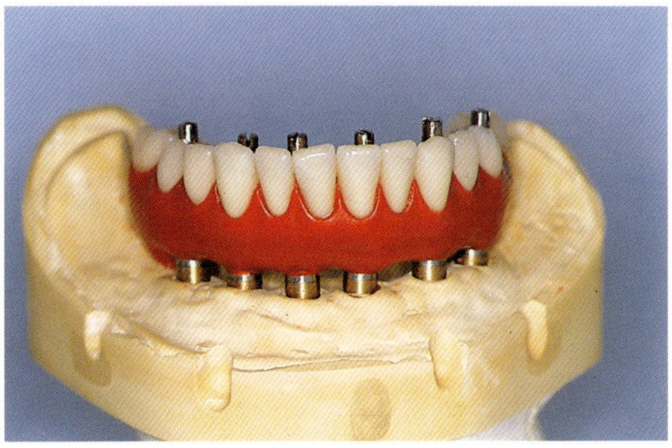

Fig. 472. After the inlay wax has hardened, the labial index is removed, and any excess or shortage of wax is adjusted for. In this way, the overall shape of the prosthesis is determined.

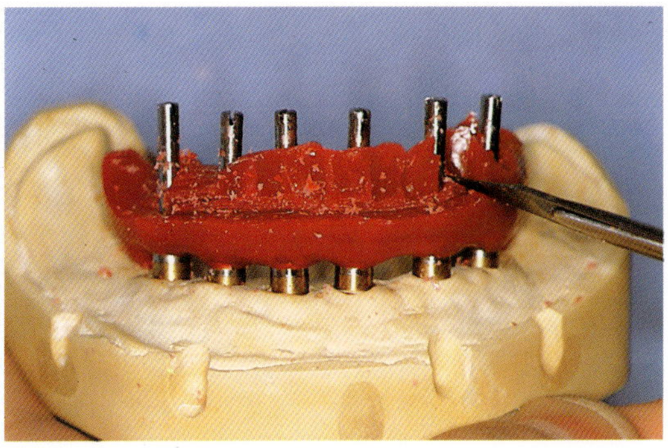

Fig. 473. The artificial teeth are removed, and the outer wax is trimmed to form the framework.

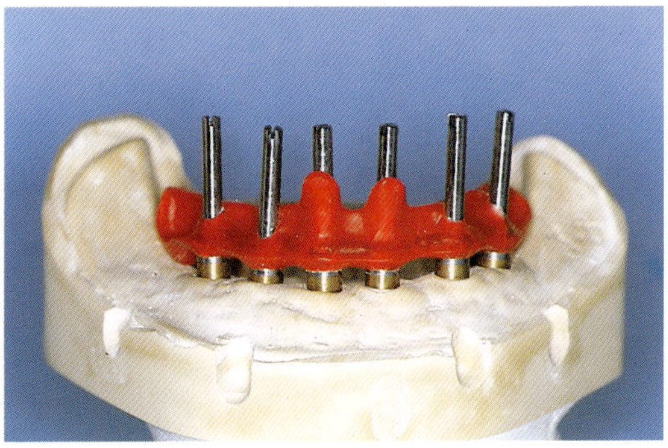

Fig. 474. The central region of the framework, when viewed horizontally, is given a concave form. The design of the labial side is created with attention given to esthetics.

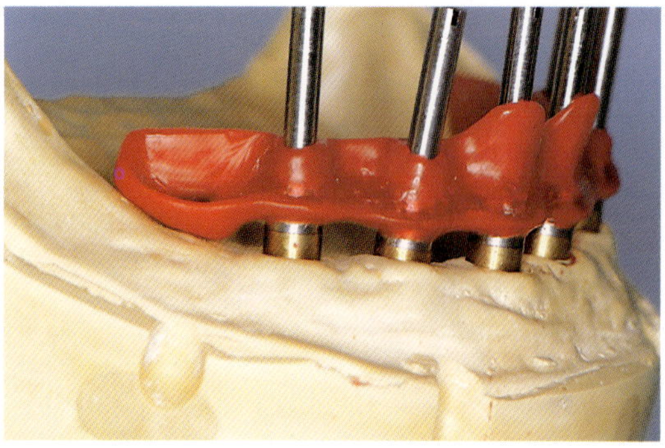

Fig. 475. The base of the framework must be U-shaped, with the gold cylinders being exposed 1 mm. The framework, within the abutment region, must be about 2–3 mm away from the mucosal surface of the alveolar crest to allow for easy cleaning. The base of the free end saddles of the framework structure is designed so that it is U-shaped and in slight contact with the alveolar crest.

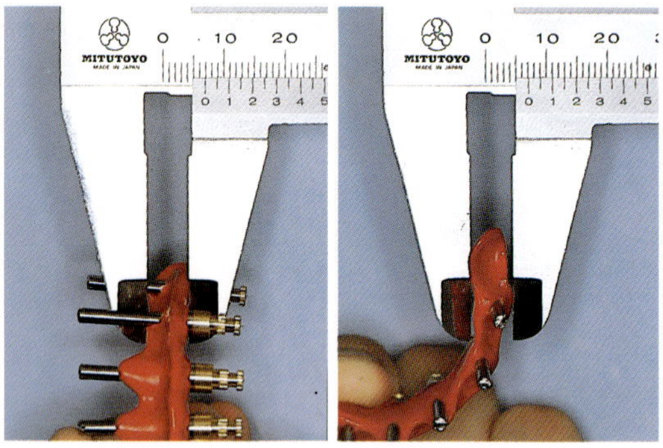

Fig. 476. As a rule, the width and height of the framework must be at least 5 mm, in order to create sufficient vertical and horizontal strength of the structure.

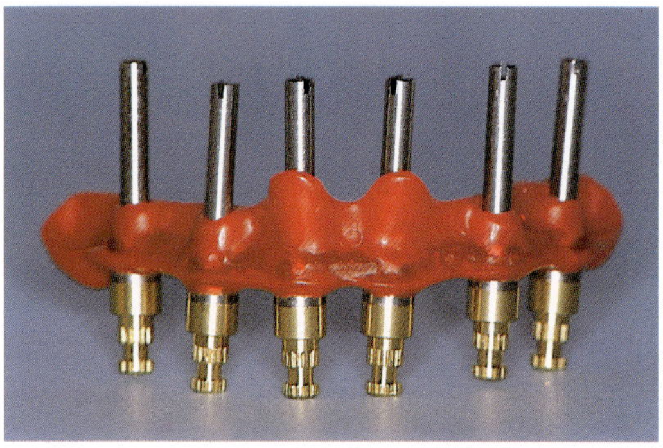

Fig. 477. The completed wax-up of the framework together with guide pins and abutment replicas.

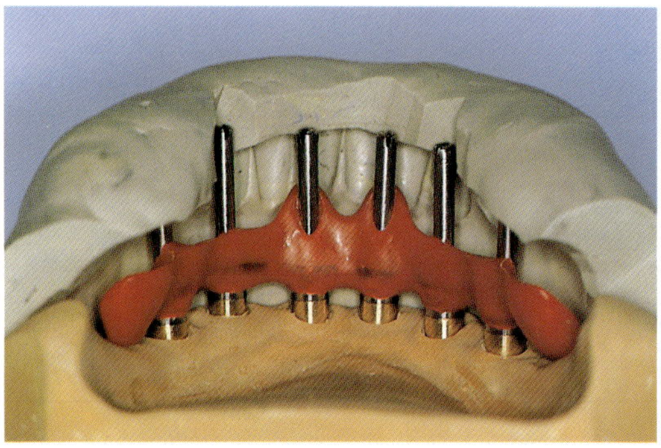

Fig. 478. After replacing the labial index to the working model, the space between the index and the framework is checked.

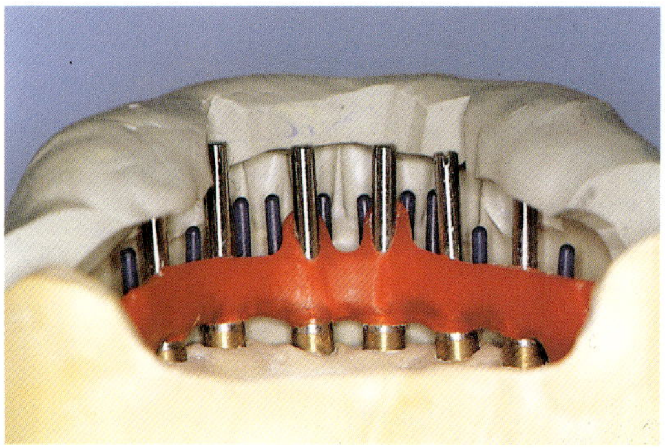

Fig. 479. Retention posts are applied to the wax framework within the areas reserved for artificial teeth, and the waxup is once again checked together with the labial index.

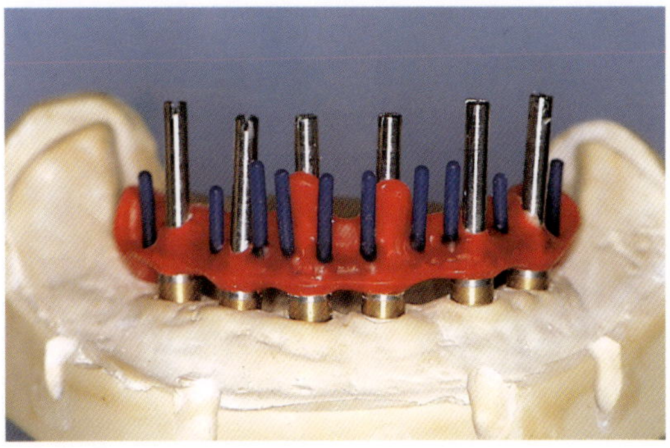

Fig. 480. One retention post is created for each artificial tooth.

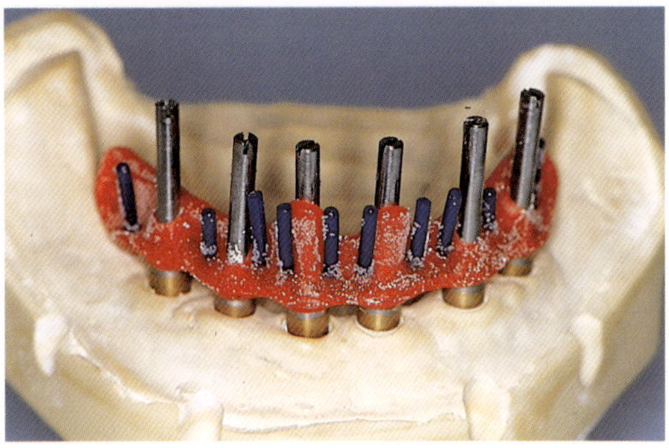

Fig. 481. Retention beads are attached to complete the wax-up of the framework.

Investing, Casting and Polishing of the Framework

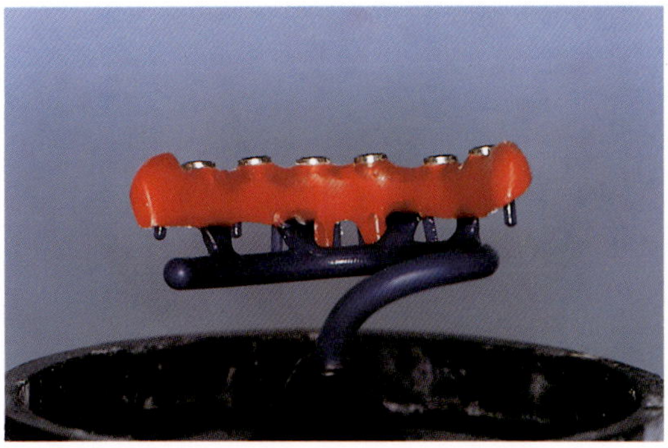

Fig. 482. The framework is produced via one-piece casting or split-casting, followed by soldering.

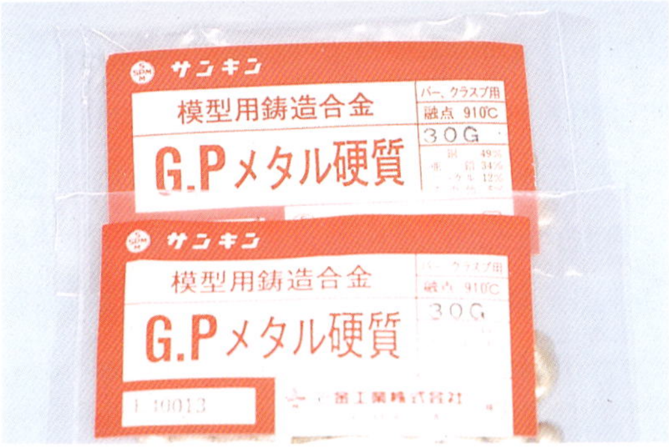

Fig. 483. In clinical situations, Type III or IV gold alloys are used for framework casting. In this trial, the substitute alloy metal (a GP metal®) is utilized.

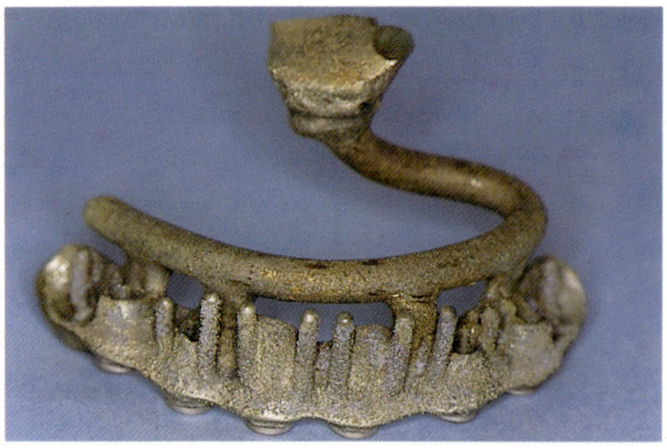

Fig. 484. After casting, the framework is washed with an acid.

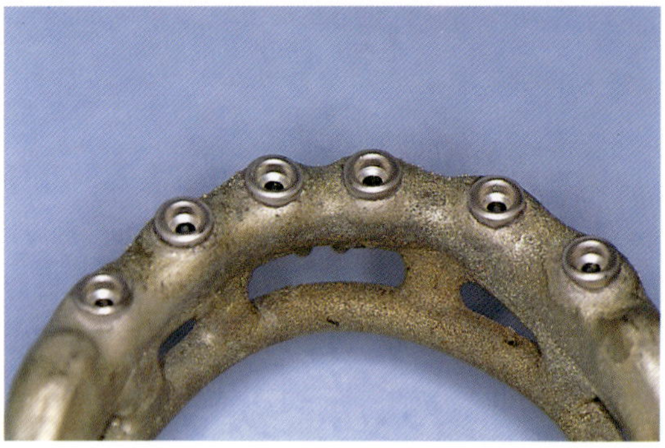

Fig. 485. During investing and casting, care is taken to avoid invasion of metal into the area around the gold cylinders.

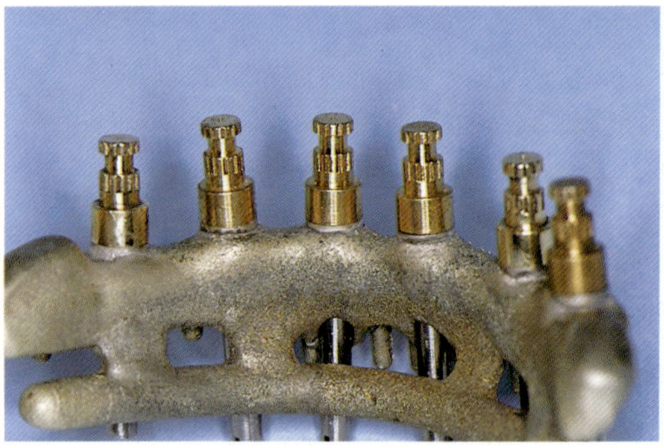

Fig. 486. When polishing the framework, the margin of the gold cylinders is protected by connecting the abutment replicas or the protection caps (see Fig. 511) to the cylinders via the guide pins.

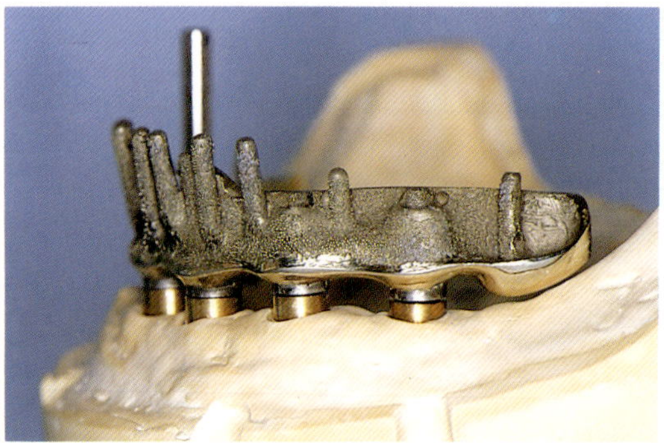

Fig. 487. After the framework has been polished, it is important to check that investment material does not remain on the inner surface of the gold cylinders. The fit between the abutment replicas and gold cylinders on the working model should also be carefully checked. Improper framework fit will cause abnormal stress within the anchorage unit, which might lead to fracture of the components or even a loss of the osseointegration. If the fit is judged to be poor, the framework must be cut into sections, which are replaced on the model for new control of their fit. The sections are thereafter resoldered.

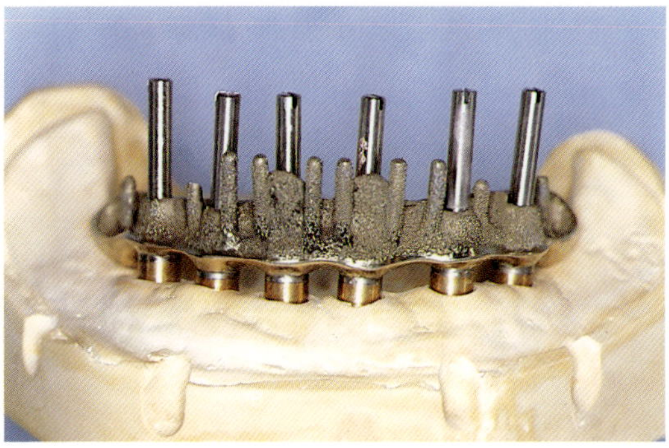

Fig. 488. A complete cast framework in position on the working model.

Resin Polymerization, Polishing and Completion

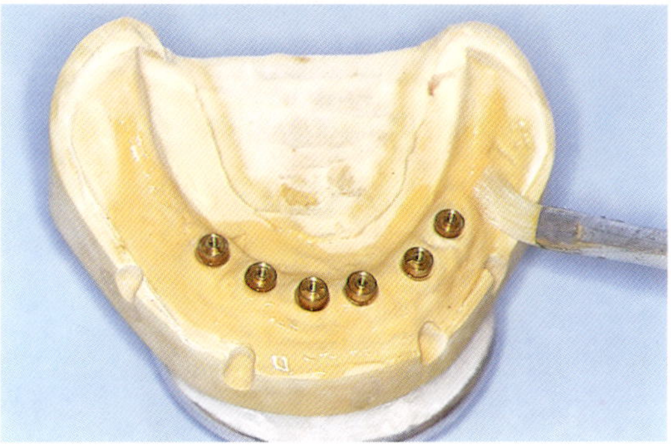

Fig. 489. A sufficient amount of resin-separating agent is applied to the plaster model.

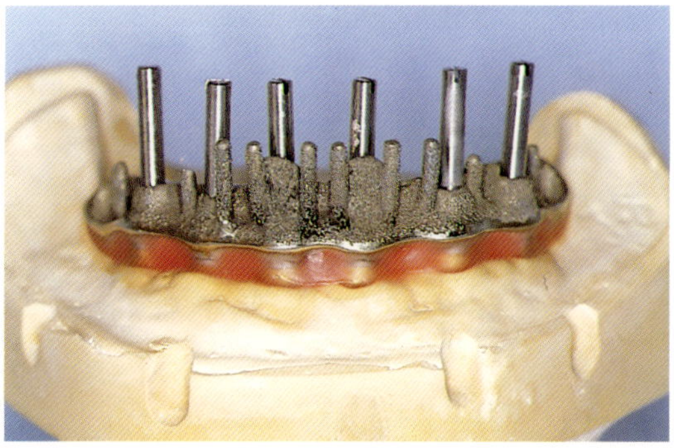

Fig. 490. The framework is fixed on the working model, using the guide pins. The space between the framework and the model is blocked with paraffin wax. This is done in a downward direction, starting from the highest labio-lingual process of the framework. Vaseline is applied to the guide pins.

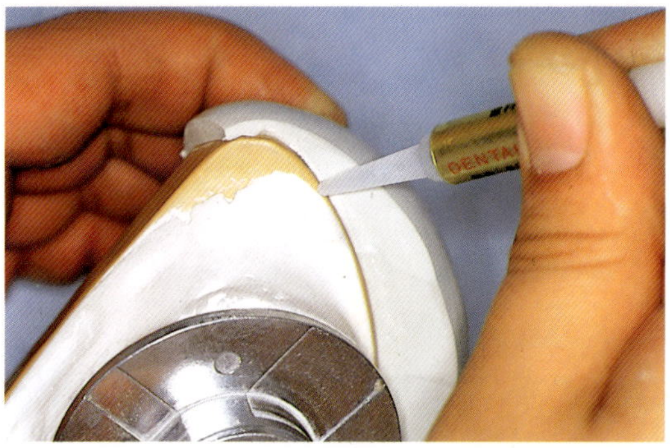

Fig. 491. The artificial teeth are returned to the working model, using the labial index which is fixed to the model, using an adhesive material (*Dental Cyanon*®).

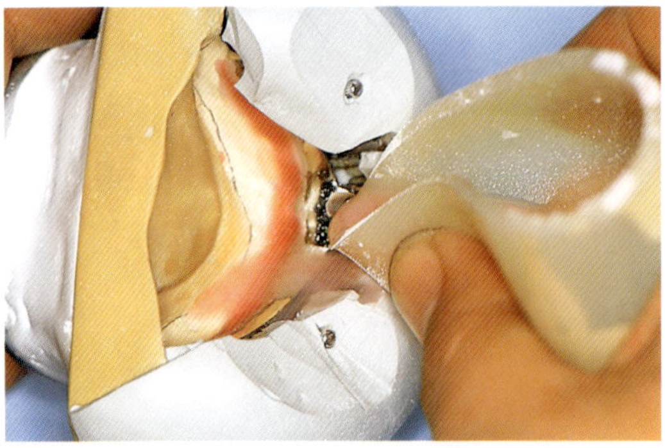

Fig. 492. Fluid resin is poured into the spaces between the artificial teeth and the framework, and the resin is allowed to polymerize.

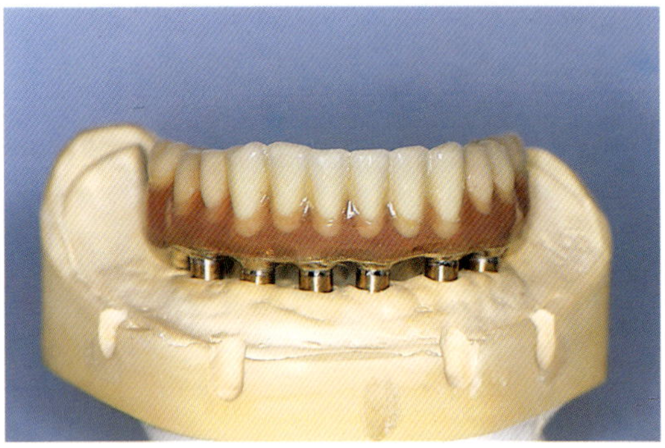

Fig. 493. When resin polymerization has been completed, polishing is performed, using usual methods.

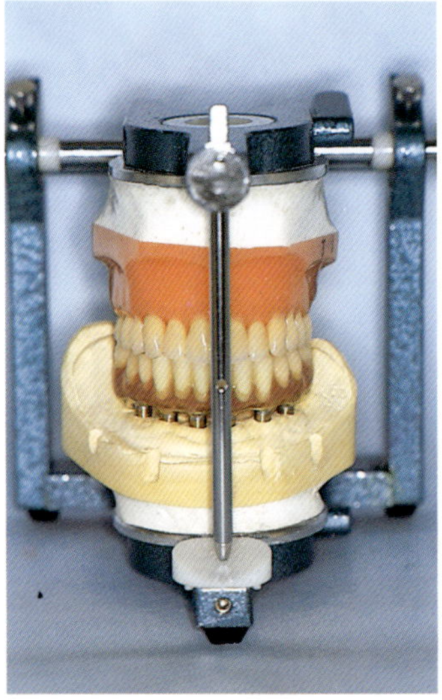

Fig. 494. Finally, the occlusal relationship is adjusted in the articulator.

CHAPTER IX

BASIC TRAINING IN LABORATORY PROCEDURES PART 2

In part 2 of the training manual, procedures for preparing implant dentures using acrylic wings are studied. For training purposes, the model represented in Fig. 495 is used as a totally edentulous jaw.

Preparation of the Occlusion Rim

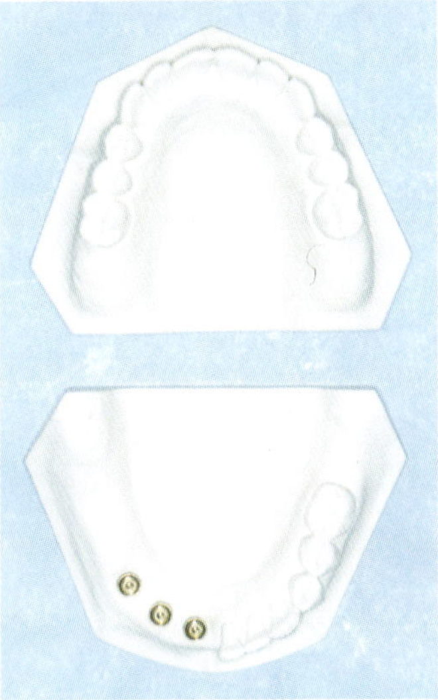

Fig. 495. A training model.

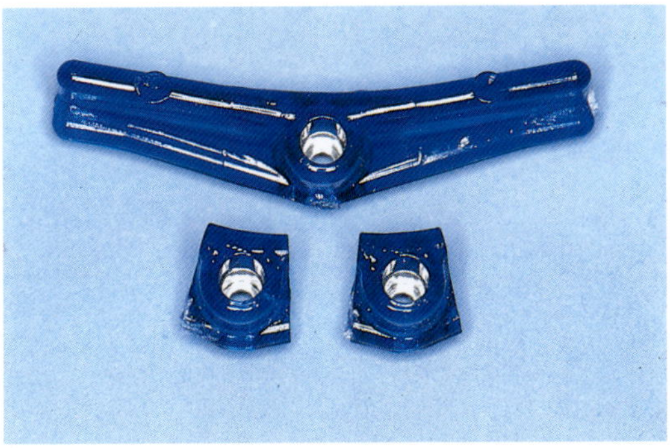

Fig. 496. Acrylic wings. Long and short wings are shown.

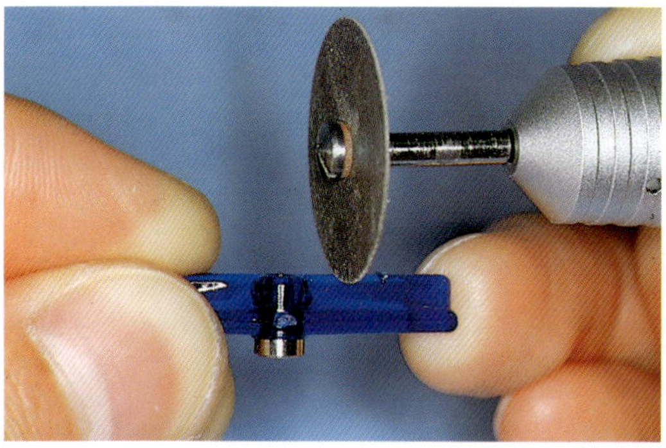

Fig. 497. Acrylic wings of desired lengths are selected and placed on the abutments. The wings can be cut with a resin disc at any point needed.

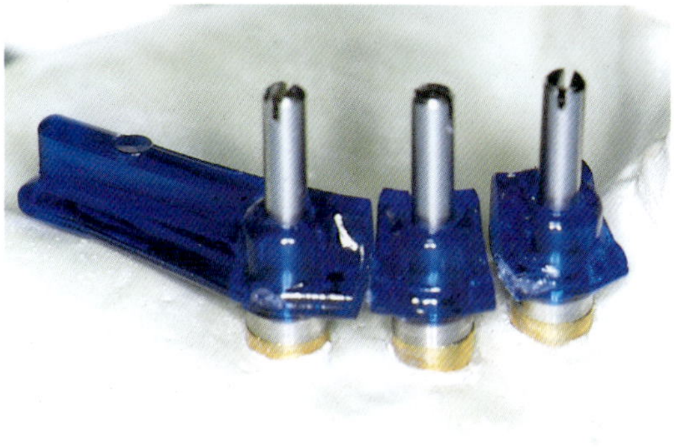

Fig. 498. Short acrylic wings. The space between the neighboring wings is adjusted to 0.5–1.0 mm to secure a space for connection and fixation.

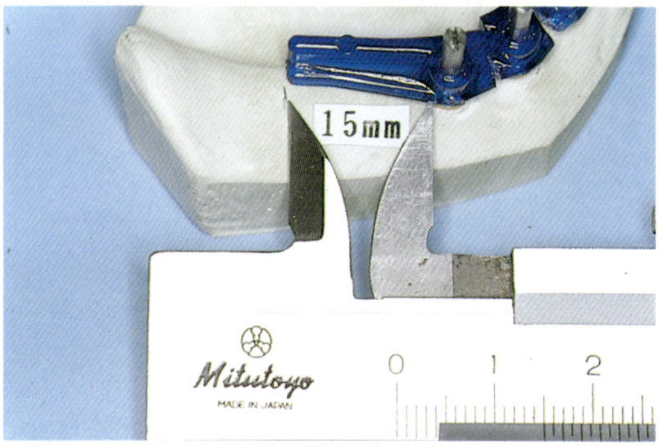

Fig. 499. The position of the posterior margin of the occlusion rim is determined, referring to Fig. 453. In this training procedure, the extention is accepted to be 15 mm from the most distal abutment.

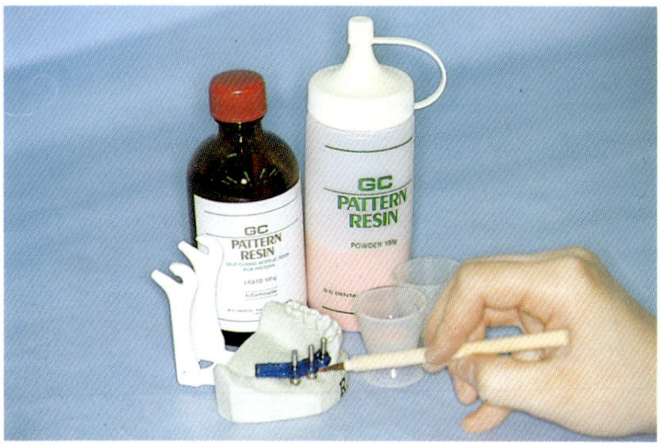

Fig. 500. After the acrylic wings have been designed, they are connected and fixed, using a low temperature burn-out resin.

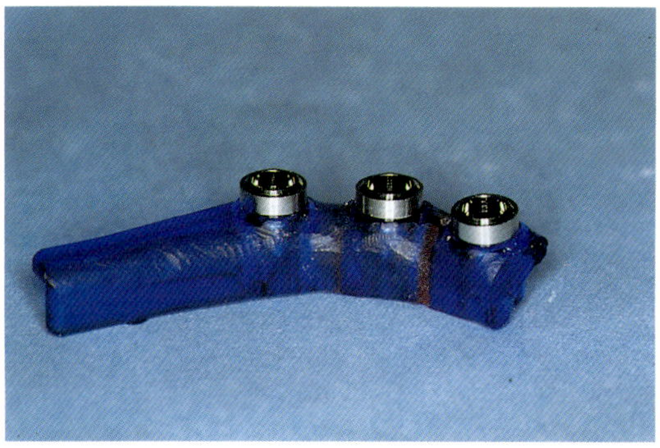

Fig. 501. The bottom of the base plate is U-shaped, and the center is concave, when viewed horizontally.

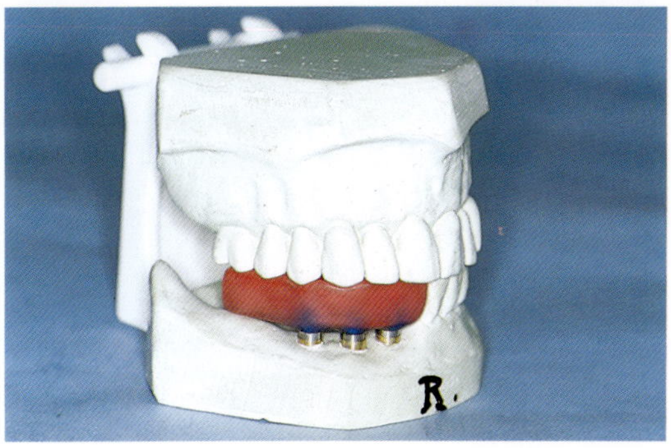

Fig. 502. An occlusion rim is formed over the base plate, using paraffin wax.

Arrangement of Artificial Teeth

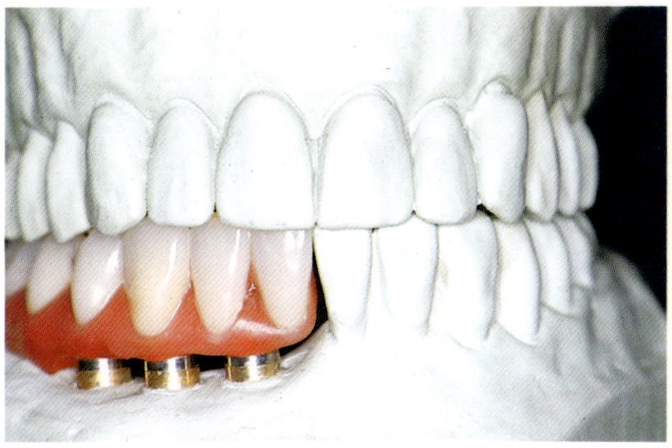

Fig. 503. Arrangement of artificial teeth.

As a rule, the mode of occlusion during lateral movement is cuspid protected, if the antagonistic teeth are natural teeth. It is full-balanced, if a removable denture is used in the opposite jaw.

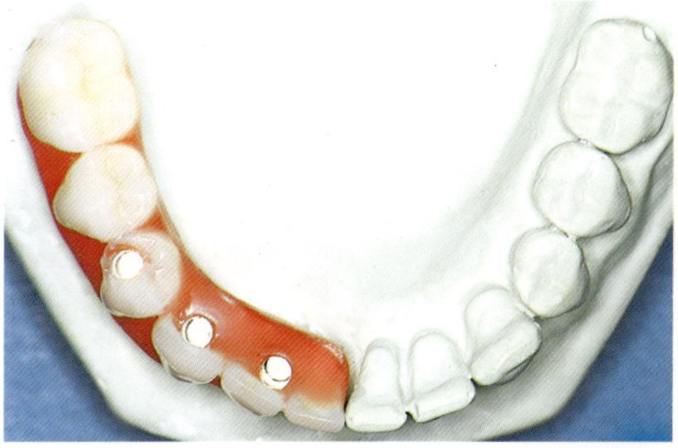

Fig. 504. Relationship between guide pins and artificial teeth.

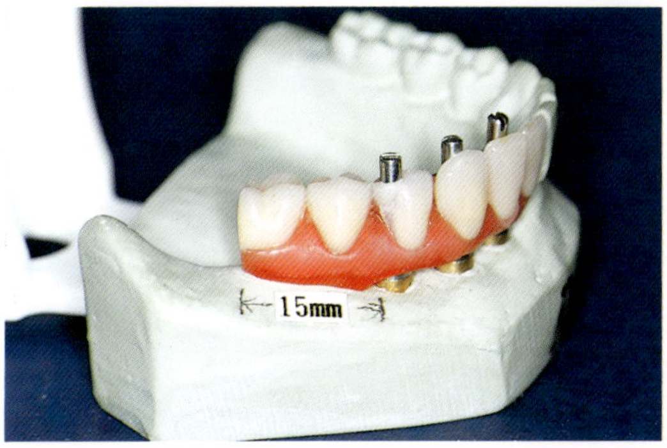

Fig. 505. Artificial teeth on the free end saddle are applied after their shape has been modified.

Preparation of a Labial Index

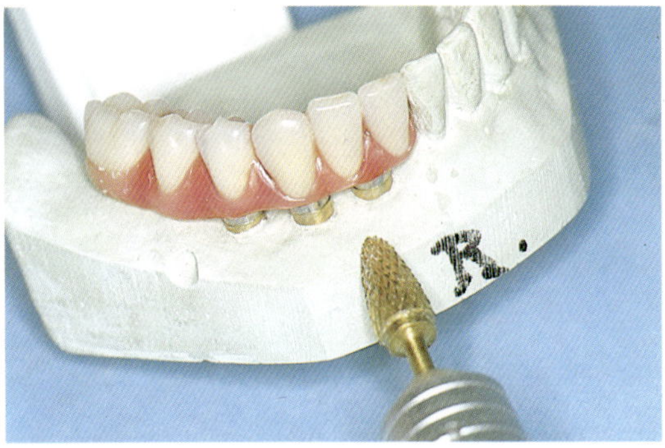

Fig. 506. Upon completion of the try-in bridge, grooves which determine the position of the labial index are formed on the bucco-labial side of the working model.

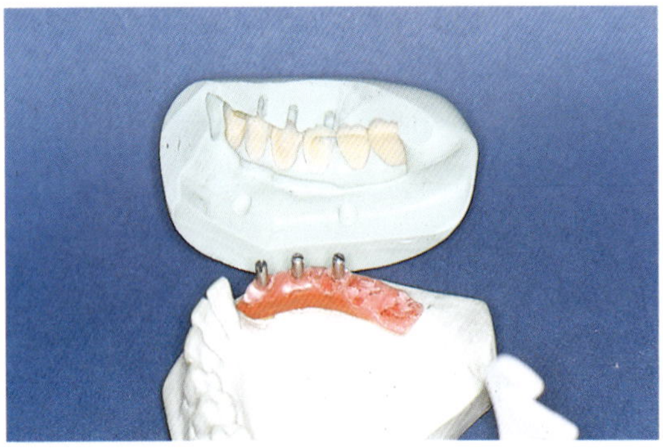

Fig. 507. A labial index for the artificial teeth and bucco-labial gum is made with a silicon impression putty material. The artificial teeth of the denture are placed back into the labial index after removal of the adhering wax.

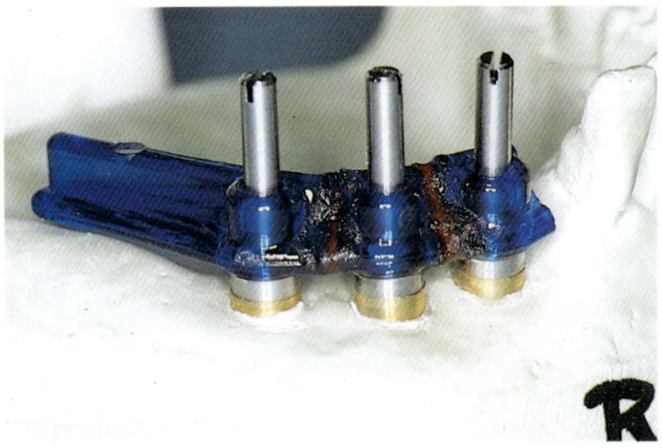

Fig. 508. After removing the wax from the occlusion rim, a wax-separating agent is applied to the plaster model.

Formation of a Wax Framework

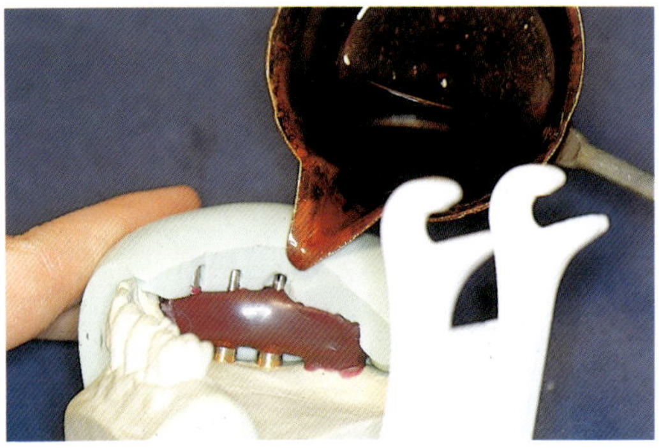

Fig. 509. After the labial index is placed back onto the model, an inlay wax is applied from the lingual side into the framework region.

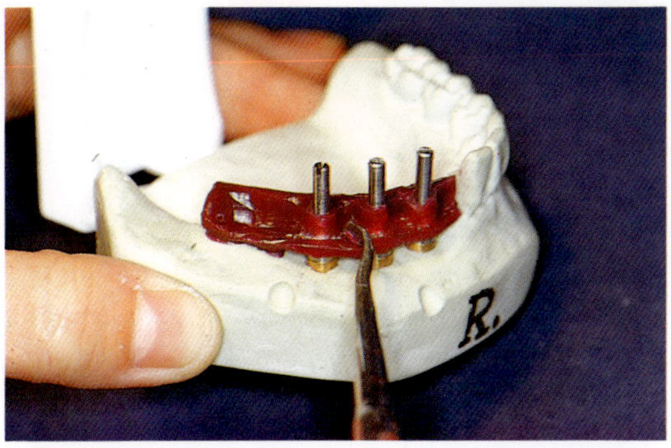

Fig. 510. After the inlay wax has hardened, the labial index and the artificial teeth are removed. In this way, the framework shape is created, whereafter the outer wax can be trimmed.

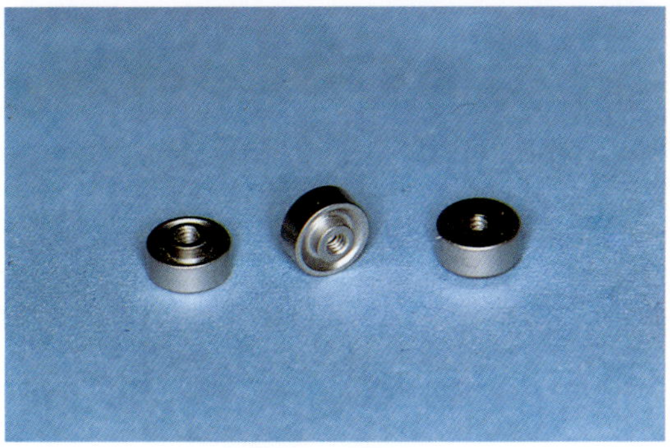

Fig. 511. Protection cap for standard gold cylinder. Protection caps are connected to the gold cylinders by guide pins.

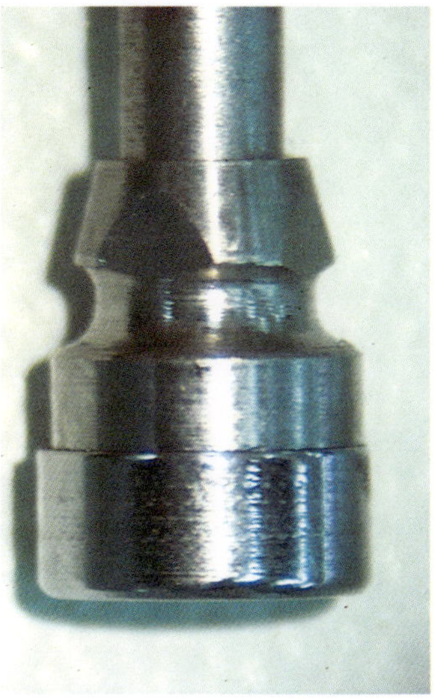

Fig. 512. Protection caps are safely protecting the gold cylinders from injury, because their outer diameter is larger than that of the gold cylinders.

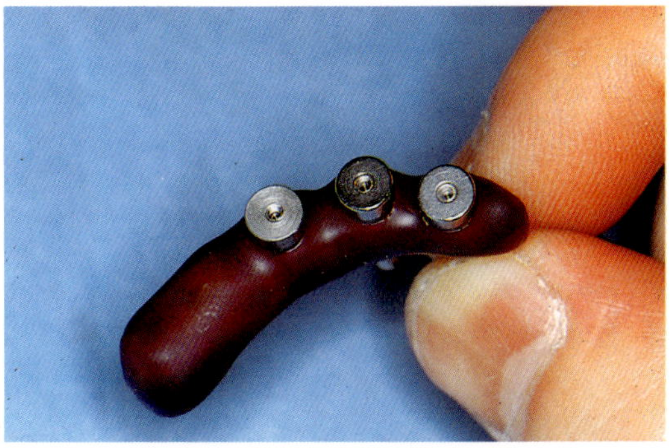

Fig. 513. The base of the framework is shaped after connecting the protection caps to the gold cylinders with the guide pins.

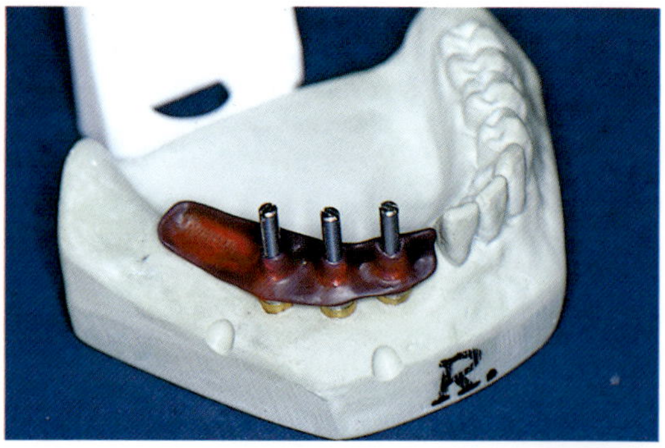

Fig. 514. The mucosal surface of the free end saddle must be U-shaped and be in slight contact with the alveolar crest mucosa. See Fig. 476 for the width and height of the framework.

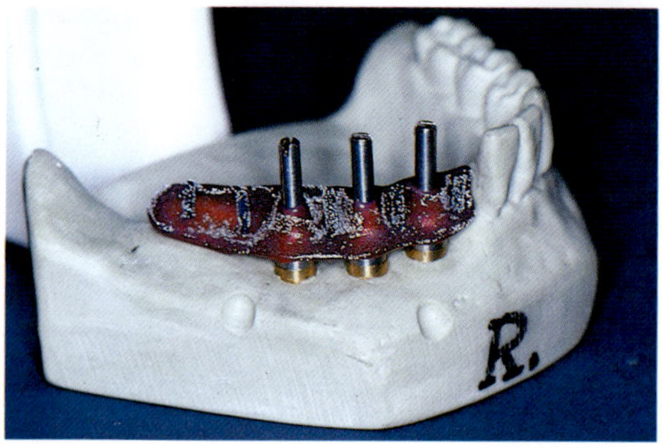

Fig. 515. The labial index is applied to the working model, and the space between the labial index and the framework is checked. Retention elements are created in the region for the artificial teeth. Finally, retention beads are then attached to the wax-frame to complete the formation of the framework.

Investing, Casting and Polishing of Framework

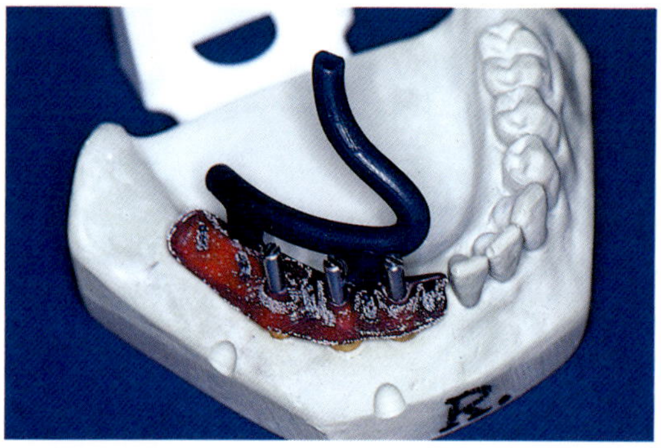

Fig. 516. Sprue formation.

The framework is cast by a one-piece casting technique.

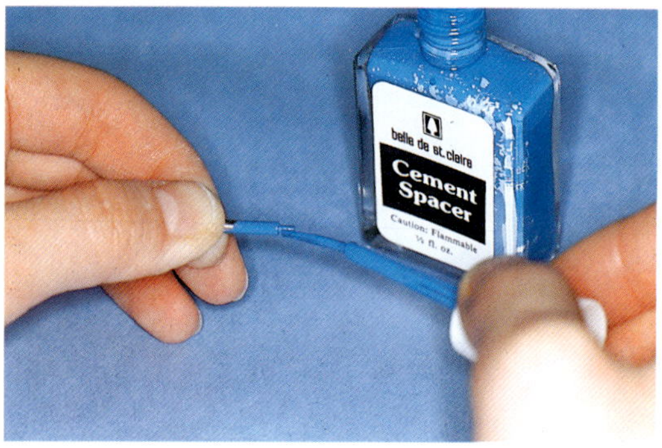

Fig. 517. A spacer is applied to the guide pins to avoid spaces between them and the wax.

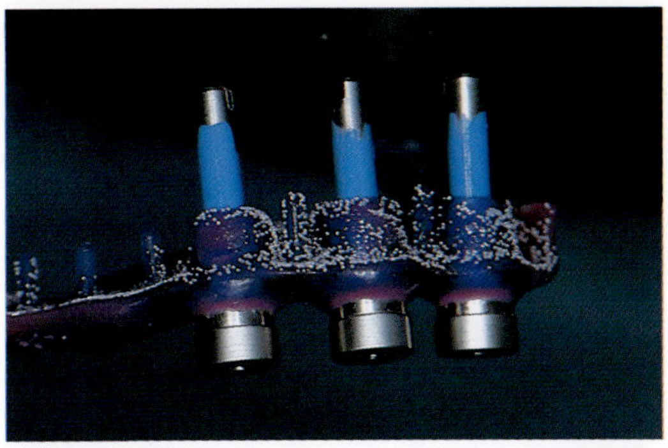

Fig. 518. To prevent melted metal from flowing around the gold cylinders during casting, the gold cylinders are covered with protection caps.

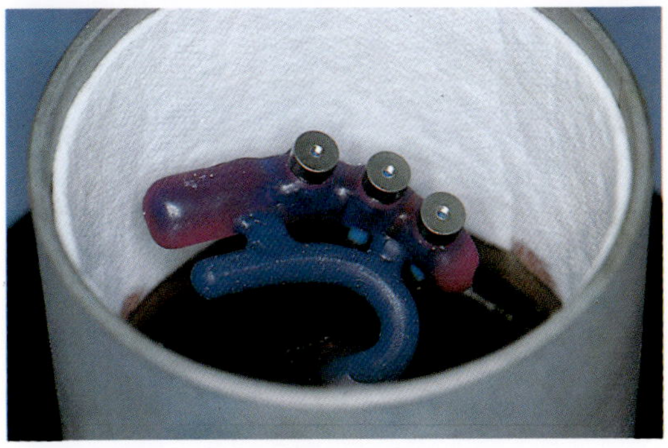

Fig. 519. Investing is performed by routin method.

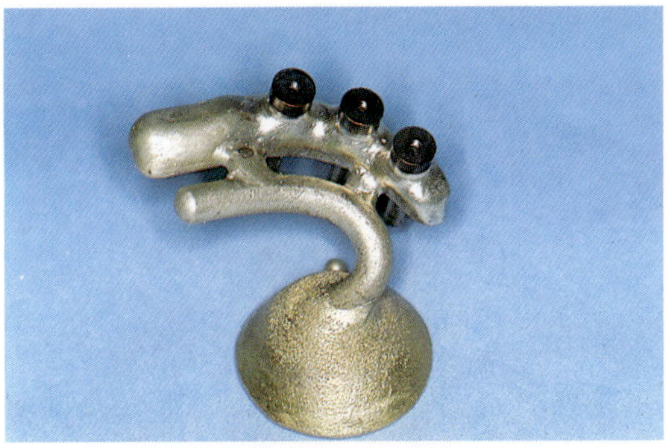

Fig. 520. Upon completion of casting, the investing material is removed, and the framework is washed in acid and sandblasted.

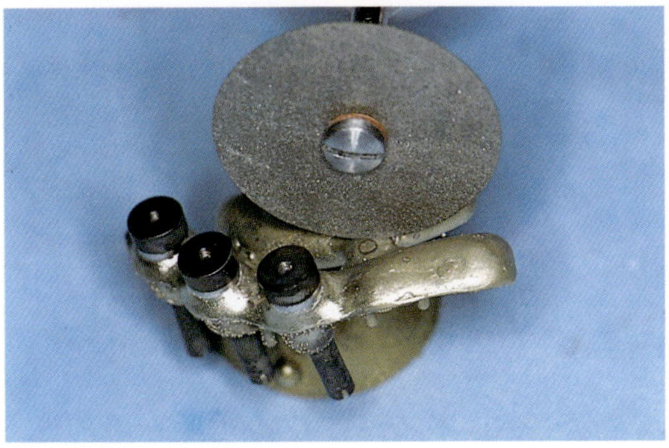

Fig. 521. Routine polishing is performed and the sprue is cut.

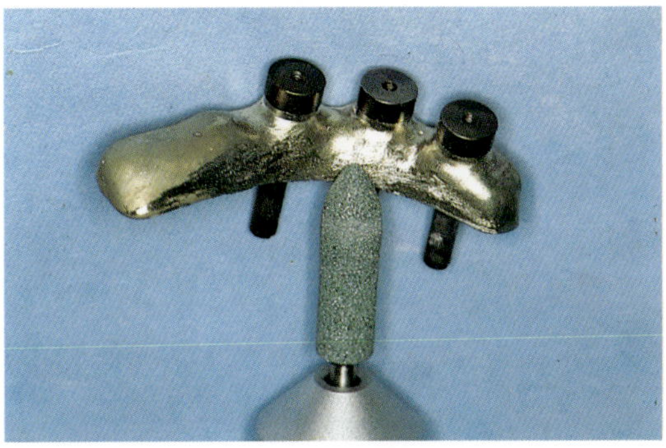

Fig. 522. Rough polishing with a carborundum point is carried out.

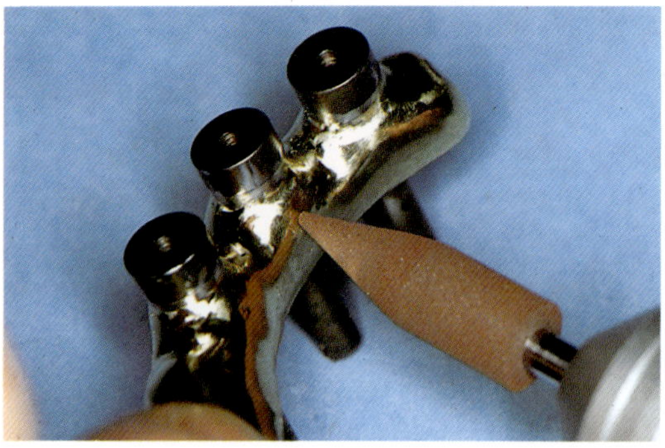

Fig. 523. Polishing with a silicon point follows.

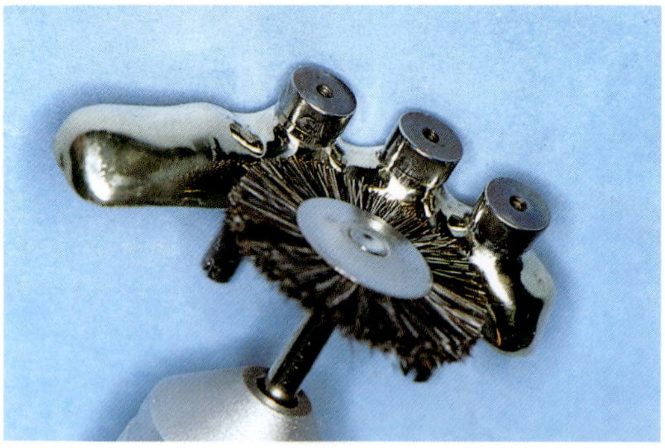

Fig. 524. Fine polishing with a soft brush and skin wheel ends this procedure.

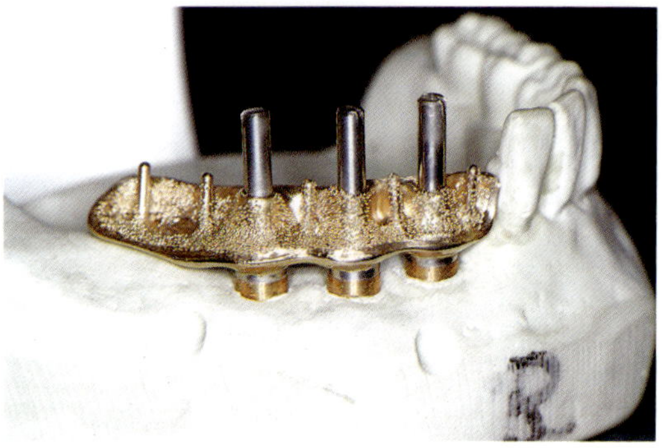

Fig. 525. After the framework has been polished, the fit of the abutment replicas to the gold cylinders is carefully checked on the working model. If seated well, the cast framework is completed. See Figs. 422 through 425 for how to check the fit.

Resin Polymerization, Polishing and Completion of Bridge-Work

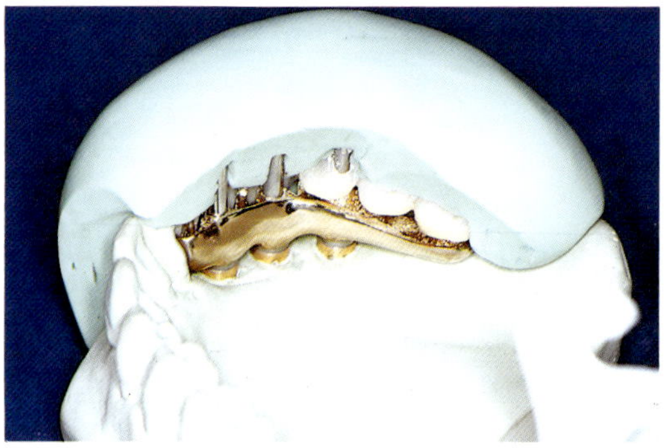

Fig. 526. A resin-separating agent is applied to the plaster model, and the cleaned artificial teeth are placed back into the labial index. Guide pins are treated with vaseline.

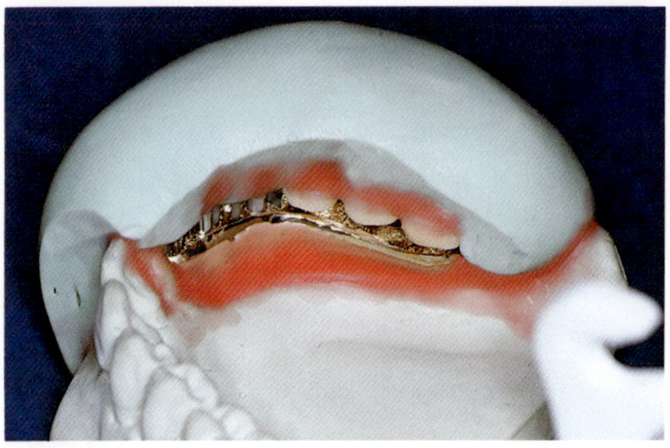

Fig. 527. The labial index is fixed on the working model with an adhesive material (*Dental Cyanon*®). Paraffin wax is thereafter applied as a relief so that the resin does not flow into the area of the artificial teeth. In addition, the space between the framework and the model is blocked out with paraffin wax.

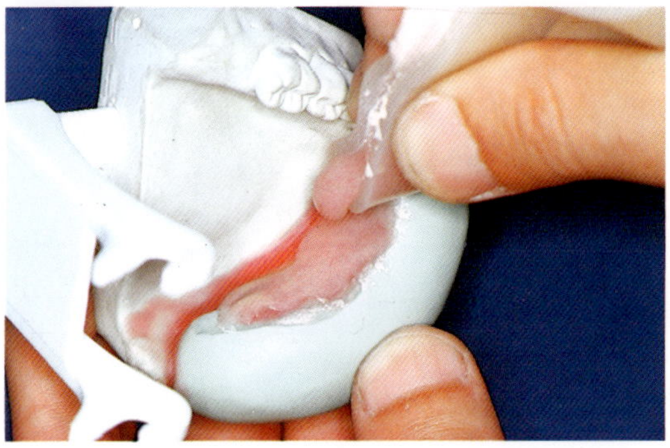

Fig. 528. Soft resin material is poured into the space between the artificial teeth and the framework and is left to polymerize.

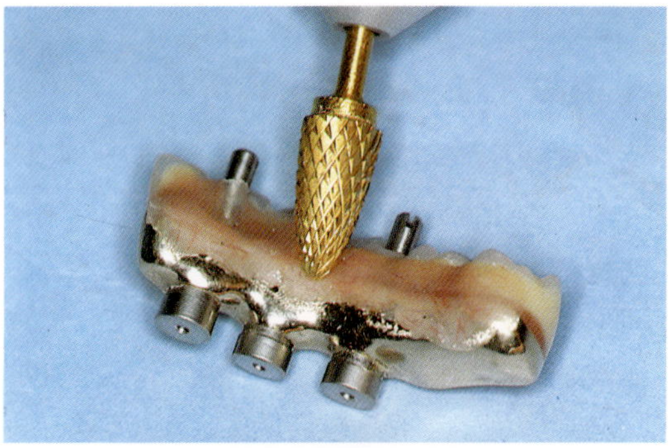

Fig. 529. When the resin has set, it is polished by routine methods. The flash is removed with a carbide bur.

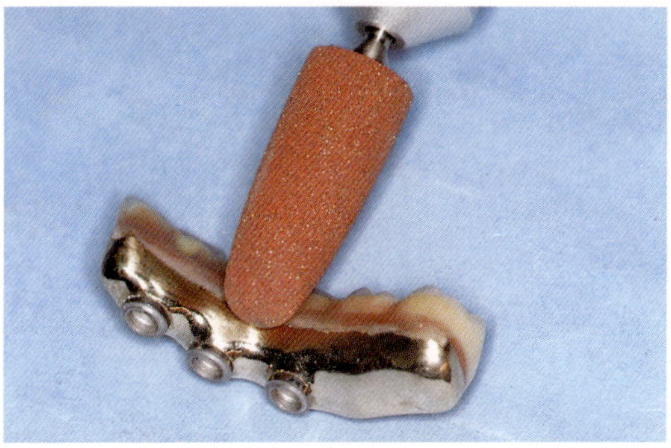

Fig. 530. Polishing with a silicon point is performed.

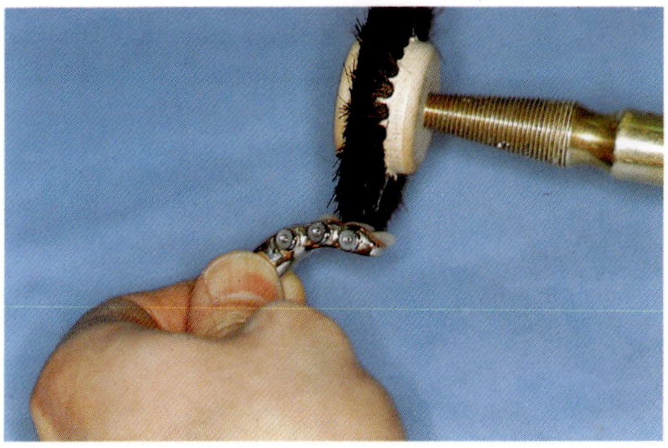

Fig. 531. Polishing with a hard hair brush follows.

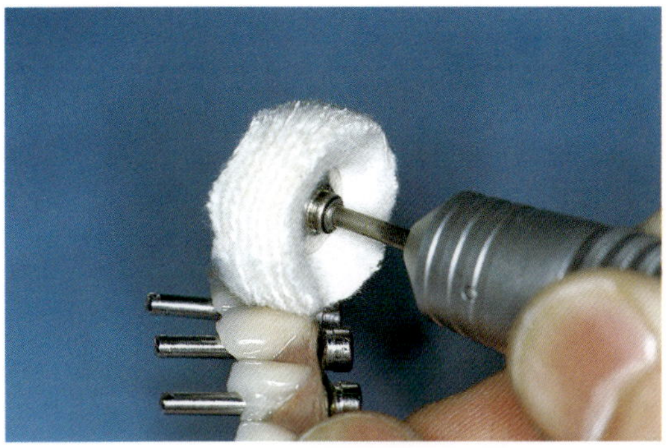

Fig. 532. Fine polishing with a cloth buff is the last step in the polishing procedure.

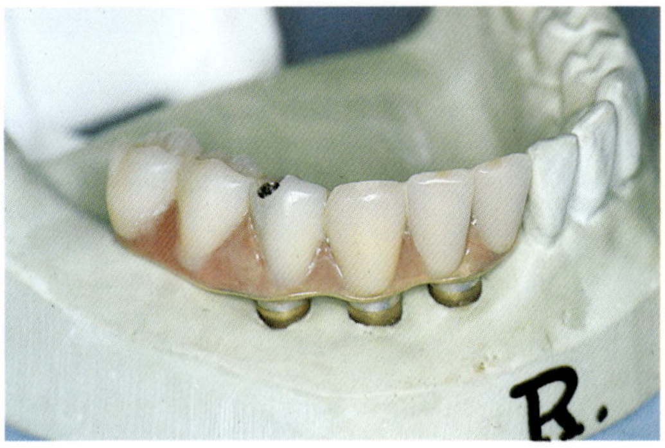

Fig. 533. Polishing has been completed.

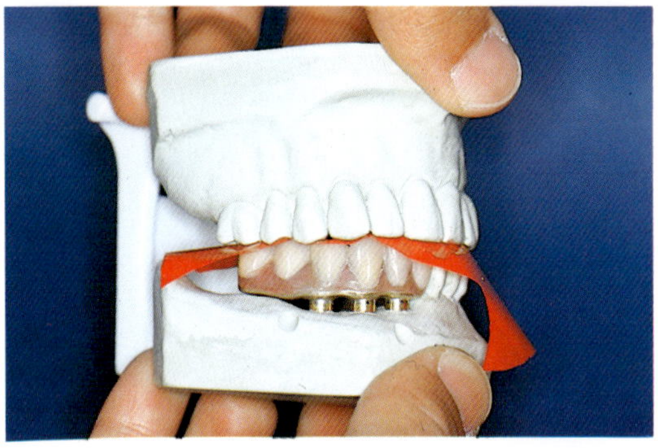

Fig. 534. The occlusal relationship is checked in an articulator and adjusted if needed.

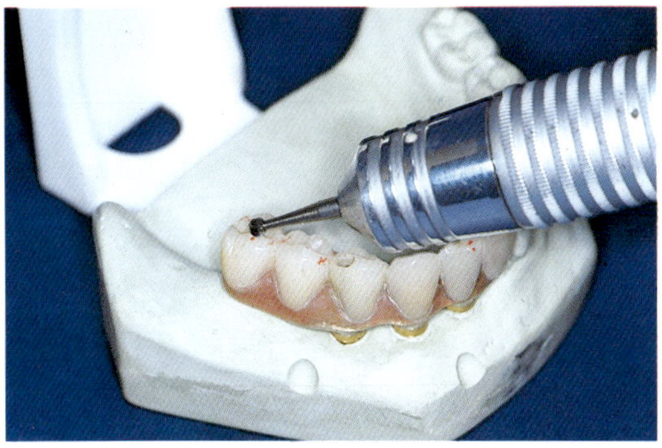

Fig. 535. Grinding with a small bur or stone is performed to correct the occlusion.

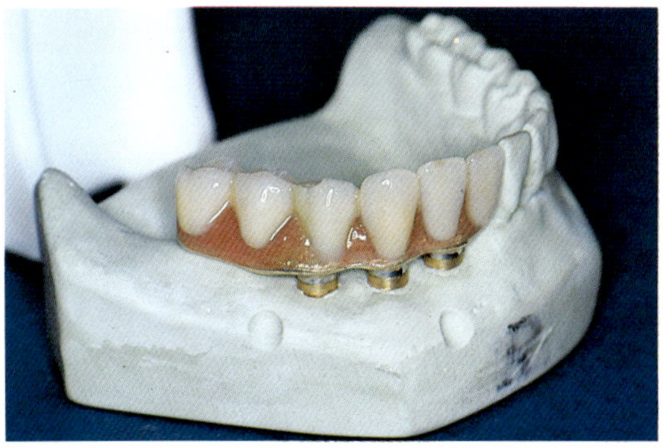

Fig. 536. A buccal view after completion of the bridge work.

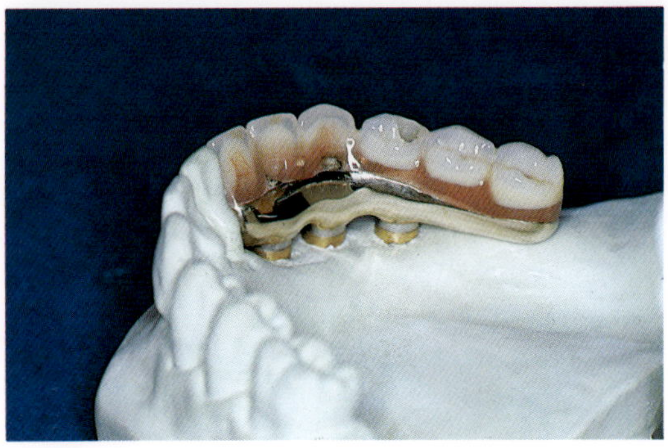

Fig. 537. A lingual view after completion of the construction.

REFERENCES

Brånemark, P-I. et al. : Surgical Procedure Manual, Nobelpharma AB, Göteborg, Sweden, 1992.

Brånemark, P-I. et al. : Tissue-Integrated Prostheses Osseointegration in Clinical Dentistry, Quintessence, Publishing Co, Chicago, U. S. A., 1987.

Ishikawa, T., and Kobayashi, Y. : Clinical Studies on Diagnosis of Condylar Position Using Lateral Radiographs of Temporomandibular Joint, Shigaku (Odontology), 72 : 493-540, 1984. (text in Japanese).

Kobayashi, Y. : Full Denture Occlusion in Old Age Patients, Dental Journal, 30 : 577-597, 1992. (text in Japanese).

Kobayashi, Y. : Future Trend of Implants : A Thought on the Future of Dental Implants, Shigaku (Odontology), 77 : 1246-1256, 1989.

Kobayashi, Y. : Osseointegrated Implants Clinical Dentistry-From the Point of View of Prosthodontics-, Shigaku (Odontology), 77 : 1223-1234, 1989.

Miyamoto, Y. et al. : Complication of Osseointegrated Implants Related to Follow up Maintenance —Two Cases of Hyperplasia Formation and Gingivitis—, J. Japanese Ass. Periodontol, 30 : 967-976, 1988.

Nakaya, Y. et al. : The Concepts of Dental Implants in Periodontology, the Quintessence, 10 : 1547-1554, 1990. (in Japanese).

Orton, Q. S. et al. : The Dental Professional's Role in Monitoring and Maintenance of Tissue-integrated Prostheses, Int. J. Oral Maxillofac. Impl, 4 : 305-310, 1989.

Sumitomo, M. : The Pain Control in Dental Practice-Psycho-sedation and Local Anesthesia-, Dental Forum, Tokyo, 1991. (in Japanese).

Sumitomo, M. et al. : Handbook of Local Anesthesia, Nagasue-Shoten, Kyoto, 1987. (in Japanese).

Yanagida, S., and Kobayashi, Y. : The Effect of Treatment Denture with Cuspless Teeth on Restoring Mandibular Displacement, Shigaku (Odontology), 80 : 840-864, 1992.